Liver Metabolism and Diseases

Liver Metabolism and Diseases

Editor: Joseph Curtis

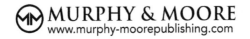

MURPHY & MOORE
www.murphy-moorepublishing.com

www.murphy-moorepublishing.com

ⓂⓂ MURPHY & MOORE

Cataloging-in-Publication Data

Liver metabolism and diseases / edited by Joseph Curtis.
    p. cm.
Includes bibliographical references and index.
ISBN 978-1-63987-785-0
1. Liver--Metabolism. 2. Liver--Diseases. I. Curtis, Joseph.
RC845 .L58 2023
616.362--dc23

Murphy & Moore Publishing
1 Rockefeller Plaza,
New York City,
NY 10020, USA

ISBN 978-1-63987-785-0

Contents

Preface

It is often said that books are a boon to mankind. They document every progress and pass on the knowledge from one generation to the other. They play a crucial role in our lives. Thus I was both excited and nervous while editing this book. I was pleased by the thought of being able to make a mark but I was also nervous to do it right because the future of students depends upon it. Hence, I took a few months to research further into the discipline, revise my knowledge and also explore some more aspects. Post this process, I begun with the editing of this book.

Liver is an integral part of the process of metabolism. It helps in the preservation and regulation of the lipid and glucose levels in the body, as well as in energy metabolism. The most common metabolic diseases which can affect the liver are Wilson disease, hereditary hemochromatosis, and Alpha-I antitrypsin deficiency (AATD). Some of the other types of disorders which affect the liver are infections, immune system issues, cancers, and heritable conditions. One of the upcoming methods of study which is used to study the cell metabolism within the liver is metabolomics. It refers to the scientific study of chemical processes involving metabolites, the small molecule substrates, intermediates, and products of cell metabolism. Metabolomics has a very high potential to detect biomarker candidates for the prospective advancement of new therapeutics. The book aims to shed light on some of the unexplored aspects of liver metabolism and the recent researches in this field with respect to liver diseases. It will provide comprehensive knowledge to both medical students and professionals.

I thank my publisher with all my heart for considering me worthy of this unparalleled opportunity and for showing unwavering faith in my skills. I would also like to thank the editorial team who worked closely with me at every step and contributed immensely towards the successful completion of this book. Last but not the least, I wish to thank my friends and colleagues for their support.

Editor

Metabolomic Salivary Signature of Pediatric Obesity Related Liver Disease and Metabolic Syndrome

Jacopo Troisi [1,2,3,4,*], Federica Belmonte [1], Antonella Bisogno [1], Luca Pierri [1], Angelo Colucci [1,2], Giovanni Scala [4], Pierpaolo Cavallo [5](ID), Claudia Mandato [6](ID), Antonella Di Nuzzi [1], Laura Di Michele [1], Anna Pia Delli Bovi [1], Salvatore Guercio Nuzio [1] and Pietro Vajro [1,7](ID)

[1] Department of Medicine and Surgery and Dentistry, "Scuola Medica Salernitana", Pediatrics Section University of Salerno, 84081 Baronissi (Salerno), Italy; fecu91@gmail.com (F.B.); a.bisogno91@gmail.com (A.B.); luca.pierri@hotmail.com (L.P.); angelocolucci2@gmail.com (A.C.); antonelladinuzzi@gmail.com (A.D.N.); lauradimichele05091993@gmail.com (L.D.M.); dellilboviannapia@gmail.com (A.P.D.B.); sguercio.nuzio@gmail.com (S.G.N.); pvajro@unisa.it (P.V.)
[2] Theoreo srl, Via degli Ulivi 3, 84090 Montecorvino Pugliano (SA), Italy
[3] European Biomedical Research Institute of Salerno (EBRIS), Via S. de Renzi, 3, 84125 Salerno, Italy
[4] Hosmotic srl, Via R. Bosco 178, 80069 Vico Equense (NA), Italy; scala@hosmotic.com
[5] Department of Physics, University of Salerno, 84084 Fisciano (Salerno), Italy; pcavallo@unisa.it
[6] Department of Pediatrics, Children's Hospital Santobono-Pausilipon, 80129 Naples, Italy; cla.mandato@gmail.com
[7] European Laboratory of Food Induced Intestinal Disease (ELFID), University of Naples Federico II, 80100 Naples, Italy
[*] Correspondence: troisi@theoreosrl.com

Abstract: Pediatric obesity-related metabolic syndrome (MetS) and nonalcoholic fatty liver disease (NAFLD) are increasingly frequent conditions with a still-elusive diagnosis and low-efficacy treatment and monitoring options. In this study, we investigated the salivary metabolomic signature, which has been uncharacterized to date. In this pilot-nested case-control study over a transversal design, 41 subjects (23 obese patients and 18 normal weight (NW) healthy controls), characterized based on medical history, clinical, anthropometric, and laboratory data, were recruited. Liver involvement, defined according to ultrasonographic liver brightness, allowed for the allocation of the patients into four groups: obese with hepatic steatosis ([St+], $n = 15$) and without hepatic steatosis ([St–], $n = 8$), and with ($n = 10$) and without ($n = 13$) MetS. A partial least squares discriminant analysis (PLS-DA) model was devised to classify the patients' classes based on their salivary metabolomic signature. Pediatric obesity and its related liver disease and metabolic syndrome appear to have distinct salivary metabolomic signatures. The difference is notable in metabolites involved in energy, amino and organic acid metabolism, as well as in intestinal bacteria metabolism, possibly reflecting diet, fatty acid synthase pathways, and the strict interaction between microbiota and intestinal mucins. This information expands the current understanding of NAFLD pathogenesis, potentially translating into better targeted monitoring and/or treatment strategies in the future.

Keywords: pediatric obesity; nonalcoholic fatty liver disease; metabolic syndrome; saliva; metabolomics; gas-chromatography mass spectrometry

1. Introduction

The incidence of obesity and its related conditions, including metabolic syndrome (MetS) and non-alcoholic fatty liver disease (NAFLD), has dramatically increased worldwide in all age groups including pediatrics [1]. Pediatric obesity definitely is an early risk factor for adult morbidity and mortality [2,3]. Due to the existence of a well-established tracking phenomenon, the early detection and treatment of MetS and fatty liver in childhood represents a valuable tool to prevent further health complications and to minimize the global socioeconomic burden of hepato-metabolic and cardiovascular obesity-associated complications in adulthood [4]. Although the exact definition of MetS is still debated regarding the pediatric population, most researchers agree (a) that it includes hypertension, hyperglycemia, dyslipidemia together with visceral obesity, and (b) that NAFLD has to be considered its hepatic component.

Metabolomics has recently started to pave the way to a better pathomechanistic understanding of these hepatometabolic complications, leading to a more efficient diagnosis and better therapeutic approaches. In this regard, studies have shown that high urinary/blood levels of aromatic (AAA) ± branched chain (BCAA) amino acids are known to be associated with insulin resistance (IR) and the risk of obesity-related MetS [5–8].

Lipid metabolism, tyrosine [9], alanine and the urea cycle [5], acylcarnitine catabolism ± changes in nucleotides, lysolipids, and inflammation markers [10], and several other components [11–13] also appear to be implicated in obesity and its related disorders.

We have recently shown a complex network of urinary molecules prevalently represented by intestinally-derived bacterial products [14] which are correlated with the clinical phenotype and can differentiate between normal weight and obese children, distinguishing between those with and without liver involvement, based also on the characteristics of their gut-liver axis (GLA) function [15].

To identify an even more easily accessible and readily obtained biofluid for possible minimally invasive disease recognition [16], few studies have shown saliva suitability for investigations of individual metabolites of oxidative stress in obesity [17] and obesity-related MetS/NAFLD [4,18]. We showed that salivary testing of uric acid, glucose, insulin and HOMA together with selected anthropometric parameters may help to identify noninvasively obese children with hepatic steatosis and/or having MetS components [4]. However, salivary metabolomics studies in this respect are lacking.

Based on these and a few other urine-and/or plasma-based metabolomic studies of pediatric obesity and MetS [15,19–21], we hypothesized that differences in the metabolite profiling of lean and obese children with and without NAFLD/MetS might also be evident in saliva, which might be ideal to screen noninvasively obese children at a higher risk of hepatometabolic complications. Prospectively, better delineation of individual or clusters of specific metabolites could serve as diagnostic biomarkers to be further investigated in future studies appraising even early stages of these comorbidities.

2. Materials and Methods

2.1. Population and Study Design

Among 46 consecutive subjects (aged 7–15 years) seen at our obesity clinic or planned for only minor surgery, 41 with verified good oral health and not taking medications were enrolled in a nested case-control study over a transversal design. Eighteen had a normal weight (NW; body mass index (BMI) < 85th percentile) and 23 were obese (BMI > 95th percentile). The patients were characterized based on clinical, anthropometric (blood pressure, BMI, waist circumference (WC), and neck circumference (NC)), laboratory (serum alanine aminotransferase (ALT), aspartate aminotransferase (AST), total and high-density lipoprotein (HDL) cholesterol, triglycerides, uric acid (UA), glucose, and insulin) parameters. An ultrasound (US) was used to determine the presence [St+] or absence [St−] of hepatic steatosis [22,23]. Blood tests were performed using a standard laboratory analyzer (Abbott Diagnostics, Santa Clara, CA, USA).

ALT upper normal values referred either to the customary normal range cut-off value of 40 IU/L or more precise SAFETY study cut-off pediatric values of 25.8 and 22.0 IU/L for boys and girls, respectively [24].

Patients with hepatic steatosis and/or transaminases >1.5 times the upper customary normal values were screened for celiac disease, Wilson disease, autoimmune hepatitis, and major and minor hepatotropic viruses [25]. According to the International Diabetes Foundation (IDF), MetS was defined as the presence of at least three of the following parameters: WC >95th percentile; triglycerides >150 mg/dL; blood glucose >100 mg/dL; systolic blood pressure (SBP) >95th percentile; and HDL cholesterol <40 mg/dL [26].

2.2. Saliva Samples

Each subject was asked to refrain from eating, drinking and brush tooting procedures for at least 1 h before saliva collection. Then he/she underwent a morning, whole saliva sampling using a saliva cotton roll commercial collection device (Salivette®; Sarstedt, Nümbrecht, Germany). As recommended by the manufacturer, to stimulate salivation patients, patients were asked to roll and gently chew the cotton swab in their mouth for 60–90 s. Then the swab was spitted in the collection tube of the kit and centrifuged within 1 h at 2000× g for 2 min. The collected clear, fluid saliva sample was aliquoted without any further processing and frozen at −80 °C until samples' analysis, as previously described [4].

2.3. Ethical Approval

The study complied with the terms of the Declaration of Helsinki of 1975 (as revised in 2013) [27] for the investigation of human subjects, with written informed consent from patients and their families. All participants agreed to participate in this study and contribute saliva samples for metabolomic analysis. All samples were collected in accordance with the ethical guidelines mandated by and approved by our institutional Health Research Ethics Board. The study protocol was approved by the Ethics Review Committee of the University Hospital S. Giovanni di Dio e Ruggi d'Aragona of Salerno (Prot. No 18.02.2013/98).

2.4. Untargeted Metabolomics Analysis

2.4.1. Metabolites Extraction and Derivatization

Metabolome extraction, purification and derivatization were carried out using the MetboPrep GC kit (Theoreo srl, Montecorvino Pugliano (SA), Italy) according to the manufacturer's instructions.

2.4.2. GC-MS Analysis

GC-MS analysis was performed on the derivatized extracted metabolome according to Troisi et al. [15] with a few minor changes. Briefly, 2 μL of the sample solution was injected into the GC-MS system (GC-2010 Plus gas chromatograph coupled to a 2010 Plus single quadrupole mass spectrometer; Shimadzu Corp., Kyoto, Japan) equipped with a 30-m, 0.25-mm ID CP-Sil 8 CB fused silica capillary GC column with 1.00-μm film thickness from Agilent (Agilent, J&W Scientific, Folsom, CA, USA), using He as a carrier gas. The initial oven temperature of 100 °C was maintained for 1 min and then raised by 6 °C/min to 320 °C with a further 2.33 min of hold time. The gas flow was set to obtain a constant linear velocity of 39 cm/s, and injections were performed in the splitless mode. The mass spectrometer was operated in electron impact (70 eV) in the full-scan mode in the interval of 35–600 m/z with a scan velocity of 3333 amu/s and a solvent cut-off time of 4.5 min. The complete GC analysis duration was 40 min. Untargeted metabolites were identified by comparing the mass spectrum of each peak with the NIST library collection (NIST, Gaithersburg, MD, USA).

2.4.3. Metabolites Identification

Of the over 240 signals per sample produced by GC-MS analysis, only 222 were investigated further because they were consistently found in at least 85% of samples.

To identify metabolites under the peaks, the Kovats' index [28] difference max tolerance was set at 10, while the minimum matching for the NIST library search was set at 85%. The results were summarized in a comma-separate matrix file and loaded in the appropriate software for statistical manipulation. The chromatographic data for PLS-DA analysis were tabulated with one sample per row and one variable (metabolite) per column. The normalization procedures consisted of data transformation and scaling. Data transformation was made by generalized log transformation and data scaling by autoscaling (mean-centered and divided by standard deviation of each variable) [29]. Relevant metabolites selected using statistical analysis were further confirmed with an analytical standard purchased from Sigma-Aldrich (Milan, Italy) as indicated in the Metabolomic Standard Initiative reports [30].

2.5. Statistical Analysis

2.5.1. Demographical and Clinical Data

Statistical analysis was performed using Statistica software (StatSoft, Tulsa, OK, USA) and Minitab (Minitab Inc., State College, PA, USA). The normal distribution of data was verified using the Shapiro–Wilks test. Because the data were normally distributed, we used one-way ANOVA with Tukey's post-hoc test for intergroup comparisons. A result with $p < 0.05$ was considered statistically significant.

2.5.2. Metabolomics Univariate Data Analysis

Metabolite concentration differences among the classes (NW, OB[St+] and OB[St−]) were evaluated in terms of fold change (FC) and p-value (assessed using Student's t-test because the metabolite amount was previously normalized).

The volcano plot representation was used to encounter both criteria. Metabolites with high FC (>1 or <−1) and lower p-value (<0.05) were selected as the most relevant.

2.5.3. Metabolomic Multivariate Data Analysis

Partial least squares discriminant analysis (PLS-DA) was performed on the internal standard peak area [31] normalized chromatogram using R (Foundation for Statistical Computing, Vienna, Austria). Mean centering and unit variance scaling were applied for all analyses. Class separation was archived by PLS-DA, which is a supervised method that uses multivariate regression techniques to extract, via linear combinations of original variables (X), the information that can predict class membership (Y). PLS regression was performed using the *plsr* function included in the R pls package [32]. Classification and cross-validation were performed using the wrapper function included in the caret package [33]. A permutation test was performed to assess the significance of class discrimination. In each permutation, a PLS-DA model was built between the data (X) and permuted class labels (Y) using the optimal number of components determined by cross validation for the model based on the original class assignment. Two types of test statistics were used to measure class discrimination. The first is based on prediction accuracy during training. The second used separation distance based on the ratio of the between groups sum of the squares and the within group sum of squares (B/W-ratio). If the observed test statistics were part of the distribution based on the permuted class assignments, class discrimination cannot be considered significant from a statistical point of view [34]. Variable importance in projection (VIP) scores were calculated for each component. A VIP score is a weighted sum of squares of the PLS loadings, considering the amount of explained Y-variation in each dimension.

The metabolic pathway was constructed using the MetScape application [35] of the software Cytoscape [36].

3. Results

The demographic and clinical laboratory characteristics of the case and control subjects are reported in Table 1. None of the NW controls had either biochemical or US hepato-metabolic abnormalities.

Table 1. Characteristics of the study population.

Anthropometric and Laboratory Parameters	Controls ($n = 18$)	Obese with Steatosis ($n = 15$)	Obese without Steatosis ($n = 8$)	All Obese ($n = 23$)
Gender (M/F)	13/5	10/5	4/4	14/9
Age (years)	10.53 ± 2.57	12.48 ± 2.77 *	12.51 ± 2.79 *	12.49 ± 2.71 *
Weight (kg)	37.42 ± 11.26	79.99 ± 28.76 *	71.9 ± 17.31 *	77.18 ± 25.24 *
Height (cm)	140.17 ± 15.17	153.41 ± 19.27 *	157.45 ± 11.97 *	154.52 ± 16.88 *
BMI (kg/cm^2)	18.52 ± 2.92	32.80 ± 6.94 *	28.93 ± 5.58 *	31.45 ± 6.65 *
BMI percentile	23.75 ± 34.25	95.14 ± 0.53 *	95.67 ± 1.03 *	95.40 ± 1.05 *
Waist circumference (cm)	61.14 ± 7.11	93.27 ± 12.68 *	86.00 ± 14.53 *	90.74 ± 13.49 *
WC percentile	65.85 ± 24.58	94.98 ± 0.97 *	94.38 ± 1.77 *	94.78 ± 1.04 *
Cm WC > 95th percentile	0	21.03 ± 10.57 *	14.00 ± 10.99 *	18.59 ± 11.01 *
WtHR	0.43 ± 0.03	0.61 ± 0.05 *	0.55 ± 0.08 *	0.59 ± 0.07 *
Neck circumference (cm)	27.67 ± 2.41	36.05 ± 4.33 *	34.69 ± 4.08 *	35.58 ± 4.20 *
NC percentile	44.12 ± 33.22	95.57 ± 5.35 *	92.61 ± 3.15	94.09 ± 4.26 *
Cm NC > 95th percentile	0	3.71 ± 2.77 *	2.41 ± 2.75 *	3.26 ± 2.77 *
SBP (mmHg)	95.98 ± 11.95	127.47 ± 8.95 *	125.63 ± 20.23 *	126.83 ± 13.49 *
SBP percentile	50.00 ± 0	86.93 ± 19.36 *	83.50 ± 20.96 *	85.74 ± 19.52 *
DBP (mmHg)	55.00 ± 10.77	61.53 ± 10.42 *	60.75 ± 11.70 *	61.26 ± 10.62 *
DBP percentile	50.00 ± 0	56.00 ± 15.83 *	55.00 ± 14.14 *	55.65 ± 14.95 *
ALT (U/L)	17.33 ± 4.31	50.17 ± 28.75 *	34.50 ± 37.74 *	44.72 ± 32.21 *
AST (U/L)	24.72 ± 4.87	46.19 ± 28.58 *	19.75 ± 5.85	37.00 ± 26.39 *
Total cholesterol (mg/dL)	148.78 ± 16.38	158.17 ± 21.91 *	162.00 ± 24.20 *	159.50 ± 22.26 *
HDL (mg/dL)	56.94 ± 14.45	45.07 ± 10.21 *	48.00 ± 5.50 *	46.09 ± 8.83 *
Triglyceride (mg/dL)	Not available	90.59 ± 26.97	138.63 ± 91.90	107.30 ± 60.80
Blood glucose (mg/dL)	83.17 ± 6.61	88.59 ± 10.36 *	90.00 ± 10.34 *	89.08 ± 10.14 *
Salivary glucose (μM)	3338.36 ± 1274.73	3167.86 ± 1192.75	2647.09 ± 1227.77	2986.70 ± 1203.86
Blood insulin (U/L)	10.27 ± 5.22	24.24 ± 10.95 *	19.60 ± 6.63 *	22.62 ± 9.77 *
Salivary insulin (nM)	5.79 ± 2.85	20.89 ± 8.69 *	17.26 ± 6.37 *	19.60 ± 8.00 *
Blood HOMA-IR	2.01 ± 1.16	5.34 ± 2.60 *	4.11 ± 2.16 *	4.91 ± 2.48 *
Salivary HOMA-IR	119.7 ± 73.99	401.81 ± 231.17 *	278.79 ± 162.48 *	358.20 ± 215.35 *
Blood uric acid (mg/dL)	4.04 ± 0.76	5.06 ± 1.23 *	4.42 ± 0.92 *	4.84 ± 1.15 *
Salivary uric acid (μM)	143.46 ± 4.53	157.29 ± 13.04 *	156.45 ± 15.31 *	157.00 ± 13.53 *

Abbreviations = ALT: alanine transaminase; AST: aspartate transaminase; BMI: Body Mass Index; DBP: diastolic blood pressure; HDL: high density lipoproteins; HOMA-IR: Homeostasis Assessment Model—Insulin Resistance WC: waist circumference; NC: neck circumference; SBP: systolic blood pressure; WtHR: Waist to Height Ratio; * p value < 0.05 compared to controls.

More than 50% of obese children ($n = 15$) had ultrasonographic (US) signs of NAFLD and hypertransaminasemia not due to the most common causes of liver diseases, as well as significantly higher values of systolic blood pressure (127 ± 9 vs. 96 ± 11 mm Hg, $p = 0.0003$) and glycemia (88.6 ± 10.4 vs. 83.2 ± 6.6 mg/dL, $p = 0.002$) compared with NW subjects. Twenty-one patients had no component of MetS, 7 had at least one component, 10 had two or three components, and only 3 had more than three components (Table 2).

As shown in Figure 1, the PLS-DA score plots clearly differentiated between obese (OB) and normal weight (NW) children (Figure 1A1) and between OB with and without steatosis and NW controls (Figure 1B1). Twelve and 13 metabolites with a VIP-score > 2 separated NW/OB and NW/OB[St+]/OB[St−], respectively (Figure 1A2,B2). A third PLS-DA model (Figure 1C1) separated children according to MetS via five metabolites that had a VIP-score >2 (Figure 1C2).

As shown in Figure 1 and Table 3, compared with NW subjects, the saliva of obese children had higher levels of palmitic acid, myristic acid, urea, N-acetyl galactosamine, maltose, gluconic acid and isoleucine and lower levels of hydroxy butyric acid and malic acid, which were prevalent in those without steatosis and lauric acid, maltose and methyl maleic acid, which were prevalent in those with steatosis.

Table 2. Metabolic Syndrome components in obese patients with and without hepatic steatosis.

	Number (%) of Obese Patients with Hepatic Steatosis	Number (%) of Obese Patients without Hepatic Steatosis	Total (%)
Sample size	15(65%)	8(35%)	23(100%)
Waist circumference >90th percentile	15(65%)	7(30%)	22(95%)
Glucose blood levels >100 mg/dL	4(17%)	2(9%)	6(26%)
Blood pressure >95th percentile	10(43%)	4(17%)	14(60%)
HDL <40 mg/dL	3(13%)	0(0%)	3(13%)
TG >150 mg/dL	2(9%)	3(13%)	5(22%)
HOMA-IR > 3	13(57%)	5(22%)	18(79%)
Numbers of patients fulfilling MetS Criteria: (WC > 90th percentile and more than two out of four other criteria)	7(30%)	3(13%)	10(43%)

Abbreviations = HDL: high density lipoproteins; HOMA-IR: Homeostasis Assessment Model – Insulin Resistance; MetS: Metabolic Syndrome; TG: Triglycerides; WC: waist circumference

Table 3. Variables important in projection (VIP) metabolites fold changes in patients versus controls' saliva.

VIP	NW (n = 18) [a]	OB[St−] (n = 15)	OB[St+] (n = 8)	p-Value [b]	MetS− (n = 38) [a]	MetS+ (n = 3)	p-Value [c]
Hydroxy butyric acid	0.00697	−0.14	−0.62 *	NS	0.00622	−1.02	NS
Palmitic acid [d]	0.00088	4.46 ***	8.06 **	NS	0.00398	−0.74	NS
Myristic acid	0.00092	3.71 **	7.58 *	NS	0.00375	−0.66	NS
Lauric acid	0.00061	−7.21 **	−3.35	NS	0.00267	0.73	NS
Urea	0.00093	4.15 **	7.65 **	NS	0.00404	−0.71	NS
N-acetyl galactosamine	0.00088	3.72 **	7.60 *	NS	0.00375	−0.66	NS
Malic acid	0.17825	−0.98	−0.98	NS	0.09066	0.96	NS
Methyl maleic acid	0.01375	−0.72	−0.24	NS	0.01164	0.81	NS
Maltose	0.07047	−0.54	−0.25	NS	0.05846	0.24	NS
Xylose	0.00864	−0.62	−0.34	NS	0.00681	0.27	NS
Butanediol	0.00070	−6.16 **	−2.79	NS	0.00272	0.34	NS
Proline	0.00999	−0.56	−0.25	NS	0.00752	−1.02	NS
Tartaric acid	0.06401	0.52	0.40	NS	0.04729	−0.40	NS

* indicates a p-value < 0.05 compared to NW, ** indicates a p-value < 0.01 compared to NW, *** indicates a p-value < 0.001 compared to NW, NS indicates a p-value > 0.05. [a] Normalized chromatographic peak area; [b] p-values of OB[St+]/OB[St−] comparison; [c] p-values of MetS−/MetS+ comparison; [d] Metabolite selected by both PLS-DA models. Abbreviations: MetS−: No metabolic syndrome diagnosis; MetS+: Diagnosis of metabolic syndrome; NW: Normal Weight; OB[St+]: Obese without steatosis; OB[St+]: Obese with Steatosis; PLS-DA: Partial Least Squares Discriminant Analysis; VIP: Variable Important in Projections

The volcano plot representation and histogram of the metabolites selected using volcano plot analysis (FC > 1 or < −1, p < 0.05) of the OB patients compared with NW (Figure S1-A1) and of the OB[St+] patients compared with the OB[St−] patients (Figure S1-A2) is reported in supplementary Figure S1.

The levels of valine, mannose, acetopyruvic acid, palmitic acid, triethylene glycol, gluconic acid, citric acid, scyllo-inositol, deoxyglucose, psicopyranose, myo-inositol and cycloserine were higher in OB patients (Figure 2B1). Conversely, the levels of 1,2,3-butanetriol, 2-oxovaleric acid, 2-palmitoylglycerol, Di-n-octyl phthalate, itaconic acid, methyl galactoside, stearic acid, 2-piperidinone, maltose, 2-deoxy-D-ribose, pentane dioic acid, glycerol, pentitol, glyceric acid, methyl maleic acid, 2-deoxypentofuranose, β-hydroxy pyruvic acid, 2-hydroxy- methylcyclopentanol, and L-serine were higher in NW patients (Figure S1-B1). OB[St+] patients had higher levels of D-glucuronic acid γ-lactone, 2′-deoxyribolactone, 2-hydroxyisocaproic acid, pyroglutamic acid, and propanoic acid. Instead, OB[St−] patients had higher levels of butanoic acid, maltose, thiamine, glucopyranose, 2-hydroxybutyric acid, and mannose (Figure S1-B).

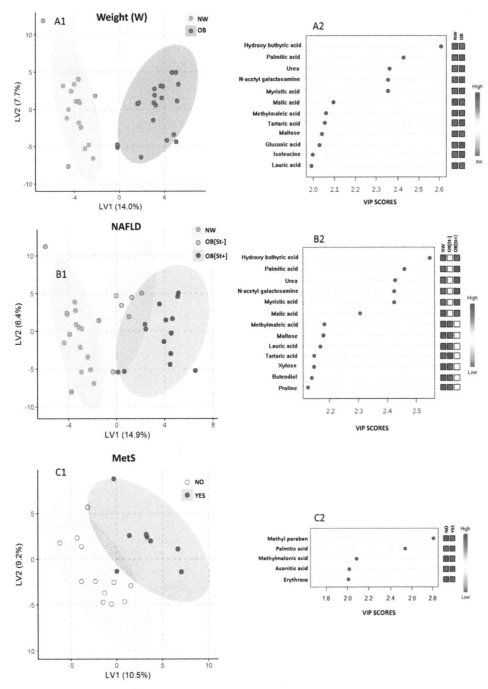

Figure 1. Partial least square discriminant analysis (PLS-DA) models to discriminate children according to Body Mass Index (BMI) (**A1**) and Non Alcoholic Fatty Liver Disease (NAFLD) (**B1**), as unique parameters investigated. The explained variance of each component is shown in parenthesis on the corresponding axis. In panel **A1**, the green ellipse contains normal weight children, while the red one contains the obese children. In panel **B1**, the purple circles represent the obese children with NAFLD (OB[St+]), the pink circles represent obese children without NAFLD (OB[St−]), while green circles represent the normal weight controls (NW). In panel **C1**, the blue circles represent the children with a diagnosis of metabolic syndrome (MetS), while the yellow ones represent the children without MetS diagnosis. The first 12, 13 and 5 variables important in projection (VIP) identified by the corresponding PLS-DA are shown in Panels **A2**, **B2** and **C2** respectively. The number of VIPs was established by setting the VIP-score ≥ 2 as a cut off value. In all cases, the colored boxes on the right indicate the relative amount of the corresponding metabolite in each group under study.

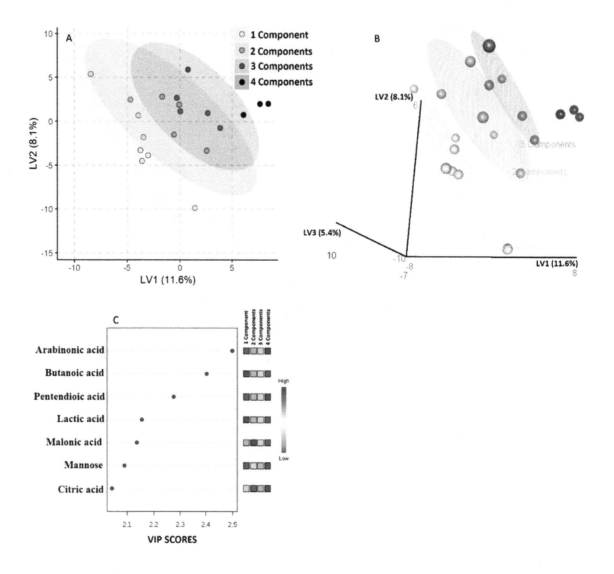

Figure 2. Partial least squares discriminant analysis (PLS-DA) model to discriminate obese children according to the number of Metabolic Syndrome (MetS) components. The explained variance of each component is shown on the corresponding axis. In panels **A** and **B**, the color darkness progression denotes the MetS components increase. The seven metabolites with a variable important in projection score (VIP-score) higher than 2 are shown in Panel **C**.

Figure 2 represents the PLS-DA model regarding the aggregation of saliva samples by the number of MetS components.

A clear-cut class separation was achieved, following the increase in the number of MetS components (Figure 2A,B). The metabolites with a VIP-score > 2 were as follows: arabinoic, butanoic, pentendioic, lactic, malonic and citric acid and mannose (Figure 2C).

Obese patients were also aggregated considering the serum ALT concentration. Figure 3A reports on the PLS-DA model when the serum ALT level higher than 40 mg/mL was considered hypertransaminasemia. Nine metabolites (butentriol, methyl valeric acid, pentanedioic acid, valine, hydroxy butanoic acid, mannose, di-n-octyl-phthalate and stearic and glyceric acid) showed a VIP-score higher than 2 (Figure 3C).

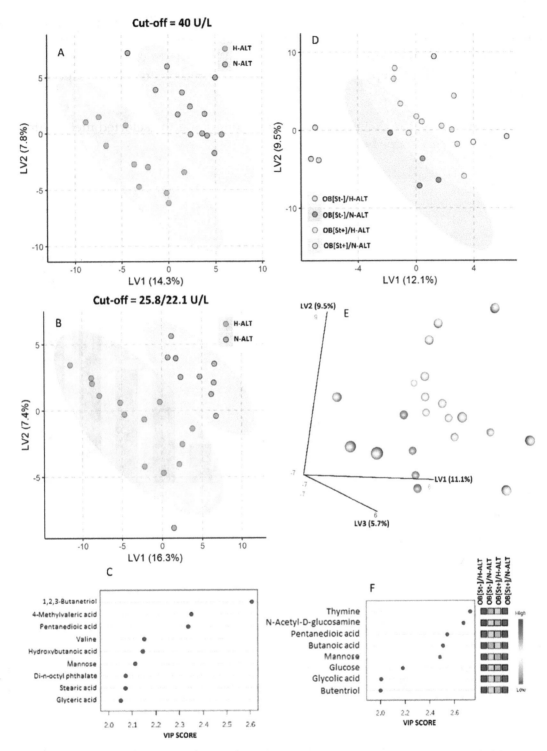

Figure 3. Partial least squares discriminant analysis (PLS-DA) model to discriminate children according to the presence/absence of hypertransaminasemia. Panel **A**: Serum Alanine transaminase (ALT) > 40 U/L was considered as hypertransaminasemia for both boys and girls. The explained variance of each component is shown on the corresponding axis. Panel **B**. Serum ALT > 25.8 U/L for boys and 22.1 U/L for girls was considered as hypertransaminasemia. In panels **A** and **B**, the cyan ellipse contains children with ALT > cut off values, while gray circles represent the children with serum ALT lower than cut off values. The nine metabolites with a VIP-score higher than 2 are shown in Panel **C**. PLS-DA shown in Panels **D/E** cumulates information on the status of both hepatic steatosis and transaminases values with respective variable important in projection scores (VIP-scores) shown in Panel **F**.

When the serum ALT level >25.8U/L for boys and 22.1 U/L for girls were considered hypertransaminasemia [24], the PLS-DA model remained discriminant (panel 3B), and the metabolites showing a VIP score >2 remained unchanged (panel 3C). PLS-DA shown in Panel 3D/E cumulates information on the status of both hepatic steatosis and transaminase values with respective VIP-scores shown in Panel F.

Figure 4 illustrates the UpSet [37] representation summarizing the selected metabolites in several classifications and the relationships between sets.

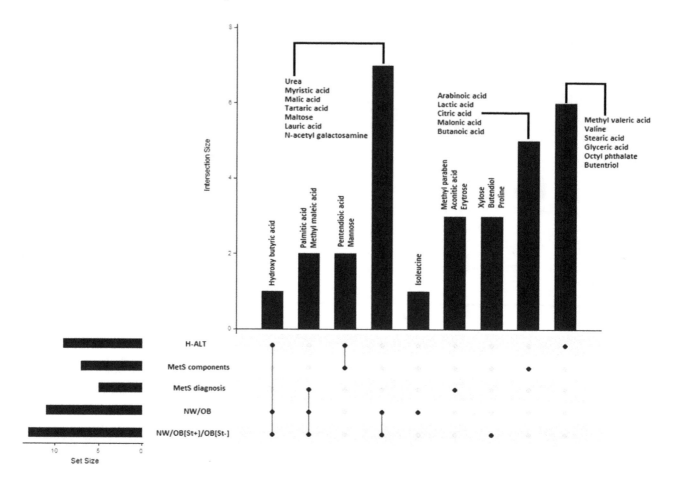

Figure 4. UpSet representation of the metabolites selected in the different classification models. H-ALT: Hypertransaminasemia; MetS: Metabolic Syndrome; NW: normal weight, OB: obese, [St]: hepatic steatosis.

Overall, as shown in the metabolic systemic map (Figure 5), there is a definite interplay of several pathways involving the following processes: de novo fatty acid biosynthesis; saturated fatty acid beta-oxidation; butanoate metabolism; glycolysis and gluconeogenesis; tricarboxylic acid cycle; urea cycle and metabolism of proline, glutamate, aspartate and asparagine; valine, leucine and isoleucine (BCCA) degradation; amino sugar metabolism; purine metabolism; and glycerophospholipid metabolism.

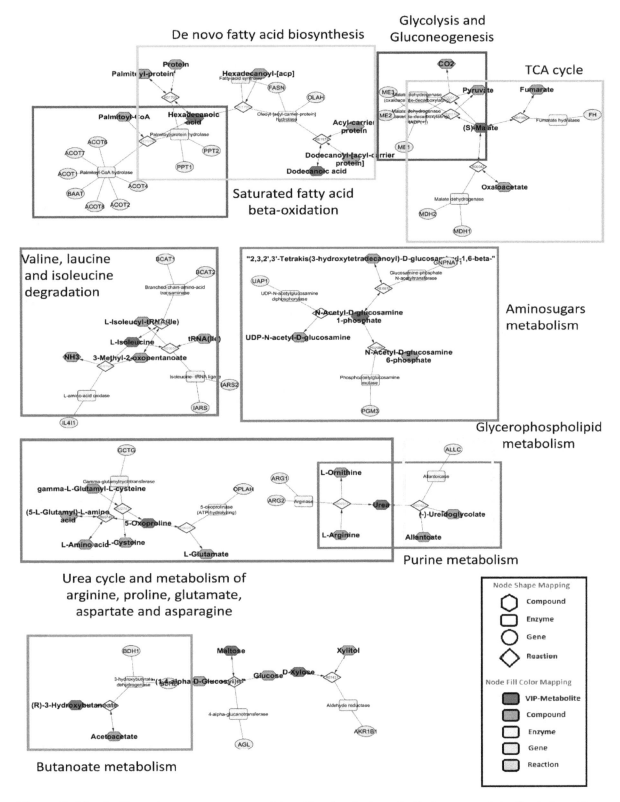

Figure 5. Metabolic systems map summarizing the shortest route that may explain the interactions among the metabolites with a variable important in projection scores higher than 2. There is a clear interplay of several pathways involving: de novo fatty acid biosynthesis; saturated fatty acid beta-oxidation; butanoate metabolism; glycolysis and gluconeogenesis; tricarboxylic acid cycle (TCA); urea cycle and metabolism of proline, glutamate, aspartate and asparagine; valine, and isoleucine (branched chain amino acids) degradation; aminosugars metabolism; purine metabolism; glycerophospholipid metabolism.

4. Discussion

As in a few other conditions (pediatric celiac disease [38], mild cognitive impairment [2], sport performance/fatigue [3,39], T2D [5,40]/T1D [41], and some neurological conditions [42]), our study shows that salivary metabolomics may represent a useful tool to obtain additional pathomechanistic information and serve as a possible clue to individuate novel disease diagnostic biomarkers data also in pediatric obesity. From our results, overall it appears that several salivary metabolites and metabolic pathways contribute to a complex metabolic fingerprint of obesity, obesity-related NAFLD and obesity-related MetS. Some of these metabolites were easily predictable based on obesity pathophysiology whereas others were not.

In line with blood and urinary metabolomic results obtained by others [43–45], the BCAAs valine and isoleucine were among the AAs more prevalently involved in the obesity-deranged pathways, but they did not appear to accurately reflect specific hepatic [43] or metabolic [44,45] involvement. The network of salivary molecules separating the lean and obese groups in obese individuals (independently from having or not MetS/NAFLD comorbidities) was also notably characterized by higher levels of two saturated fatty acids, palmitic acid and myristic acid, which tended to be prevalent in those with steatosis. Interestingly, this finding is in line with recently reported data suggesting that elevated total serum ceramide, as well as specific concentrations of myristic, palmitic, palmitoleic, stearic, oleic, behenic and lignoceric ceramide, with insulin resistance and play a potential role in the development of NAFLD in obese children [46]. The correlation of the lipid profile with glucose and insulin levels has been reported to probably mirror a still preserved ability to adapt to a caloric challenge compared with metabolically unhealthy individuals [47,48], in line with recent suggestions that propose a fatty acid profile is a useful tool to explain part of the heterogeneity between abdominal obesity and MetS [11,48,49]. Others have reported that, in addition to palmitic and stearic acid, other FAs are deranged and that increased activity of C16 Δ9-desaturase and C18 Δ9-desaturase in parallel with decreased Δ5-desaturase activity may be a causative factor in disturbed fatty acid metabolism [50]. In line with recent mouse model studies [51] where chronic oral administration of myristic acid improved hyperglycemia by decreasing insulin-responsive glucose levels and reducing body weight, myristic acid in our enrichment pathway is a fatty acid that appears to be associated with obesity but not with MetS. Finally, patients with fatty liver had higher levels of salivary pyroglutamic acid, a metabolite that has recently been proposed as a possible diagnostic biomarker for more severe liver disease [52].

Even more interestingly, as seen also by others in blood [12], PLS-DA showed that the salivary metabolic profiles could correctly identify children with a fewer number of MetS criteria than those who displayed more. This suggests that metabolic profiles can stratify MetS subpopulations, therefore, paving the way for their utilization for both early disease diagnosis and monitoring in those with MetS. This appears particularly relevant as in a recent Clinical Report, the American Academy of Pediatrics (AAP) Committee on Nutrition [53] acknowledged that although several attempts have been made to define MetS in the pediatric population, the construct at this age is difficult to define and has unclear implications for clinical care. For this reason, the Committee focused on the importance of (a) screening for and treating each individual risk factor component of MetS and (b) increasing awareness of comorbid conditions including NAFLD to be addressed and referred to specialists, as needed.

Study Limitations and Strengths

Our findings should be considered in the context of several study limitations, including a relatively small sample size, methodological flaws, and the lack of liver biopsy and prospective data during follow-up. First, our sample size was somewhat limited, and we may have had insufficient power to detect significant associations, particularly for stratified analyses. Larger series with patient follow-up are needed to confirm the preliminary results of our pilot study. Second, our findings related to VIP metabolites should be interpreted with caution given that these were obtained on only one saliva sample for each of the participant children. Although saliva was revealed to be a reliable biofluid for metabolomics studies [17], neurological disorder [42], and T1D [41], the likely risks of poor reproducibility persist. In fact, possible, differences among unstimulated, stimulated (e.g., obtained with oral movements such as gentle mastication), and pure parotid saliva exist [54,55]. Third, ultrasound may be insensitive compared with biopsy or magnetic resonance imaging (MRI). Nevertheless, it is the reference test for use in pediatric clinical practice. Furthermore, liver biopsy cannot be considered a screening procedure because it is invasive, not riskless and not exempt from possible sampling errors. As a non-invasive alternative to assess hepatic steatosis, US is repeatable because it does not require sedation or the delivery of ionizing radiation [1,56]. Although it is the less robust of the numerous imaging options [57], methodological progress has shown good diagnostic specificity and sensitivity, especially if the steatosis involves at least 20% of the hepatocytes [58]. Overall, these limitations do not allow us to draw definite conclusions but strongly suggest the viability of such an approach. These limitations, however, are balanced by several important strengths, including a full auxological and biochemical characterization of our subjects' cohort that allowed us to build several classification models on the same group of patients and delineate the metabolite/metabolic pathways. Moreover, this represents the first study to show the potential usefulness of saliva to define a metabolomic signature of pediatric obesity and related hepato-metabolic comorbidities.

5. Conclusions

Using the saliva of children affected by obesity, we showed a definite interplay of several metabolic pathways with possible specific patterns capable of sorting fatty liver and MetS. The involved metabolic processes include the following: de novo fatty acid biosynthesis; saturated fatty acid beta-oxidation; butanoate metabolism; glycolysis and gluconeogenesis; tricarboxylic acid cycle; urea cycle; metabolism of proline, glutamate, aspartate and asparagine; valine, leucine and isoleucine (BCAA) degradation; aminosugar metabolism; purine metabolism; and glycerophospholipid metabolism. Overall, this information, along with that of other recent progress regarding the study of salivary simple analytes [4], trace elements [59], major adipocytokines [60,61], and specific microRNAs [62], reinforces the idea that saliva will soon represent a useful tool for deepening pathomechanismistic aspects, noninvasive diagnosis and monitoring of pediatric and adult individuals with obesity. The early and non-invasive detection of incipient MetS/fatty liver in childhood through salivary metabolomics as described here, therefore, appears as a promising helpful tool to prevent further health hepato-metabolic and cardiovascular complications in adulthood, and ultimately serves to minimize their related global socioeconomic burden.

Supplementary Materials: Figure S1: Panels (A) show the selected metabolites with fold change (FC) values <-1 or >+1 with a simultaneous p-value < 0.05 (red dot). (A1) Normal weight (NW) versus Obese (OB) metabolite. (A2) Steatosis obese patients (OB[St+]) versus non-steatosis obese patients (OB[St−]). FC of the selected metabolites are shown in the corresponding panel (B1 and B2).

Author Contributions: J.T. and P.V. conceived and designed the experimental study, and contributed equally; F.B., A.B., L.P., C.M., A.D.N., A.G.D.A, L.D.M., A.P.D.B. and S.G.N. characterized clinical/lab features of the patients; J.T., A.C. and G.S. performed GC/MS experiments; P.C., G.S. and J.T. analyzed the data; J.T and G.S. contributed reagents/materials/analysis tools and to the development of the analytical methods; J.T. and P.V. wrote the paper which was integrated and fully agreed by all authors.

Funding: The research work was partially funded to PV by University of Salerno UNISA/FARB 2016 and 2017 and to GS by "POR FESR CAMPANIA 2014/2020-O.S. 1.1—Avviso pubblico per il sostegno alle imprese nella realizzazione di studi di fattibilità (Fase 1) e progetti di trasferimento tecnologico (Fase 2) coerenti con la RIS 3—Concessione contributo in forma di sovvenzione—Soggetto proponente: HOSMOTIC Srl—Progetto: Strumenti di supporto alla prevenzione, diagnosi e monitoraggio dell'obesità in età pediatrica—CUP:B73D18000100007".

References

1.   Clemente, M.G.; Mandato, C.; Poeta, M.; Vajro, P. Pediatric non-alcoholic fatty liver disease: Recent solutions, unresolved issues, and future research directions. *World J. Gastroenterol.* **2016**, *22*, 8078–8093. [CrossRef] [PubMed]

2. Zheng, J.; Dixon, R.A.; Li, L. Development of Isotope Labeling LC-MS for Human Salivary Metabolomics and Application to Profiling Metabolome Changes Associated with Mild Cognitive Impairment. *Anal. Chem.* **2012**, *84*, 10802–10811. [CrossRef] [PubMed]

3. Ra, S.-G.; Maeda, S.; Higashino, R.; Imai, T.; Miyakawa, S. Metabolomics of salivary fatigue markers in soccer players after consecutive games. *Appl. Physiol. Nutr. Metab.* **2014**, *39*, 1120–1126. [CrossRef] [PubMed]

4. Troisi, J.; Belmonte, F.; Bisogno, A.; Lausi, O.; Marciano, F.; Cavallo, P.; Guercio Nuzio, S.; Landolfi, A.; Pierri, L.; Vajro, P. Salivary markers of hepato-metabolic comorbidities in pediatric obesity. *Dig. Liver Dis.* **2018**. [CrossRef] [PubMed]

5. Martos-Moreno, G.A.; Sackmann-Sala, L.; Barrios, V.; Berrymann, D.E.; Okada, S.; Argente, J.; Kopchick, J.J. Proteomic analysis allows for early detection of potential markers of metabolic impairment in very young obese children. *Int. J. Pediatr. Endocrinol.* **2014**, *2014*, 9. [CrossRef] [PubMed]

6. Miccheli, A.; Capuani, G.; Marini, F.; Tomassini, A.; Pratico, G.; Ceccarelli, S.; Gnani, D.; Baviera, G.; Alisi, A.; Putignani, L.; et al. Urinary (1)H-NMR-based metabolic profiling of children with NAFLD undergoing VSL#3 treatment. *Int. J. Obes.* **2015**, *39*, 1118–1125.

7. Wiklund, P.K.; Pekkala, S.; Autio, R.; Munukka, E.; Xu, L.; Saltevo, J.; Cheng, S.; Kujala, U.M.; Alen, M.; Cheng, S. Serum metabolic profiles in overweight and obese women with and without metabolic syndrome. *Diabetol. Metab. Syndr.* **2014**, *6*, 40. [CrossRef]

8. Wurtz, P.; Makinen, V.-P.; Soininen, P.; Kangas, A.J.; Tukiainen, T.; Kettunen, J.; Savolainen, M.J.; Tammelin, T.; Viikari, J.S.; Ronnemaa, T.; et al. Metabolic signatures of insulin resistance in 7098 young adults. *Diabetes* **2012**, *61*, 1372–1380. [CrossRef]

9. Jin, T.; Yu, H.; Huang, X.-F. Selective binding modes and allosteric inhibitory effects of lupane triterpenes on protein tyrosine phosphatase 1B. *Sci. Rep.* **2016**, *6*, 20766. [CrossRef]

10. Butte, N.F.; Liu, Y.; Zakeri, I.F.; Mohney, R.P.; Mehta, N.; Voruganti, V.S.; Goring, H.; Cole, S.A.; Comuzzie, A.G. Global metabolomic profiling targeting childhood obesity in the Hispanic population. *Am. J. Clin. Nutr.* **2015**, *102*, 256–267. [CrossRef]

11. Baek, S.H.; Kim, M.; Kim, M.; Kang, M.; Yoo, H.J.; Lee, N.H.; Kim, Y.H.; Song, M.; Lee, J.H. Metabolites distinguishing visceral fat obesity and atherogenic traits in individuals with overweight. *Obesity* **2017**, *25*, 323–331. [CrossRef] [PubMed]

12. Zhong, F.; Xu, M.; Bruno, R.S.; Ballard, K.D.; Zhu, J. Targeted high performance liquid chromatography tandem mass spectrometry-based metabolomics differentiates metabolic syndrome from obesity. *Exp. Biol. Med.* **2017**, *242*, 773–780. [CrossRef]

13. Pujos-Guillot, E.; Brandolini, M.; Pétéra, M.; Grissa, D.; Joly, C.; Lyan, B.; Herquelot, É.; Czernichow, S.; Zins, M.; Goldberg, M. Systems metabolomics for prediction of metabolic syndrome. *J. Proteome Res.* **2017**, *16*, 2262–2272. [CrossRef] [PubMed]

14. Pierri, L.; Saggese, P.; Guercio Nuzio, S.; Troisi, J.; Di Stasi, M.; Poeta, M.; Savastano, R.; Marchese, G.; Tarallo, R.; Massa, G.; et al. Relations of gut liver axis components and gut microbiota in obese children with fatty liver: A pilot study. *Clin. Res. Hepatol. Gastroenterol.* **2018**, *42*, 387–390. [CrossRef]

15. Troisi, J.; Pierri, L.; Landolfi, A.; Marciano, F.; Bisogno, A.; Belmonte, F.; Palladino, C.; Guercio Nuzio, S.; Campiglia, P.; Vajro, P. Urinary Metabolomics in Pediatric Obesity and NAFLD Identifies Metabolic Pathways/Metabolites Related to Dietary Habits and Gut-Liver Axis Perturbations. *Nutrients* **2017**, *9*, E485. [CrossRef] [PubMed]

16. Dame, Z.T.; Aziat, F.; Mandal, R.; Krishnamurthy, R.; Bouatra, S.; Borzouie, S.; Guo, A.C.; Sajed, T.; Deng, L.; Lin, H.; et al. The human saliva metabolome. *Metabolomics* **2015**, *11*, 1864–1883. [CrossRef]

17. Hartman, M.-L.; Goodson, J.M.; Barake, R.; Alsmadi, O.; Al-Mutawa, S.; Ariga, J.; Soparkar, P.; Behbehani, J.; Behbehani, K. Salivary Biomarkers in Pediatric Metabolic Disease Research. *Pediatr. Endocrinol. Rev.* **2016**, *13*, 602–611.

18. Belmonte, F.; Bisogno, A.; Troisi, J.; Landolfi, A.M.; Lausi, O.; Lamberti, R.; Nuzio, S.G.; Pierri, L.; Siano, M.; Viggiano, C.; et al. Salivary levels of uric acid, insulin and HOMA: A promising field of study to non-invasively identify obese children at risk of metabolic syndrome and fatty liver. *Dig. Liver Dis.* **2017**, *49*, e247. [CrossRef]

19. Cho, K.; Moon, J.S.; Kang, J.-H.; Jang, H.B.; Lee, H.-J.; Park, S.I.; Yu, K.-S.; Cho, J.-Y. Combined untargeted and targeted metabolomic profiling reveals urinary biomarkers for discriminating obese from normal-weight adolescents. *Pediatr. Obes.* **2017**, *12*, 93–101. [CrossRef]

20. Ho, J.E.; Larson, M.G.; Ghorbani, A.; Cheng, S.; Chen, M.-H.; Keyes, M.; Rhee, E.P.; Clish, C.B.; Vasan, R.S.; Gerszten, R.E.; et al. Metabolomic Profiles of Body Mass Index in the Framingham Heart Study Reveal Distinct Cardiometabolic Phenotypes. *PLoS ONE* **2016**, *11*, e0148361. [CrossRef]

21. Zheng, H.; Yde, C.C.; Arnberg, K.; Molgaard, C.; Michaelsen, K.F.; Larnkjaer, A.; Bertram, H.C. NMR-based metabolomic profiling of overweight adolescents: An elucidation of the effects of inter-/intraindividual differences, gender, and pubertal development. *Biomed. Res. Int.* **2014**, *2014*, 537157. [CrossRef] [PubMed]

22. Vajro, P.; Lenta, S.; Pignata, C.; Salerno, M.; D'Aniello, R.; De Micco, I.; Paolella, G.; Parenti, G. Therapeutic options in pediatric non alcoholic fatty liver disease: Current status and future directions. *Ital. J. Pediatr.* **2012**, *38*, 55. [CrossRef]

23. Schwenzer, N.F.; Springer, F.; Schraml, C.; Stefan, N.; Machann, J.; Schick, F. Non-invasive assessment and quantification of liver steatosis by ultrasound, computed tomography and magnetic resonance. *J. Hepatol.* **2009**, *51*, 433–445. [CrossRef] [PubMed]

24. Schwimmer, J.B.; Dunn, W.; Norman, G.J.; Pardee, P.E.; Middleton, M.S.; Kerkar, N.; Sirlin, C.B. SAFETY study: Alanine aminotransferase cutoff values are set too high for reliable detection of pediatric chronic liver disease. *Gastroenterology* **2010**, *138*, 1357–1364. [CrossRef] [PubMed]

25. Vajro, P.; Maddaluno, S.; Veropalumbo, C. Persistent hypertransaminasemia in asymptomatic children: A stepwise approach. *World J. Gastroenterol.* **2013**, *19*, 2740–2751. [CrossRef] [PubMed]

26. Zimmet, P.; Alberti, K.G.M.; Kaufman, F.; Tajima, N.; Silink, M.; Arslanian, S.; Wong, G.; Bennett, P.; Shaw, J.; Caprio, S. The metabolic syndrome in children and adolescents—An IDF consensus report. *Pediatr. Diabetes* **2007**, *8*, 299–306. [CrossRef] [PubMed]

27. World Medical Association. World medical association declaration of helsinki: Ethical principles for medical research involving human subjects. *JAMA* **2013**, *310*, 2191–2194. [CrossRef]

28. Kovats, E.S. Gas-chromatographische charakterisierung organischer verbindungen. Teil 1: Retentionsindices aliphatischer halogenide, alkohole, aldehyde und ketone. *Helv. Chim. Acta* **1958**, *41*, 1915–1932. [CrossRef]

29. van den Berg, R.A.; Hoefsloot, H.C.; Westerhuis, J.A.; Smilde, A.K.; van der Werf, M.J. Centering, scaling, and transformations: Improving the biological information content of metabolomics data. *BMC Genom.* **2006**, *7*, 142. [CrossRef]

30. Sumner, L.W.; Amberg, A.; Barrett, D.; Beale, M.H.; Beger, R.; Daykin, C.A.; Fan, T.W.-M.; Fiehn, O.; Goodacre, R.; Griffin, J.L.; et al. Proposed minimum reporting standards for chemical analysis Chemical Analysis Working Group (CAWG) Metabolomics Standards Initiative (MSI). *Metabolomics* **2007**, *3*, 211–221. [CrossRef]

31. Sysi-Aho, M.; Katajamaa, M.; Yetukuri, L.; Oresic, M. Normalization method for metabolomics data using optimal selection of multiple internal standards. *BMC Bioinformatics* **2007**, *8*, 93. [CrossRef] [PubMed]

32. Mevik, B.-H.; Wehrens, R. The pls Package: Principal Component and Partial Least Squares Regression in R. *J. Stat. Softw.* **2007**. [CrossRef]

33. Kuhn, M. Building Predictive Models in R Using the caret Package. *J. Stat. Softw.* **2008**, *28*, 1–26. [CrossRef]

34. Bijlsma, S.; Bobeldijk, I.; Verheij, E.R.; Ramaker, R.; Kochhar, S.; Macdonald, I.A.; van Ommen, B.; Smilde, A.K. Large-scale human metabolomics studies: A strategy for data (pre-) processing and validation. *Anal. Chem.* **2006**, *78*, 567–574. [CrossRef] [PubMed]

35. Karnovsky, A.; Weymouth, T.; Hull, T.; Tarcea, V.G.; Scardoni, G.; Laudanna, C.; Sartor, M.A.; Stringer, K.A.; Jagadish, H.V.; Burant, C.; et al. Metscape 2 bioinformatics tool for the analysis and visualization of metabolomics and gene expression data. *Bioinformatics* **2012**, *28*, 373–380. [CrossRef] [PubMed]

36. Nishida, K.; Ono, K.; Kanaya, S.; Takahashi, K. KEGGscape: A Cytoscape app for pathway data integration. *F1000Research* **2014**, *3*, 144. [CrossRef] [PubMed]

37. Lex, A.; Gehlenborg, N.; Strobelt, H.; Vuillemot, R.; Pfister, H. UpSet: Visualization of Intersecting Sets. *IEEE Trans. Vis. Comput. Gr.* **2014**, *20*, 1983–1992. [CrossRef] [PubMed]

38. Francavilla, R.; Ercolini, D.; Piccolo, M.; Vannini, L.; Siragusa, S.; De Filippis, F.; De Pasquale, I.; Di Cagno, R.; Di Toma, M.; Gozzi, G.; et al. Salivary microbiota and metabolome associated with celiac disease. *Appl. Environ. Microbiol.* **2014**, *80*, 3416–3425. [CrossRef]

39. Santone, C.; Dinallo, V.; Paci, M.; D'Ottavio, S.; Barbato, G.; Bernardini, S. Saliva metabolomics by NMR for the evaluation of sport performance. *J. Pharm. Biomed.* **2014**, *88*, 441–446. [CrossRef]

40. Rao, P.V.; Reddy, A.P.; Lu, X.; Dasari, S.; Krishnaprasad, A.; Biggs, E.; Roberts, C.T.; Nagalla, S.R. Proteomic identification of salivary biomarkers of type-2 diabetes. *J. Proteome Res.* **2009**, *8*, 239–245. [CrossRef]

41. Pappa, E.; Vastardis, H.; Mermelekas, G.; Gerasimidi-Vazeou, A.; Zoidakis, J.; Vougas, K. Saliva Proteomics Analysis Offers Insights on Type 1 Diabetes Pathology in a Pediatric Population. *Front. Physiol.* **2018**, *9*, 444. [CrossRef] [PubMed]

42. Walton, E.L. Saliva biomarkers in neurological disorders: A "spitting image" of brain health? *Biomed. J.* **2018**, *41*, 59–62. [CrossRef] [PubMed]

43. Goffredo, M.; Santoro, N.; Tricò, D.; Giannini, C.; D'Adamo, E.; Zhao, H.; Peng, G.; Yu, X.; Lam, T.T.; Pierpont, B. A branched-chain amino acid-related metabolic signature characterizes obese adolescents with non-alcoholic fatty liver disease. *Nutrients* **2017**, *9*, 642. [CrossRef] [PubMed]

44. Wu, N.; Wang, W.; Yi, M.; Cheng, S.; Wang, D. *Study of the Metabolomics Characteristics of Patients with Metabolic Syndrome Based on Liquid Chromatography Quadrupole Time-Of-Flight Mass Spectrometry*; Elsevier: Amsterdam, The Netherlands, 2018; Volume 79, pp. 37–44.

45. Reddy, P.; Leong, J.; Jialal, I. Amino acid levels in nascent metabolic syndrome: A contributor to the pro-inflammatory burden. *J. Diabetes Complicat.* **2018**, *32*, 465–469. [CrossRef] [PubMed]

46. Wasilewska, N.; Bobrus-Chociej, A.; Harasim-Symbor, E.; Tarasów, E.; Wojtkowska, M.; Chabowski, A.; Lebensztejn, D. Serum concentration of ceramides in obese children with nonalcoholic fatty liver disease. *J. Pediatr. Gastroenterol. Nutr.* **2018**, *66*, S2. [CrossRef] [PubMed]

47. Badoud, F.; Lam, K.P.; Perreault, M.; Zulyniak, M.A.; Britz-McKibbin, P.; Mutch, D.M. Metabolomics reveals metabolically healthy and unhealthy obese individuals differ in their response to a caloric challenge. *PLoS ONE* **2015**, *10*, e0134613. [CrossRef] [PubMed]

48. Aristizabal, J.C.; Barona, J.; Gonzalez-Zapata, L.I.; Deossa, G.C.; Estrada, A. Fatty acid content of plasma triglycerides may contribute to the heterogeneity in the relationship between abdominal obesity and the metabolic syndrome. *Metab. Syndr. Relat. Disord.* **2016**, *14*, 311–317. [CrossRef] [PubMed]

49. Aristizabal, J.C.; González-Zapata, L.I.; Estrada-Restrepo, A.; Monsalve-Alvarez, J.; Restrepo-Mesa, S.L.; Gaitán, D. Concentrations of plasma free palmitoleic and dihomo-gamma linoleic fatty acids are higher in children with abdominal obesity. *Nutrients* **2018**, *10*, 31. [CrossRef]

50. Kang, M.; Lee, A.; Yoo, H.J.; Kim, M.; Kim, M.; Shin, D.Y.; Lee, J.H. Association between increased visceral fat area and alterations in plasma fatty acid profile in overweight subjects: A cross-sectional study. *Lipids Health Dis.* **2017**, *16*, 248. [CrossRef]

51. Takato, T.; Iwata, K.; Murakami, C.; Wada, Y.; Sakane, F. Chronic administration of myristic acid improves hyperglycaemia in the Nagoya–Shibata–Yasuda mouse model of congenital type 2 diabetes. *Diabetologia* **2017**, *60*, 2076–2083. [CrossRef]

52. Qi, S.; Xu, D.; Li, Q.; Xie, N.; Xia, J.; Huo, Q.; Li, P.; Chen, Q.; Huang, S. Metabonomics screening of serum identifies pyroglutamate as a diagnostic biomarker for nonalcoholic steatohepatitis. *Clin. Chim. Acta* **2017**, *473*, 89–95. [CrossRef]

53. Magge, S.N.; Goodman, E.; Armstrong, S.C. The Metabolic Syndrome in Children and Adolescents: Shifting the Focus to Cardiometabolic Risk Factor Clustering. *Pediatrics* **2017**, *24*, e20171603. [CrossRef]

54. Denny, P.; Hagen, F.K.; Hardt, M.; Liao, L.; Yan, W.; Arellanno, M.; Bassilian, S.; Bedi, G.S.; Boontheung, P.; Cociorva, D. The proteomes of human parotid and submandibular/sublingual gland salivas collected as the ductal secretions. *J. Proteome Res.* **2008**, *7*, 1994–2006. [CrossRef]

55. Tiwari, M. Science behind human saliva. *J. Nat. Sci. Biol. Med.* **2011**, *2*, 53–58. [CrossRef]

56. Vajro, P.; Lenta, S.; Socha, P.; Dhawan, A.; McKiernan, P.; Baumann, U.; Durmaz, O.; Lacaille, F.; McLin, V.; Nobili, V. Diagnosis of nonalcoholic fatty liver disease in children and adolescents: Position paper of the ESPGHAN Hepatology Committee. *J. Pediatr. Gastroenterol. Nutr.* **2012**, *54*, 700–713. [CrossRef]

57. Vos, M.B.; Abrams, S.H.; Barlow, S.E.; Caprio, S.; Daniels, S.R.; Kohli, R.; Mouzaki, M.; Sathya, P.; Schwimmer, J.B.; Sundaram, S.S. NASPGHAN clinical practice guideline for the diagnosis and treatment of nonalcoholic fatty liver disease in children: Recommendations from the Expert Committee on NAFLD (ECON) and the North American Society of Pediatric Gastroenterology, Hepatology and Nutrition (NASPGHAN). *J. Pediatr. Gastroenterol. Nutr.* **2017**, *64*, 319–334.

58. Koot, B.G.; van der Baan-Slootweg, O.H.; Bohte, A.E.; Nederveen, A.J.; van Werven, J.R.; Tamminga-Smeulders, C.L.; Merkus, M.P.; Schaap, F.G.; Jansen, P.L.; Stoker, J. Accuracy of prediction scores and novel biomarkers for predicting nonalcoholic fatty liver disease in obese children. *Obesity* **2013**, *21*, 583–590. [CrossRef]

59. Marin Martinez, L.; Molino Pagan, D.; Lopez Jornet, P. Trace Elements in Saliva as Markers of Type 2 Diabetes Mellitus. *Biol. Trace Elem. Res.* **2018**, *186*, 354–360. [CrossRef]

60. Abdalla, M.M.I.; Soon, S.C. Salivary adiponectin concentration in healthy adult males in relation to anthropometric measures and fat distribution. *Endocr. Regul.* **2017**, *51*, 185–192. [CrossRef]

61. Ibrahim Abdalla, M.M.; Siew Choo, S. Salivary Leptin Level in Young Adult Males and its Association with Anthropometric Measurements, Fat Distribution and Muscle Mass. *Eur. Endocrinol.* **2018**, *14*, 94–98. [CrossRef]

62. Vriens, A.; Provost, E.B.; Saenen, N.D.; De Boever, P.; Vrijens, K.; De Wever, O.; Plusquin, M.; Nawrot, T.S. Children's screen time alters the expression of saliva extracellular miR-222 and miR-146a. *Sci. Rep.* **2018**, *8*, 8209. [CrossRef]

2

Comprehensive Dipeptide Analysis Revealed Cancer-Specific Profile in the Liver of Patients with Hepatocellular Carcinoma and Hepatitis

Hitoshi Ozawa [1,2], Akiyoshi Hirayama [1,2,*], Futaba Shoji [1], Midori Maruyama [1], Kumi Suzuki [1], Hisami Yamanaka-Okumura [3], Hiroshi Tatano [3,4], Yuji Morine [5], Tomoyoshi Soga [1,2], Mitsuo Shimada [5] and Masaru Tomita [1,2]

[1] Institute for Advanced Biosciences, Keio University, Tsuruoka, Yamagata 997-0052, Japan; 038hts@sfc.keio.ac.jp (H.O.); dofla20mingo@yahoo.co.jp (F.S.); green12@ttck.keio.ac.jp (M.M.); ksuzuki@ttck.keio.ac.jp (K.S.); soga@sfc.keio.ac.jp (T.S.); mt@sfc.keio.ac.jp (M.T.)

[2] Systems Biology Program, Graduate School of Media and Governance, Keio University, Fujisawa, Kanagawa 252-0882, Japan

[3] Department of Clinical Nutrition and Food Management, Graduate School of Biomedical Sciences, Tokushima University Graduate School, Tokushima 770-8503, Japan; okumurah@tokushima-u.ac.jp (H.Y.-O.); h-tatano@u-shimane.ac.jp (H.T.)

[4] Department of Health and Nutrition, Faculty of Nursing and Nutrition, The University of Shimane, Izumo, Shimane 693-8550, Japan

[5] Department of Digestive and Pediatric Surgery, Graduate School of Medical Sciences, Tokushima University, Tokushima 770-8503, Japan; ymorine@tokushima-u.ac.jp (Y.M.); mitsuo.shimada@tokushima-u.ac.jp (M.S.)

* Correspondence: hirayama@ttck.keio.ac.jp

Abstract: As the physical properties and functionality of dipeptides differ from those of amino acids, they have attracted attention in metabolomics; however, their functions in vivo have not been clarified in detail. Hepatocellular carcinoma (HCC) is the most common type of primary liver cancer, and its major cause is chronic hepatitis. This study was conducted to explore tumor-specific dipeptide characteristics by performing comprehensive dipeptide analysis in the tumor and surrounding nontumor tissue of patients with HCC. Dipeptides were analyzed by liquid chromatography tandem mass spectrometry and capillary electrophoresis tandem mass spectrometry. Principal component analysis using 236 detected dipeptides showed differences in the dipeptide profiles between nontumor and tumor tissues; however, no clear difference was observed in etiological comparison. In addition, the N- and C-terminal amino acid compositions of the detected dipeptides significantly differed, suggesting the substrate specificity of enzyme proteins, such as peptidase. Furthermore, hepatitis-derived HCC may show a characteristic dipeptide profile even before tumor formation. These results provide insight into HCC pathogenesis and may help identify novel biomarkers for diagnosis.

Keywords: dipeptide; hepatocellular carcinoma; hepatitis B virus; hepatitis C virus; liquid chromatography tandem mass spectrometry; capillary electrophoresis tandem mass spectrometry; metabolomics

1. Introduction

Hepatocellular carcinoma (HCC) is the third leading cause of cancer-related deaths worldwide [1]. A major cause of HCC is chronic hepatitis caused by hepatitis virus infection. Infection with hepatitis B virus (HBV) or C virus (HCV) causes hepatitis, and long-term destruction and regeneration of hepatocytes leads to cirrhosis and, finally, HCC [2]. The most characteristic feature of HCC is that tumor growth is rapid and initial symptoms are unlikely to be detected. When a tumor is found, it has often spread to other organs [3].

An important approach to understanding the characteristics of liver cancer is metabolome analysis, which can reveal the metabolite profile in vivo. Metabolome analysis has been applied to various tumor tissues such as gastric cancer [4], liver cancer [5,6], prostate cancer [7,8], breast cancer [9], oral cancer [10], and lung cancer [7,11]. Additionally, several studies have reported the discovery of potential serum biomarkers of HCC by metabolome analysis using gas chromatography-mass spectrometry (GC-MS) and liquid chromatography-mass spectrometry (LC-MS) [12–15].

As post-amino acids, dipeptides are highly diverse with different physical and functional properties from amino acids [16]. In recent years, dipeptides have attracted attention as functional biomaterials, particularly as potential disease biomarkers [17]. For instance, carnosine and anserine containing an imidazole group derived from histidine can remove reactive oxygen and thus play a role as endogenous antioxidants [18,19]. In addition, leucine-histidine suppresses microglia activity, reduces proinflammatory cytokine production, and ameliorates depression and depression-related emotional disturbances [20]. It has also been reported that dipeptides consisting of aromatic amino acids and leucine, such as Tyr-Leu, Phe-Leu, and Trp-Leu, have anxiolytic-like activity in mice [21]. The physiological activity of artificially synthesized dipeptides has also been reported [22,23].

Some dipeptides have also been used as biomarkers of disease. For example, prolyl-4-hydroxyproline, a dipeptide produced when collagen is degraded, is used as a urinary biomarker of bone resorption [24,25]. Furthermore, we found that the concentration of γ-glutamyl dipeptides in the serum fluctuates in nine types of liver diseases such as hepatitis, cirrhosis, and HCC, indicating the potential of these biomarkers for liver disease screening [26,27].

Thus, analyzing dipeptides in a biological sample may lead to the discovery of new functional components and various disease biomarkers. Although some dipeptides have been measured, few comprehensive dipeptide analyses have been performed. One reason for this is that all dipeptides, except those composed of the same amino acid, have structural isomers with opposite amino acid binding orders. As these isomers have the same molecular weight, it is difficult to distinguish them by mass spectrometry. Therefore, these isomers must be separated by chromatography before being introduced into a mass spectrometer, but it is difficult to separate many dipeptides by a single analytical method. To overcome this limitation, we recently developed a comprehensive dipeptide analytical method using liquid chromatography tandem mass spectrometry (LC-MS/MS) and capillary electrophoresis tandem mass spectrometry (CE-MS/MS), which enabled simultaneous quantitation of 335 types of dipeptides [16].

In this study, we applied LC-MS/MS and CE-MS/MS to compare the dipeptide profiles of tumors and surrounding nontumor tissues of patients with liver cancer. The characteristics of the amino acids constituting the dipeptide detected in the tissues were also examined. Furthermore, the dipeptide profiles in HCC with different etiologies were compared. It was found that the dipeptide profiles in non-tumor and tumor tissues differed, and hepatitis-derived cancer has a characteristic dipeptide profile before tumor onset.

2. Results

2.1. Study Population and Data Analysis

Tumor and surrounding nontumor liver tissues were surgically resected from 13 patients with HCC and 3 patients with metastatic liver cancer. The clinical information of the patients is listed in Table 1. All liver cancer cases were the first instance of cancer, and the patients had no treatment history prior to surgery. The mean ± standard deviation of the patients' age and body mass index were 67.6 ± 9.3 years and 22.6 ± 3.6, respectively. The HCC group contained 6 non-B/C samples, 2 HBV samples, and 5 HCV samples. The stages of cancer in HCC varied from I to IVB.

Table 1. Clinical characteristics of patients in this study.

ID	Age	Sex	BMI	Type	Virus	Stage
1	68	Female	31.9	HCC	Non B/C	III
2	73	Female	23.1	HCC	Non B/C	II
3	73	Male	17.3	HCC	Non B/C	II
4	72	Male	24.7	HCC	Non B/C	II
5	63	Male	18.2	HCC	Non B/C	II
6	67	Male	- *	HCC	Non B/C	III
7	44	Male	22.3	HCC	HBV	II
8	65	Male	19.0	HCC	HBV	III
9	61	Male	21.8	HCC	HCV	II
10	57	Male	21.5	HCC	HCV	I
11	78	Female	20.5	HCC	HCV	III
12	75	Male	25.4	HCC	HCV	II
13	60	Male	21.8	HCC	HCV	IVB
14	78	Female	22.1	MLC	Non B/C	
15	68	Female	23.3	MLC	Non B/C	
16	80	Male	26.7	MLC	Non B/C	

BMI, body mass index; HCC, hepatocellular carcinoma; MLC, metastatic liver cancer; Non B/C, Non B-Non C hepatitis; HBV, hepatitis B virus; HCV, hepatitis C virus. *, missing value.

In this study, 140 and 96 dipeptides were detected in the liver by LC-MS/MS and CE-MS/MS, respectively (quantitative results are shown in Supplementary Table S1). Among the total of 236 dipeptides detected in both methods, the peak of 14 dipeptides could not be distinguished by MRM transition and retention time. The amount of each dipeptide was standardized to nmol/g liver tissue, and subsequent analysis was performed using this value. Additionally, the amino acids comprising the dipeptides were expressed as one-letter codes.

2.2. Outlier Analysis

First, principal component analysis (PCA) was performed to identify trends in the dipeptide profiles of all samples measured in this study (Figure 1). The results of the PCA score plots (Figure 1a) suggested that two tumor tissues were supposed outliers. Therefore, outlier analysis was carried out to investigate whether outliers were included in the measured samples. Figure 1b shows the results of outlier analysis using Hotelling's T^2 statistics in PCA. As Hotelling's T^2 statistics of two tumor tissues (No. 4T and 6T) exceeded the upper control limit at a significance level of 0.01, these samples were considered outliers and excluded from subsequent analysis.

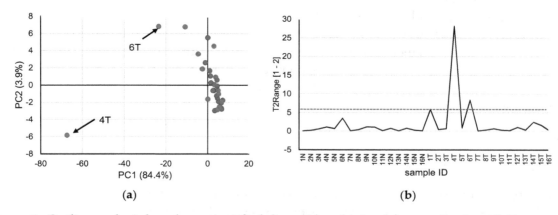

(a)   (b)

Figure 1. Outlier analysis based on quantified dipeptides obtained from patients with liver cancer. (**a**) principal component analysis score plots using the auto-scaled dipeptide data of paired non-tumor (blue) and tumor (red) tissues. The contribution ratios were 84.4% and 3.9% for PC1 and PC2, respectively. (**b**) Hotelling's T^2 range plot of all samples. The red dashed line indicates the upper control limit ($\alpha = 0.01$).

2.3. Principal Component Analysis

Next, PCA based on Pareto scaling was performed using the remaining 14 samples (each sample contained non-tumor and tumor tissues, respectively), excluding samples showing outliers (Figure 2). In the PCA score plot (Figure 2a), nontumor and tumor tissues were sufficiently separated mainly by principal component 2. In addition, QE (Gln-Glu) + EQ (Glu-Gln) + EK (Glu-Lys) + KE (Lys-Glu) (overlapped peak) and TY (The-Tyr), IK (Ile-Lys), and EN (Glu-Asn) showed relatively large values in principal component 2 of the loading plot (Figure 2b), suggesting that these dipeptides contributed to the separation of nontumor and tumor tissues.

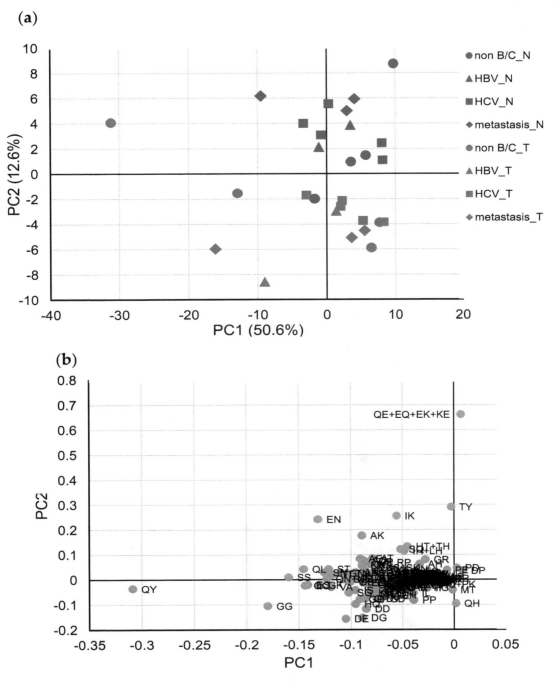

Figure 2. Principal component analysis (PCA) using the Pareto-scaled dipeptide data. (a) PCA score plots of paired nontumor (blue) and tumor (red) tissues in different types of liver cancers. The contribution ratios were 50.6% and 12.6% for PC1 and PC2, respectively. (b) PCA loading plots of dipeptides on the first two principal components.

2.4. *Characteristics of Dipeptides Detected in Liver Tissue*

To determine the characteristics of the dipeptides detected in each sample, grouping was performed for each amino acid constituting the N-terminus (Figure 3a) and C-terminus (Figure 3b). A relatively high accumulation of dipeptide was observed in the nontumor tissue of sample ID14 and tumor tissues of samples ID1, 2, and 15, but no obvious difference was observed in the amino acid composition of these samples compared to the other samples. This trend was similar between nontumor and tumor tissues. The amino acid compositions at the C- and N-termini significantly differed (Figure 3c). For example, dipeptides containing alanine (A), aspartic acid (D), and isoleucine (I) were predominant at the N-terminus, whereas dipeptides containing lysine (K), asparagine (N), proline (P), and tyrosine (Y) were increased at the C-terminus.

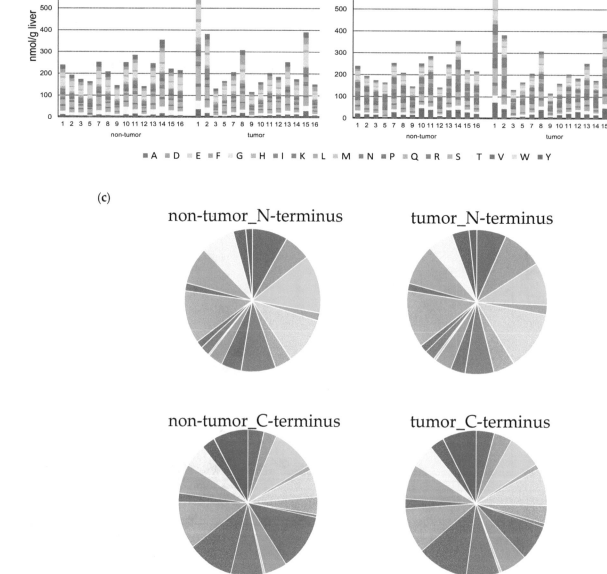

Figure 3. Amino acid composition of N-terminus (**a**) and C-terminus (**b**) in dipeptide detected from each liver tissue. The columns represent the number of moles (nmol/g liver). (**c**) The difference in the average composition ratio of N-terminal and C-terminal amino acids in each tissue.

2.5. Changes in Dipeptide Profile with and Without Hepatitis in HCC

The dipeptide profiles of non-hepatitis- and hepatitis-derived HCC were compared. Volcano plots were prepared using the quantitated values of dipeptides detected in non-hepatitis (non B/C, $n = 4$) and hepatitis (HBV or HCV, $n = 7$) samples from the tumor (Figure 4a) and nontumor tissues (Figure 4b) of HCC, respectively. In tumor tissues, only the amount of HT + TH was significantly decreased ($p < 0.05$, fold-change < 0.67) in hepatitis samples compared to non-hepatitis samples. Additionally, a significant increase ($p < 0.05$, fold-change > 1.5) in 6 dipeptides in hepatitis samples, including VI, IY, IE, TI, VN, and VT, was observed in the nontumor tissues. According to the results of the volcano plot, the number of dipeptides that was increased in hepatitis samples was slightly higher in nontumor tissues, whereas this number was mostly decreased in tumor tissues.

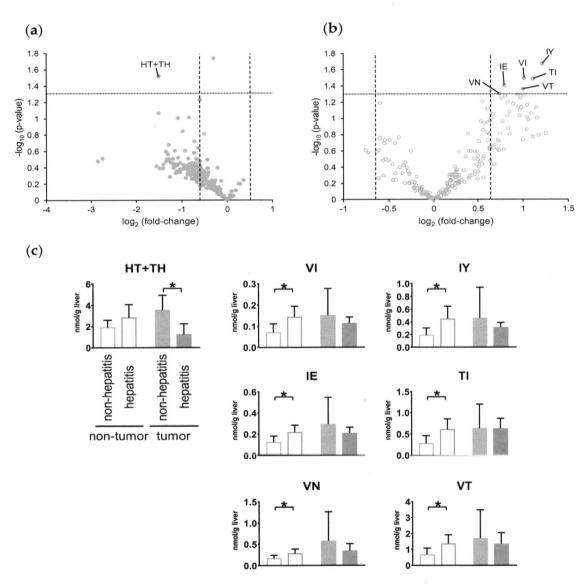

Figure 4. Volcano plot of differential dipeptides in the tumor (**a**) and nontumor (**b**) tissues with and without hepatitis in hepatocellular carcinoma. For each dipeptide, the $-\log_{10}$ (p-value) was plotted vs. $\log_2$ (fold-change). (**c**) Dipeptides showing a significant difference in the volcano plot ($p < 0.05$ and fold-change < 0.67 or > 1.5). The columns represent the average number of moles (nmol/g tissue), and error bars indicate the standard deviation. * $p < 0.05$.

Finally, we investigated the relationship of the dipeptide abundance between non-tumor and tumor tissues with and without hepatitis. Figure 4c shows the number of dipeptides in both tissues, showing significant differences in either tissue. One of the dipeptides that showed significance in tumor tissue showed no significance in nontumor tissue, whereas six of the dipeptides that showed significance in nontumor tissue showed no significance in tumor tissue.

3. Discussion

In this study, we performed a comprehensive dipeptide analysis of paired tumors and surrounding nontumor liver tissues obtained from 13 patients with HCC and three patients with metastatic liver cancer. We successfully quantified 236 dipeptides (14 overlapped) with our previously developed method using LC-MS/MS and CE-MS/MS [16]. This study reports the largest number of dipeptides detected in the liver tissue to date.

Unlike the analysis of body fluids such as blood and urine, it is necessary to consider variability between samples when performing metabolome analysis of tissues. Particularly, tumor tissues exhibit cancer heterogeneity, and the amounts of metabolites and dipeptides may greatly differ depending on the sample location. Therefore, effectively removing outliers is useful for searching for effective biomarkers in subsequent analyses. In this study, PCA using auto-scaled dipeptide data revealed that the score plots of samples 4T and 6T tended to deviate from the score plots of the other samples. Therefore, in outlier analysis with Hotelling's T^2 statistics, these two samples exceeded the upper control limit at a significance level of 0.01 and were therefore excluded from subsequent analysis.

PCA was performed again on the remaining 14 nontumor and tumor tissues using Pareto-scaled dipeptide data, which showed that nontumor and tumor tissues were separated for principal component 2. In contrast, no significant difference was observed depending on the factors causing liver cancer. These results demonstrate that the difference in the dipeptide profile in the liver depends on whether it is a nontumor- or tumor-derived tissue and does not depend on the factors causing cancer. This finding is similar to the serum metabolic profiles obtained by LC-MS from two HCC cohorts infected with HBV or HCV [28].

The characteristics of the detected dipeptides were also examined. A comparison of the total amount of dipeptides in nontumor and tumor tissues in each specimen showed that 7 of 14 specimens showed an increase, and the others showed a decrease in the amounts of dipeptides in the tumor tissue. When amino acids in various tumor tissues were measured by metabolome analysis [7,29], the samples showed different tendencies, possibly because of the heterogeneity of cancer. In addition, no significant difference was found in the amino acid composition between nontumor and tumor tissues, whereas a significant difference was observed at the N- and C-termini. One possible cause for this is the substrate specificity of the peptidase. For example, chymotrypsin, a serine protease, specifically cleaves the C-terminal of aromatic amino acids. In addition, elastase, which has a shallow bottom in the substrate-binding pocket, specifically cleaves the peptide bond at the C-terminus of amino acids with small side chains. However, various factors require further analysis, such as where the dipeptides detected in the liver tissue are produced.

Although there are several routes to HCC development, HBV and HCV infections are the most important risk factors [30]. Therefore, investigating the differences in dipeptide profiles depending on the presence or absence of hepatitis is important for understanding the process of HCC development. In addition, determining the differences in dipeptide profiles will enable identifying the biomarker candidates for future evaluation using biofluids. Nevertheless, there are limited numbers of studies searching for biomarkers by measuring dipeptides in body fluids. Recently, the dipeptides, such as hydroxyproline-Leu, EW, and FF, have been selected as promising predictive biomarkers for the diagnosis of epithelial ovarian cancer [31].

In this study, analysis of dipeptides with and without hepatitis revealed that seven dipeptides were significantly changed ($p < 0.05$, fold-change < 0.67 or >1.5). Among the tumor tissues, HT + TH was significantly decreased in hepatitis samples, and most other dipeptides also tended to decrease. In contrast, in nontumor tissues, VI, IY, IE, TI, VN, and VT were significantly increased in hepatitis samples, and many other dipeptides also tended to increase. For the seven dipeptides showing significant differences, the amounts in corresponding tissues were also examined, but none of the dipeptides showed a common change between tissues. Thus, hepatitis-derived HCC showed a characteristic tendency, with the amount of dipeptide increased in the surrounding nontumor tissue but decreased in the tumor tissue. This suggests that the change in the dipeptide profile due to the presence or absence of hepatitis already occurred before tumor formation and was maintained throughout the production of different dipeptides and metabolic mechanisms even after tumor generation.

There were several limitations to this study. First, because the number of samples used in this study was relatively small, the power of statistical analysis may not have been sufficient. In addition, as only liver cancer was analyzed, it is necessary to investigate other liver diseases such as cirrhosis and nonalcoholic steatohepatitis. Further studies of larger sample sizes are needed to examine the roles of dipeptides in liver cancer in detail.

In conclusion, we detected 236 dipeptides in liver cancer tissue using a comprehensive dipeptide analytical method involving CE-MS/MS and LC-MS/MS. Similar to previously reported metabolite results, the dipeptide profiles in nontumor and tumor tissues differed, although no clear difference was observed in the etiological comparison. We also found that the N- and C-terminal amino acid compositions of the detected dipeptides significantly differed in both tissues, suggesting the substrate specificity of enzyme proteins, such as peptidase. A comparison of the dipeptide profiles depending on the presence or absence of hepatitis suggested that hepatitis-derived cancer has a characteristic dipeptide profile before tumor onset.

4. Materials and Methods

4.1. Sample Collection and Dipeptide Extraction

This study was approved by the Tokushima University Hospital Ethics Committee (Approved no. 1815), and the corresponding regulatory agencies and all experiments were carried out in accordance with approved guidelines. All patients involved in the study signed an informed consent form.

Tumor and surrounding nontumor tissues were surgically resected from 13 patients with HCC and 3 patients with metastatic liver cancer. The resected tissue samples were quickly frozen at −80 °C until sample preparation.

Liver tissues were weighed (~100 mg) and homogenized in methanol (500 μL) containing internal standards (20 μM methionine sulfone and 50 μM Phe-Gly-$^{13}C_9$-$^{15}N_1$) using a Shake Master NEO instrument (Biomedical Science Co., Ltd., Tokyo, Japan). The homogenates were mixed with chloroform (500 μL) and Milli-Q water (200 μL), and the mixture was centrifuged at 4600× g for 15 min at 4 °C. The upper aqueous layer (300 μL) was centrifugally filtered through a 5-kDa cutoff filter (Human Metabolome Technologies, Tsuruoka, Japan) to remove proteins. The filtrate was centrifugally concentrated in a vacuum evaporator and dissolved in Milli-Q water (25 μL) immediately before CE-MS/MS analysis. This sample was diluted by 5-fold with Milli-Q water and subjected to LC-MS/MS analysis.

4.2. Dipeptide Analysis

Comprehensive dipeptide analysis was performed by CE-MS/MS and LC-MS/MS, as described previously [16]. The CE-MS/MS system was composed of an Agilent 1600 CE system (Agilent Technologies, Santa Clara, CA, USA), Agilent 6490 triple quadrupole mass spectrometer, Agilent 1200 series isocratic HPLC pump, and Agilent G1607A CE-ESI-MS sprayer kit. The separation was carried out on a fused-silica capillary (50 μm I.D., 360 μm O.D., 135 cm total length, Polymicro Technologies, Phoenix, AZ, USA) using 200 mM of aqueous acetic acid as a background electrolyte. Prior to the first use, a new capillary was rinsed with background electrolyte for 20 min. Equilibration was performed for 4 min by flushing with background electrolyte before each run. The sample solution was injected at 5 kPa for 15 s (~15 nL), and a positive voltage of 30 kV was applied. The capillary was maintained at 20 °C, and the sheath liquid (methanol: water = 1:1, v/v) was delivered at 10 μL/min.

ESI-MS/MS analysis was conducted in positive ion mode using the following source parameters: dry gas temperature, 280 °C; dry gas flow rate, 11 L/min; nebulizer pressure, 10 psi; capillary voltage, 4 kV; fragmentor voltage, 380 V; cell accelerator voltage, 7 V; high- and low-pressure radiofrequency voltage of ion funnel, 150 and 60 V, respectively; and dwell time, 5 ms.

LC-MS/MS analysis was carried out using an Agilent 1290 Infinity HPLC system coupled to an Agilent 6490 triple quadrupole mass spectrometer with an Agilent jet stream ESI interface. Dipeptides were separated on an Acquity UPLC HSS PFP column (2.1 × 150 mm, 1.8 μm; Waters, Milford, MA, USA). The mobile phase was composed of 0.1 vol% aqueous formic acid (A) and 0.1 vol% formic acid in 95 vol% aqueous acetonitrile (B). The flow rate was 0.2 mL/min, and the following linear gradient was used: 0–3 min, 1% B; 3–30 min, 1% to 50% B; 30–30.1 min, 50% to 99% B; 30.1–35 min, 99% B; 35–35.1 min, 99% to 1% B, followed by equilibration with 1% B for 15 min. The injection volume was 1 μL, and the column temperature was maintained at 45 °C.

Agilent jet stream-ESI-MS/MS analysis was performed in positive ion mode using the following source parameters: dry gas temperature, 280 °C; dry gas flow rate, 12 L/min; nebulizer pressure, 30 psi; sheath gas temperature, 380 °C; sheath gas flow rate, 12 L/min; capillary voltage, 3.5 kV; nebulizer voltage, 2.0 kV; fragmentor voltage, 380 V; cell accelerator voltage, 7 V; high- and low-pressure radiofrequency voltage of the ion funnel, 150 and 60 V, respectively; and dwell time, 2 ms.

The molar amount of each dipeptide in 1 g of liver tissue was determined by normalizing the peak area of each dipeptide with respect to the area of the internal standard and by using the single-point standard calibration curves (CE-MS/MS; 20 μM, LC-MS/MS; 15 μM).

4.3. Outlier Analysis

To examine the outliers, the T^2 statistic and upper control limit were used to evaluate the results of PCA with autoscaling [32]. The T^2 statistic in each sample was evaluated using Equation (1).

$$T_i^2 = M_i^2 = X_{ci} P_A L^{-1} P_A{}^t X_{ci}{}^t \tag{1}$$

where M_i is the Mahalanobis distance, X_{ci} is the line vector of the standardized data of dipeptide amount, P_A is the matrix including the eigenvector of principal component A, and L is the diagonal matrix of the eigenvalue of principal component A.

The control limit was evaluated using Equation (2).

$$CL_{1-\alpha} = \frac{(n-1)^2}{n} x_{1-\alpha}^{\beta} \left[\frac{A}{2}, \frac{n-A-1}{2} \right] \tag{2}$$

where n is the number of specimens, A is the number of principal components, α is the significance level ($\alpha = 0.01$), and $x_{1-\alpha}^{\beta}$ is the $(1 - \alpha)$-quantile of the beta distribution of parameter $[A/2, (n - A - 1)/2]$.

4.4. Data Analysis

The acquired data were analyzed using the MassHunter software (version B.06.00, Agilent Technologies). PCA was performed using the SIMCA software (version 13, Umetrics AB, Umeå, Sweden). The Mann-Whitney U-test was used for statistical analysis. A p-value of less than 0.05 was considered statistically significant.

Supplementary Materials: Table S1: Amount of dipeptide quantified in non-tumor and tumor tissues of patients with HCC and MLC (nmol/g liver).

Author Contributions: Conceptualization, H.O. and A.H.; methodology, H.O. and A.H.; formal analysis, H.O.; investigation, H.O., A.H., F.S., M.M., H.Y.-O., H.T. and Y.M.; resources, H.Y.-O., Y.M. and M.S.; data curation, H.O.; writing—original draft preparation, H.O. and A.H.; writing—review and editing, H.O., A.H., H.Y.-O., Y.M., T.S., M.S. and M.T.; visualization, A.H. and K.S.; supervision, T.S., M.S. and M.T.; project administration, A.H.; funding acquisition, A.H., H.Y.-O., M.S. and M.T. All authors have read and agreed to the published version of the manuscript.

Funding: This research was funded by the Japan Agency for Medical Research and Development (AMED) GAPFREE programs 18ak0101043h0104, 18ak0101043s1404, and 18ak0101043h0004 (A.H.); AMED research program on hepatitis 19fk0210048 and 20fk0210048 (Y.M., M.S.); JSPS KAKENHI JP18H04804 (A.H.), JP18K08219 (A.H.), JP19K11742 (H.Y.-O.) and JP18H02871 (A.H., Y.M., M.S.), and grants from the Yamagata prefectural government and the city of Tsuruoka.

References

1. Yang, J.D.; Roberts, L.R. Hepatocellular carcinoma: A global view. *Nat. Rev. Gastroenterol. Hepatol.* **2010**, *7*, 448–458. [CrossRef] [PubMed]

2. Sakamoto, M. Early HCC: Diagnosis and molecular markers. *J. Gastroenterol.* **2009**, *44*, 108–111. [CrossRef] [PubMed]

3. Ryder, S.D. Guidelines for the diagnosis and treatment of hepatocellular carcinoma (HCC) in adults. *Gut* **2003**, *52*, iii1–iii8. [CrossRef] [PubMed]

4. Wu, H.; Xue, R.; Tang, Z.; Deng, C.; Liu, T.; Zeng, H.; Sun, Y.; Shen, X. Metabolomic investigation of gastric cancer tissue using gas chromatography/mass spectrometry. *Anal. Bioanal. Chem.* **2010**, *396*, 1385–1395. [CrossRef] [PubMed]

5. Huang, Q.; Tan, Y.; Yin, P.; Ye, G.; Gao, P.; Lu, X.; Wang, H.; Xu, G. Metabolic characterization of hepatocellular carcinoma using nontargeted tissue metabolomics. *Cancer Res.* **2013**, *73*, 4992–5002. [CrossRef] [PubMed]

6. Ferrarini, A.; Di Poto, C.; He, S.; Tu, C.; Varghese, R.S.; Kara Balla, A.; Jayatilake, M.; Li, Z.; Ghaffari, K.; Fan, Z.; et al. Metabolomic Analysis of Liver Tissues for Characterization of Hepatocellular Carcinoma. *J. Proteome Res.* **2019**, *18*, 3067–3076. [CrossRef]

7. Kami, K.; Fujimori, T.; Sato, H.; Sato, M.; Yamamoto, H.; Ohashi, Y.; Sugiyama, N.; Ishihama, Y.; Onozuka, H.; Ochiai, A.; et al. Metabolomic profiling of lung and prostate tumor tissues by capillary electrophoresis time-of-flight mass spectrometry. *Metabolomics* **2013**, *9*, 444–453. [CrossRef]

8. Sreekumar, A.; Poisson, L.M.; Rajendiran, T.M.; Khan, A.P.; Cao, Q.; Yu, J.; Laxman, B.; Mehra, R.; Lonigro, R.J.; Li, Y.; et al. Metabolomic profiles delineate potential role for sarcosine in prostate cancer progression. *Nature* **2009**, *457*, 910–914. [CrossRef]

9. Budczies, J.; Denkert, C.; Muller, B.M.; Brockmoller, S.F.; Klauschen, F.; Gyorffy, B.; Dietel, M.; Richter-Ehrenstein, C.; Marten, U.; Salek, R.M.; et al. Remodeling of central metabolism in invasive breast cancer compared to normal breast tissue—A GC-TOFMS based metabolomics study. *BMC Genom.* **2012**, *13*, 334. [CrossRef] [PubMed]

10. Ishikawa, S.; Sugimoto, M.; Kitabatake, K.; Sugano, A.; Nakamura, M.; Kaneko, M.; Ota, S.; Hiwatari, K.; Enomoto, A.; Soga, T.; et al. Identification of salivary metabolomic biomarkers for oral cancer screening. *Sci. Rep.* **2016**, *6*, 31520. [CrossRef] [PubMed]

11. Hori, S.; Nishiumi, S.; Kobayashi, K.; Shinohara, M.; Hatakeyama, Y.; Kotani, Y.; Hatano, N.; Maniwa, Y.; Nishio, W.; Bamba, T.; et al. A metabolomic approach to lung cancer. *Lung Cancer* **2011**, *74*, 284–292. [CrossRef]

12. Baniasadi, H.; Gowda, G.A.; Gu, H.; Zeng, A.; Zhuang, S.; Skill, N.; Maluccio, M.; Raftery, D. Targeted metabolic profiling of hepatocellular carcinoma and hepatitis C using LC-MS/MS. *Electrophoresis* **2013**, *34*, 2910–2917. [CrossRef] [PubMed]

13. Chen, F.; Xue, J.; Zhou, L.; Wu, S.; Chen, Z. Identification of serum biomarkers of hepatocarcinoma through liquid chromatography/mass spectrometry-based metabonomic method. *Anal. Bioanal. Chem.* **2011**, *401*, 1899–1904. [CrossRef] [PubMed]

14. Gao, R.; Cheng, J.; Fan, C.; Shi, X.; Cao, Y.; Sun, B.; Ding, H.; Hu, C.; Dong, F.; Yan, X. Serum metabolomics to identify the liver disease-specific biomarkers for the progression of hepatitis to hepatocellular carcinoma. *Sci. Rep.* **2015**, *5*, 18175. [CrossRef]

15. Han, J.; Qin, W.X.; Li, Z.L.; Xu, A.J.; Xing, H.; Wu, H.; Zhang, H.; Wang, M.D.; Li, C.; Liang, L.; et al. Tissue and serum metabolite profiling reveals potential biomarkers of human hepatocellular carcinoma. *Clin. Chim. Acta* **2019**, *488*, 68–75. [CrossRef]

16. Ozawa, H.; Hirayama, A.; Ishikawa, T.; Kudo, R.; Maruyama, M.; Shoji, F.; Doke, T.; Ishimoto, T.; Maruyama, S.; Soga, T.; et al. Comprehensive dipeptide profiling and quantitation by capillary electrophoresis and liquid chromatography coupled with tandem mass spectrometry. *Anal. Chem.* **2020**. [CrossRef]

17. Tang, Y.; Li, R.; Lin, G.; Li, L. PEP search in MyCompoundID: Detection and identification of dipeptides and tripeptides using dimethyl labeling and hydrophilic interaction liquid chromatography tandem mass spectrometry. *Anal. Chem.* **2014**, *86*, 3568–3574. [CrossRef] [PubMed]

18. Fonteh, A.N.; Harrington, R.J.; Tsai, A.; Liao, P.; Harrington, M.G. Free amino acid and dipeptide changes in the body fluids from Alzheimer's disease subjects. *Amino Acids* **2007**, *32*, 213–224. [CrossRef]

19. Saoi, M.; Percival, M.; Nemr, C.; Li, A.; Gibala, M.; Britz-McKibbin, P. Characterization of the human skeletal muscle metabolome for elucidating the mechanisms of bicarbonate ingestion on strenuous interval exercise. *Anal. Chem.* **2019**, *91*, 4709–4718. [CrossRef]

20. Ano, Y.; Kita, M.; Kitaoka, S.; Furuyashiki, T. Leucine-Histidine Dipeptide Attenuates Microglial Activation and Emotional Disturbances Induced by Brain Inflammation and Repeated Social Defeat Stress. *Nutrients* **2019**, *11*, 2161. [CrossRef]

21. Mizushige, T.; Kanegawa, N.; Yamada, A.; Ota, A.; Kanamoto, R.; Ohinata, K. Aromatic amino acid-leucine dipeptides exhibit anxiolytic-like activity in young mice. *Neurosci. Lett.* **2013**, *543*, 126–129. [CrossRef] [PubMed]

22. Gudasheva, T.A.; Deeva, O.A.; Mokrov, G.V.; Yarkov, S.A.; Yarkova, M.A.; Seredenin, S.B. The first dipeptide ligand of translocator protein: Design and anxiolytic activity. *Dokl. Biochem. Biophys.* **2015**, *464*, 290–293. [CrossRef]

23. Vasconcelos, S.N.; Drewes, C.C.; de Vinci Kanda Kupa, L.; Farsky, S.H.; Stefani, H.A. Evaluation of toxicity on epithelial and tumor cells of biaryl dipeptide tyrosines. *Eur. J. Med. Chem.* **2016**, *114*, 1–7. [CrossRef]

24. Cimlova, J.; Kruzberska, P.; Svagera, Z.; Husek, P.; Simek, P. In situ derivatization-liquid liquid extraction as a sample preparation strategy for the determination of urinary biomarker prolyl-4-hydroxyproline by liquid chromatography-tandem mass spectrometry. *J. Mass Spectrom.* **2012**, *47*, 294–302. [CrossRef] [PubMed]

25. Mazzi, G.; Fioravanzo, F.; Burti, E. New marker of bone resorption: Hydroxyproline-containing peptide. High-performance liquid chromatographic assay without hydrolysis as an alternative to hydroxyproline determination: A preliminary report. *J. Chromatogr. B Biomed. Appl.* **1996**, *678*, 165–172. [CrossRef]

26. Hirayama, A.; Igarashi, K.; Tomita, M.; Soga, T. Development of quantitative method for determination of gamma-glutamyl peptides by capillary electrophoresis tandem mass spectrometry: An efficient approach avoiding matrix effect. *J. Chromatogr. A* **2014**, *1369*, 161–169. [CrossRef] [PubMed]

27. Soga, T.; Sugimoto, M.; Honma, M.; Mori, M.; Igarashi, K.; Kashikura, K.; Ikeda, S.; Hirayama, A.; Yamamoto, T.; Yoshida, H.; et al. Serum metabolomics reveals gamma-glutamyl dipeptides as biomarkers for discrimination among different forms of liver disease. *J. Hepatol.* **2011**, *55*, 896–905. [CrossRef]

28. Zhou, L.; Ding, L.; Yin, P.; Lu, X.; Wang, X.; Niu, J.; Gao, P.; Xu, G. Serum metabolic profiling study of hepatocellular carcinoma infected with hepatitis B or hepatitis C virus by using liquid chromatography-mass spectrometry. *J. Proteome Res.* **2012**, *11*, 5433–5442. [CrossRef]

29. Hirayama, A.; Kami, K.; Sugimoto, M.; Sugawara, M.; Toki, N.; Onozuka, H.; Kinoshita, T.; Saito, N.; Ochiai, A.; Tomita, M.; et al. Quantitative metabolome profiling of colon and stomach cancer microenvironment by capillary electrophoresis time-of-flight mass spectrometry. *Cancer Res.* **2009**, *69*, 4918–4925. [CrossRef]

30. Petruzziello, A. Epidemiology of Hepatitis B Virus (HBV) and Hepatitis C Virus (HCV) Related hepatocellular carcinoma. *Open Virol. J.* **2018**, *12*, 26–32. [CrossRef]

31. Lu, X.; Li, Y.; Xia, B.; Bai, Y.; Zhang, K.; Zhang, X.; Xie, H.; Sun, F.; Hou, Y.; Li, K. Selection of small plasma peptides for the auxiliary diagnosis and prognosis of epithelial ovarian cancer by using UPLC/MS-based nontargeted and targeted analyses. *Int. J. Cancer* **2019**, *144*, 2033–2042. [CrossRef]

32. Adams, E.; De Maesschalck, R.; De Spiegeleer, B.; Vander Heyden, Y.; Smeyers-Verbeke, J.; Massart, D.L. Evaluation of dissolution profiles using principal component analysis. *Int. J. Pharm.* **2001**, *212*, 41–53. [CrossRef]

3

Transcriptional Regulation in Non-Alcoholic Fatty Liver Disease

Sandra Steensels †, Jixuan Qiao † and Baran A. Ersoy *

Joan & Sanford I. Weill Department of Medicine, Weill Cornell Medical College, New York, NY 10021, USA; sas2906@med.cornell.edu (S.S.); jiq2001@med.cornell.edu (J.Q.)
* Correspondence: bersoy@med.cornell.edu
† These authors have contributed equally to this work.

Abstract: Obesity is the primary risk factor for the pathogenesis of non-alcoholic fatty liver disease (NAFLD), the worldwide prevalence of which continues to increase dramatically. The liver plays a pivotal role in the maintenance of whole-body lipid and glucose homeostasis. This is mainly mediated by the transcriptional activation of hepatic pathways that promote glucose and lipid production or utilization in response to the nutritional state of the body. However, in the setting of chronic excessive nutrition, the dysregulation of hepatic transcriptional machinery promotes lipid accumulation, inflammation, metabolic stress, and fibrosis, which culminate in NAFLD. In this review, we provide our current understanding of the transcription factors that have been linked to the pathogenesis and progression of NAFLD. Using publicly available transcriptomic data, we outline the altered activity of transcription factors among humans with NAFLD. By expanding this analysis to common experimental mouse models of NAFLD, we outline the relevance of mouse models to the human pathophysiology at the transcriptional level.

Keywords: non-alcoholic fatty liver disease; non-alcoholic steatohepatitis; transcription factors; inflammation; metabolic stress; fibrosis; lipid homeostasis; glucose homeostasis

1. Introduction

Obesity often results in the dysregulation of lipid and glucose metabolism and is therefore the primary risk factor for the pathogenesis of metabolic disorders, including cardiovascular disease, type 2 diabetes mellitus (T2DM), and non-alcoholic fatty liver disease (NAFLD) [1]. The global prevalence of NAFLD, which was 15% in 2005, has quickly escalated to 24% by 2016 in a parallel trend to obesity [2]. NAFLD encompasses a spectrum of pathologies ranging from hepatocellular lipid accumulation (steatosis) to non-alcoholic steatohepatitis (NASH) characterized by steatosis and inflammation. In addition, chronic inflammation activates hepatic stellate cells (HSC), which promote fibrosis by secreting type I and III collagen and fibronectin into the extracellular matrix (ECM) [3]. When fibrotic NASH remains untreated, it can lead to cirrhosis and hepatocellular carcinoma (HCC) [4]. Despite alarming increases in prevalence, the treatment strategy of NAFLD remains limited to weight loss regiments and requires a more complete understanding of diet-induced pathogenesis of NAFLD in obese patients [5].

The pathogenesis of NAFLD is complex, and evolving theories have culminated in a two-hit versus multiple-hit hypotheses [6]. In the 'two-hit hypothesis', the first hit originates from the accumulation of more than 5% hepatic steatosis, during which insulin resistance emerges as a pathogenic contributor. This makes the liver more susceptible to a second hit, including oxidative stress, the production of pro-inflammatory cytokines, and apoptosis, which progress the disease to the necro-inflammatory stage defined as NASH [7]. In contrast, the 'multiple-hit' hypothesis encompasses the interplay of multiple factors whereby genetics, environment, unhealthy dietary habits, insulin resistance, adipocyte differentiation, and the intestinal microbiota together contribute to disease development and progression [8]. Regardless of the source of the hit (s), hepatic responses to extrahepatic stimuli are controlled by well-described transcriptionally regulated pathways that help transcribe the relevant biological machinery to maintain energy homeostasis. However, obesity-induced maladaptive activation or the inhibition of these transcriptional regulators often exacerbates lipid accumulation, insulin resistance, inflammation, and fibrosis [9].

The efforts toward identifying the promoters of obesity-induced NAFLD have relied heavily on rodent models due to limited access to and the variability within human samples arising from differences in disease stage, age, sex, medication, body weight, and other lifestyle choices such as alcohol consumption. However, rodent models do not capture all the features of the human pathophysiology. The rodent NAFLD models described in this review are categorized by their mode of induction using diet, chemicals, or genetic alteration (Box 1). For the diet-induced models, we highlight high-fat diet (HFD), Western diet (WD), methionine- and choline-deficient diet (MCD), choline-deficient L-amino acid-defined (CDAA) diet, and fructose-palmitate-cholesterol and trans-fat (FPC or NASH) diet. The chemically induced models include the combination of HFD with streptozotocin (STZ) supplementation or the use of carbon tetrachloride (CCl_4). For genetic models, we highlight the APOE2 knock-in (APOE2-KI) mouse [10], hepatocyte-specific phosphatase and tensin homolog (PTEN) knockout model [11], and Mice expressing urokinase-type plasminogen activator (uPA) under the control of the major urinary protein (MUP) promoter (MUP-uPA mice) [12].

In this review, we discuss our current understanding of the transcription factors that have been linked to the pathogenesis and progression of NAFLD. Transcription factors that are associated with obesity-induced liver injury and the pathogenesis and progression of NAFLD often serve essential biological functions in the maintenance of energy homeostasis and stress response. Furthermore, recent studies have indicated that the gut microbiota may contribute to NAFLD by altering the production of endogenous substrates that control the activity of hepatic transcription factors. Therefore, we have categorized these transcriptional regulators under lipid and glucose metabolism, inflammation, metabolic stress, fibrosis, and microbiome dysbiosis. Key transcriptional regulators that play significant roles in multiple metabolic responses have been addressed in all relevant categories.

Box 1. Mouse models of non-alcoholic fatty liver disease (NAFLD).

Diet-based models

High-fat diet (HFD, 60 kcal% fat) and Western diet (WD, 40% kcal fat and 40% kcal carbohydrates)—HFD feeding of mice (8–12 weeks) leads to a phenotype similar to simple steatosis in humans, which is characterized by obesity, insulin resistance, and hyperlipidemia [13]. Alanine aminotransferase (ALT) and aspartate aminotransferase (AST) levels also become exacerbated after extended exposure (>8 months). However, this diet barely induces fibrosis even after extended exposure (up to 1 year) [13].

MCD diet—In the MCD diet, the absence of methionine (4–8 weeks) leads to hepatic injury, inflammation, and fibrosis, while the deficiency of choline leads to macrovesicular steatosis. Due to the nature of its pathogenesis, this model is less representative of the initiation of NAFLD in humans. Nonetheless, the diet induces progressive steatohepatitis leading to fibrosis, which is histologically similar to the human disease. The main drawback of MCD is its induction of body weight loss and decrease in plasma triglyceride levels [14].

CDAA diet—CDAA is similar to MCD due to their shared deficiency in choline. However, in CDAA, proteins are substituted with an equivalent and corresponding mixture of L-amino acids [15]. Animals fed CDAA develop the same or perhaps a more severe degree of NASH as well as a larger increase in alanine aminotransferase (ALT) levels, albeit on a longer time frame (12 weeks) [15].

FCP (NASH) diet—The FCP or NASH diet entails a HFD supplemented with 1.25% cholesterol and drinking water containing glucose and fructose (95%/45%, *w/v*). The FCP diet includes Western and American Lifestyle-Induced Obesity Syndrome model diets to achieve both metabolic and hepatic NASH features within 4 months. Fructose-supplemented drinking water for eight weeks results in simple steatosis in rodents without features of NASH and induces a significant increase in body weight and plasma triglyceride and glucose levels [16].

Pharmacological models

STAM—STZ-induced T2DM is a well-known experimental model of T2DM and is achieved by the administration of a low dose of STZ shortly after birth, which results in the apoptotic death of insulin-secreting pancreatic islets. When this approach is combined with HFD, it can be used as a model for NAFLD and NASH [17]. This model results in simple steatosis at 6 weeks of age, NASH with inflammatory foci and ballooning at 8 weeks, and progressive peri-cellular fibrosis starting between 8 and 12 weeks. Starting at 6 weeks of age, mice exhibit elevated ALT levels and fasting glycemia. Multiple hepatocellular carcinomas appear after 20 weeks of treatment [17].

CCl$_4$—Supplementation of diet with CCl$_4$ exacerbates the histological features of NASH, fibrosis, and tumor development in the setting of HFD. HFD coupled with CCl$_4$ results in advanced fibrosis at 12 weeks and HCC at 24 weeks in rodent models [18].

Genetic models

Apoe—A rodent model that replicates the early stages of NAFLD is the APOE2-KI mouse in which the mouse *Apoe* gene is replaced by the human APOE2 allele. In addition to dyslipidemia and atherosclerosis, APOE2-KI mice develop diet-induced NASH when fed WD. A major advantage of this mouse model is that it displays good responses to pharmacological treatments [10].

Pten—PTEN is a tumor suppressor gene mutated in many human cancers, and its expression is reduced or absent in almost half of hepatoma patients, making this a relevant model for human HCC [11]. Hepatocyte-specific PTEN deficiency results in steatohepatitis and HCC in mouse models [11].

MUP-uPA mice—This model is based on feeding HFD to MUP-uPA transgenic mice, which express high amounts of uPA specifically in hepatocytes during the first 6 weeks of life [12]. HFD-fed MUP-uPA mice exhibit increased HSC activation and a substantial upregulation of collagen gene expression. Key diagnostic parameters of NASH, including ballooning, inflammatory infiltrates and pericellular and bridging fibrosis, are evident following 4 months of HFD and are indistinguishable from human NASH, making this a relevant study model [12].

2. Lipid Metabolism

Hepatic steatosis is a consequence of increased hepatic lipid uptake, increased *de novo* lipogenesis, and reduced lipid clearance. Excessive nutrition, accompanied by hyperinsulinemia and hyperglycemia, drives steatosis by promoting *de novo* lipogenesis in the liver, which contributes substantially to the accumulation of triglycerides and other lipid species [19]. Hepatic lipid homeostasis is mainly regulated by peroxisome proliferator-activated receptor alpha (PPARα), PPARγ, PPARδ and sterol regulatory element binding protein 1c (SREBP1c), which coordinate transcriptional responses to altered metabolic conditions such as feeding and fasting to promote fat storage or catabolism, respectively. Other transcription factors of lipid metabolism that are altered in the setting of NAFLD include the constitutive androstane receptor (CAR), liver X receptor (LXR), Cyclic AMP-responsive element-binding protein H (CREBH), Farnesoid X receptor (FXR), signal transducer and activator of transcription 5 (STAT5), and CCAAT/enhancer binding protein alpha (C/EBPα) (Table 1).

Table 1. Changes in the activity of transcription factors that regulate glucose and lipid metabolism, inflammation and fibrosis in the setting of NAFLD in humans and mice.

Factor	Model	Pathway	Regulation	Reference
PPARα	Humans, mice	Lipid metabolism, inflammation, fibrosis	Upregulation	[20]
PPARγ	Humans, mice	Lipid metabolism, inflammation, fibrosis	Upregulation	[20]
SREBP Family	Humans, mice	Lipid metabolism	Genetic variations increase risk of NAFLD	[21]
ChREBP	Humans, mice	Lipid metabolism	Upregulation	[22]
CAR	Humans, mice	Lipid metabolism, inflammation	Upregulation	[23]
LXR	Humans	Lipid metabolism, inflammation	Upregulation	[24]
FXR	Humans	Lipid metabolism	Downregulation	[25]
STAT5	Humans	Lipid metabolism	Upregulated	[26]
C/EBPα	Mice	Lipid metabolism	Upregulation	[27]
PGC1α	Mice	Glucose homeostasis	Downregulation	[28]
FoxO	Humans	Glucose homeostasis	Upregulation	[29]
HNF4α	Humans	Central regulator, Glucose homeostasis	Downregulation	[25]
NF-κB	Humans, mice	Inflammation	Upregulation	[30]
IRFs	Mice	Inflammation	Upregulation	[31]
STAT1/3	Mice	Inflammation	Upregulation	[32]
AP-1 and c-Jun	Humans, mice	Inflammation, fibrosis	Upregulation	[30,33]
SHP	Humans, mice	Inflammation	Downregulation	[34]
Nrf2	Mice	Inflammation	Upregulation	[35]
Runx2	Mice	Inflammation	Upregulation	[36]
C/EBPβ		Inflammation		
IRE1α	Human	Metabolic stress	Upregulation	[37]
Xbp1	Mice	Metabolic stress	Upregulation	[38]
eIF2α	Mice	Metabolic stress	Upregulation	[39]
ATF4	Humans	Metabolic stress	Upregulation	[40]
ATF6	Humans	Metabolic stress	Upregulation	[41]
Smad	Humans, mice	Fibrosis	Upregulation	[42]
TGFβ	Humans, mice	Fibrosis	Upregulation	[42]
AEBP1	Humans, mice	Fibrosis	Upregulation	[43]
AATF/che-1	Humans, mice	Fibrosis	Upregulation	[44]
YAP	Humans, mice	Fibrosis	Upregulation	[45]

Abbreviations: peroxisome proliferator-activated receptor (PPAR), sterol regulatory element binding protein (SREBP), carbohydrate-responsive element-binding protein (ChREBP), constitutive androstane receptor (CAR), liver X receptor (LXR), farnesoid X receptor (FXR), signal transducer and activator of transcription (STAT), CCAAT/enhancer binding protein (C/EBP), PPARγ coactivator 1 alpha (PGC1α), forkhead protein O (FoxO), hepatocyte nuclear factor (HNF), nuclear factor of the κ light chain enhancer of B cells (NF-κB), interferon regulatory factors (IRFs), activator protein 1 (AP-1), small heterodimer partner (SHP), nuclear factor erythroid 2-related factor 2 (Nrf2), runt-related transcription factor 2 (Runx2), inositol-requiring enzyme 1α (IRE1α), X box-binding protein 1 (Xbp1), eukaryotic translation initiation factor 2α (eIF2α), activating transcription factor (ATF), transcription factors against decapentaplegic homolog (Smad), transforming growth factor β (TGFβ), adipocyte enhancer binding protein 1 (AEBP1), apoptosis antagonizing transcription factor (AATF/che-1), yes-associated protein (YAP).

2.1. PPARα

PPARα belongs to the PPAR nuclear receptor family. PPARα is mostly expressed in hepatocytes where it becomes activated upon binding by fatty acids (FAs) and promotes FA uptake and utilization through β-oxidation and ketogenesis [46]. Hepatic PPARα expression is increased in male mice and both male and female humans with NAFLD [20,46]. Suggestive of a protective function, mice lacking

PPARα expression exhibit more severe steatosis [47]. Therefore, NAFLD-induced increases in PPARα abundance can be further enhanced by its pharmacological activation: the PPARα agonist WY-14643 protects mice against steatosis and steatohepatitis by preventing intrahepatic lipid and lipoperoxide accumulation [47]. Since WY-14643 causes toxicity in humans, other fibrates have been extensively used in the treatment of hypertriglyceridemia. However, these studies failed to establish benefits against NASH, which is most likely due to the widespread extrahepatic expression of PPARα [48].

2.2. PPARγ

Another member of the PPAR family, PPARγ is also activated by FA ligands and promotes lipogenesis and lipid accumulation. In humans and mice, two isoforms of PPARγ exist: PPARγ1 is found in nearly all tissues except muscle, while PPARγ2 is mostly expressed in adipose tissue and the intestine. PPARγ2 expression is upregulated in the liver and adipose tissue of obese humans and high-fat diet (HFD)-fed mice, whereas the PPARγ1 expression remains unchanged under these conditions [49]. In hepatocytes, PPARγ1 increases the transcription of genes that are required for FA uptake and *de novo* lipogenesis [50]. Meanwhile, lipidomic analyses suggest that PPARγ2 plays an important anti-lipotoxic role when induced ectopically in liver and muscle by facilitating the deposition of lipid droplets and preventing the accumulation of reactive lipid species, such as ceramides and pro-inflammatory lysophosphatidylcholine [51]. HFD-fed mice with a hepatocyte specific loss of PPARγ expression exhibit a reduction of hepatic lipid vacuoles as well as the downregulation of genes involved in *de novo* lipogenesis [52]. Furthermore, the liver-specific ablation of PPARγ in *ob/ob* mice reduces hepatic triglycerides despite increasing serum FAs [53]. Livers of NAFLD patients have increased hepatic PPARγ expression [20,46]. Whereas increased PPARγ activity within hepatocytes would be expected to contribute to steatosis [54,55], the treatment of patients with the PPARγ agonists rosiglitazone or pioglitazone result in reduced hepatic steatosis [56–58]. This alleviation could be explained by the extrahepatic effects of PPARγ activation in the adipose tissue where it promotes the storage of excess energy in the form of lipid droplets, thereby limiting exposure of the liver to excess lipids.

2.3. PPARδ

Similar to other PPARs, PPARδ binds to the PPAR response element (PPRE) to initiate or repress the expression of target genes [59]. PPARδ is ubiquitously expressed and is activated by polyunsaturated fatty acids and their metabolites. In mouse livers, PPARδ prevents lipid accumulation by increasing β-oxidation and autophagy. In addition, the activation of PPARδ in the adipose tissue of mice upregulates the expression of genes involved in β-oxidation and energy dissipation [60,61]. Recent clinical studies using PPARδ agonists atorvastatin and cardarine reduced hepatic fat content in overweight patients with mixed dyslipidemia [61,62].

2.4. SREBP

The SREBP family transcription factors consist of three isoforms: SREBP1a, SREBP1c, and SREBP2. Each isoform exhibits a different tissue expression pattern and metabolic control [63]. SREBP1a is the predominant isoform in the intestine, spleen, and cultured cells, while SREBP1c and SREBP2 exhibit higher abundance in the liver [63]. SREBP1a is a potent activator of genes that mediate the synthesis of cholesterol, fatty acids, and triglycerides. The roles of SREBP1c and SREBP2 are more restricted than those of SREBP1a. SREBP1c promotes the transcription of genes involved in lipogenesis, such as acetyl-coenzyme A (CoA) carboxylase (ACC), FA synthase (FASN), and steroyl–CoA desaturase in response to insulin and high-energy state [64]. By contrast, hepatic markers for energy deprivation, such as glucagon signaling (protein kinase A [PKA], AMP activated protein kinase [AMPK]) and the deacetylase sirtuin1 (SIRT1) inhibit SREBP1c, suggesting that SREBP1c does not promote hepatic lipid synthesis in the setting of starvation [65]. Among the genes involved in lipogenesis, SREBP1c also promotes the transcription of patatin-like phospholipase3 (PNPLA3), which in turn stimulates lipid accumulation [66]. Independent studies in humans have confirmed that PNPLA3 variants are strongly associated with the severity of NAFLD and NASH [67–69]. SREBP1c is upregulated in the livers of humans and mice with NAFLD [70]. Interestingly, there is also a positive correlation between single nucleotide polymorphisms (i.e., rs2297508) as well as rare variants of *SREBP1* with the risk of developing NAFLD [21]. Unlike SREBP1c, SREBP2 preferentially activates cholesterol synthesis [71]. In mice, SREBP2 contributes to the onset of NASH by triggering cholesterol accumulation [72]. Increased hepatic SREBP2 is also associated with increased free cholesterol in NASH patients [73].

2.5. CAR

CAR is a member of the nuclear receptor superfamily [74]. It mainly functions as a sensor of endobiotic and xenobiotic substances, as CAR-activated genes regulate drug metabolism and enhance bilirubin clearance [74]. Unlike most nuclear receptors, this transcriptional regulator is constitutively active in the absence of a ligand. CAR activity is anti-obesogenic and improves insulin sensitivity [75]. The metabolic benefits of CAR activation stem from the combined effects of reduced lipogenesis, very low-density lipoprotein (VLDL) secretion, and gluconeogenesis, as well as increased peripheral fat mobilization for thermogenesis in brown adipose tissue [75]. The anti-steatotic effect of CAR was first demonstrated using a mouse model with the genetic ablation of cytoplasmic CAR retention protein (CCRP), which isolates CAR to the cytosol and inactivates it. Subsequent CAR activation represses lipogenic gene expression and increases β-oxidation [76]. Similar to mouse models of NAFLD, CAR is also upregulated in the livers of patients with NAFLD [23].

2.6. LXR

LXR is a member of the nuclear receptor family of transcription factors that is closely related to PPARs [77]. LXR forms heterodimers with the obligate partner retinoid X receptor (RXR), which is activated by retinoic acid and cholesterol derivatives. LXR is an important regulator of cholesterol, FA, and glucose homeostasis [77]. LXR activation increases hepatic triglyceride accumulation and cholesterol metabolism in both humans and mice and initiates bile acid degradation in mice [78]. Humans express two LXR family members, namely LXRα (*NR1H3*) and LXRβ (*NR1H2*). LXRα expression increases by 2- and 3-fold in the livers of NAFLD and NASH patients, respectively, compared to healthy controls [24]. Furthermore, LXRα expression positively correlates with the amount of hepatic fat and hepatic expression of the cholesterol transporter ATP-binding cassette sub-family G member 5 (ABCG5/8), the FA transporter cluster of differentiation 36 (CD36), and SREBP1c [24].

2.7. CREBH

CREBH is primarily expressed in the endoplasmic reticulum (ER) of cells in the liver and small intestine [79,80]. CREBH expression increases in response to fasting through glucagon signaling [81]. CREBH expression is also controlled by the binding of glucocorticoid or PPRE to its promotor region [82]. Therefore, CREBH expression can be induced by a variety of PPARα agonists such as palmitate and oleate [82]. ER-anchored CREBH becomes activated in response to hepatic lipid accumulation and VLDL assembly. The activation of CREBH requires ER-to-golgi trafficking followed by proteolytic cleavage and nuclear translocation [81,83,84]. CREBH activates a group of genes that are involved in TG and lipoprotein production [85,86]. CREBH also binds to and functions as a co-activator for both PPARα and LXRα to promote FA uptake and utilization [86]. CREBH-deficient mice are susceptible to hepatic steatosis following fasting [81] or diets with high-fat content [79,86]. Interestingly, the livers of CREBH-deficient mice exhibit the reduced expression of genes that promote *de novo* lipogenesis and FA elongation [86]. Observed steatosis most likely arises from the reduced hepatic expression of genes involved in FA oxidation and increased lipolysis in the adipose tissue, resulting in an increased flow of FA from adipose tissue to the liver [79]. Furthermore, fibroblast growth factor (FGF) 21 is a critical CREBH target that reduces hepatic lipid storage. CREBH overexpression in the livers of mice suppresses hepatic lipid accumulation by increasing FGF21 secretion [87].

2.8. FXR

FXR is a major member of the ligand-activated nuclear receptor superfamily [78]. The family consists of four isoforms namely, FXRα1, FXRα2, FXRβ1, and FXRβ2 [88]. Similar to LXR, bile acids are natural ligands for FXR, which plays an important role in regulating bile acid homeostasis, glucose and lipid metabolism, intestinal bacterial growth, and hepatic regeneration [89]. While LXR facilitates the storage of carbohydrate- and fat-derived energy, FXR decreases TG levels and improves glucose metabolism [90]. One of the primary functions of FXR activation is the suppression of CYP7A1, the rate-limiting enzyme in bile acid synthesis from cholesterol [91]. FXR expression is decreased in NASH patients [25], which can aggravate the development of steatosis and NASH: (1) FXR activation represses hepatic lipogenesis via the FXR–SHP–SREBP1c pathway (see below for more on small heterodimer partner [SHP]), (2) FXR activation promotes β-oxidation by stimulating the expression of PPARα and CPT1, and (3) FXR activation reduces hepatic FA uptake by reducing the expression of CD36 [89].

2.9. STAT5

STAT5 belongs to a family of intracellular transcription factors that are activated by membrane receptor-associated Janus kinases (JAK). The growth hormone (GH)-mediated activation of STAT5 [92] plays an important role in hepatic fat metabolism through the downregulation of CD36 [93]. The liver-specific loss of STAT5 in mice induces hepatic steatosis following a HFD [92]. These mice also exhibit hyperglycemia, hyperinsulinemia, hyperleptinemia, and elevated free FA and cholesterol concentrations following HFD. At the transcriptional stage, the loss of STAT5 results in the transcription of genes involved in lipid uptake (CD36), VLDL uptake (very low-density lipoprotein receptor), and lipogenesis (stearoyl-CoA desaturase and PPARγ) [93]. However, it is unclear whether STAT5 directly regulates the expression of these factors. In addition, its relevance in human steatosis associated with GH-deficiency is yet to be established.

2.10. C/EBPα

C/EBPα belongs to a transcription factor family of six members which are involved in a variety of cellular responses [94]. C/EBPα plays a role in lipogenic gene expression by inducing the expression of PPARγ [95]. The liver-specific ablation of C/EBPα reduces lipogenic gene expression and triglycerides in the livers of leptin-deficient *ob/ob* mice, which otherwise display severe steatosis [95]. These findings were confirmed by a similar observation of reduced hepatic gene expression following siRNA-mediated inhibition of C/EBPα expression in the livers of leptin receptor-deficient (*db/db*) mice [27].

3. Glucose Metabolism

The liver does not only play a central role in systemic lipid homeostasis but also regulates the glucose balance in circulation. This is mediated by the activation of carbohydrate-responsive element-binding protein (ChREBP) in response to increases in plasma glucose and the nuclear localization of PPARγ coactivator 1 alpha (PGC1α), cAMP response element binding protein (Creb), CREBH, forkhead protein O1 (FOXO1), and hepatocyte nuclear factor 4α (HNF4α) in response to fasting to promote hepatic glucose production [96] (Table 1). Furthermore, PPARδ also plays a role in glucose homeostasis. The exacerbation of hepatic glucose production coupled with hyperglycemia and insulin resistance play an important pathogenic role in NAFLD.

3.1. ChREBP

ChREBP consists of ChREBPα, the full-length isoform, or ChREBP-β, the truncated isoform [97]. ChREBPα is directly activated by glucose, independently from insulin signaling [98]. Little is known about ChREBPβ, which was reported to be expressed in a glucose- and ChREBP-dependent manner whereby glucose-activated ChREBPα initiates ChREBPβ transcription from an alternate promoter [99].

In the liver, ChREBP promotes glycolysis and lipogenesis. ChREBP expression is increased in the livers of NASH patients with advanced steatosis [100]. By contrast, decreased ChREBP expression is associated with severe insulin resistance [22]. This pattern indicates that ChREBP is essential for the storage of excess glucose as triglycerides. In fact, mice that overexpress ChREBP exhibit improved insulin sensitivity and glucose tolerance despite having more pronounced hepatic steatosis. Together, these studies have demonstrated that increased ChREBP activity improves insulin sensitivity by promoting simple steatosis without lipotoxicity [22].

3.2. PGC1α

The PGC1 family of transcriptional co-activators play a central role in the regulation of metabolism. The PGC1 family consists of three members, namely PGC1α, PGC1β, and the PGC-related co-activator (PRC), which interact with transcription factors and nuclear receptors to exert their biological functions. PGC1α expression is induced by metabolic cues such as exercise, cold, and fasting [101]. The activation of PGC1α in the liver drives the expression of genes that are essential to gluconeogenesis, FA oxidation, lipid transport, and mitochondrial biogenesis. The activity of PGC1α becomes impaired in the setting of liver injury and steatosis in mice, and the loss of PGC1α has been linked to the increased susceptibility to NAFLD in HFD-fed mice [102]. PGC1α haploinsufficiency in mouse liver inhibits β-oxidation and increases triglyceride synthesis, leading to hepatic steatosis and insulin resistance. Similarly, PGC1α overexpression in rat hepatocytes results in reduced concentrations of hepatic triglycerides in vitro and in vivo, due to increased β-oxidation [28].

3.3. CREB

CREB becomes activated in response to glucagon-mediated increases in cellular cAMP. The knockdown of CREB dramatically reduces fasting plasma glucose concentrations in several rodent models for obesity and type 2 diabetes, including Zucker diabetic fatty (ZDF) rats, STZ-treated/HFD-fed rats, and *ob/ob* mice. CREB does not only promote the expression of gluconeogenic genes but also increases plasma TG and cholesterol concentrations as well as hepatic steatosis by activating *de novo* lipogenesis in the liver [103].

3.4. CREBH

CREBH was reported to bind and upregulate genes that contain cAMP-responsive elements, including phosphoenolpyruvate carboxykinase 1 (*Pck1*) and glucose-6-phosphatase (G6Pase) [80,81], which are essential promoters of gluconeogenesis. CREBH also upregulates the rate-limiting enzyme for hepatic glycogenolysis, namely glycogen phosphorylase (*Pygl*) [81]. Consequently, CREBH overexpression in the livers of mice increases plasma glucose levels, while its knockdown reduces circulating glucose [81].

3.5. FOXO

The forkhead protein family comprises of more than 100 members in humans and are enumerated FOXA to FOXR based on their sequence similarity [104]. The members of the FOXO subfamily, which consists of FOXO1, FOXO3, FOXO4, and FOXO6, are regulated by insulin signaling whereby Akt-mediated phosphorylation sequesters FOXOs within the cytosol, inhibiting their transcriptional activity in the nucleus [105]. FOXO family members mediate the expression of genes that play a role in cell death, DNA repair, glucose, and energy metabolism [106]. Hepatic FOXO1 regulates the expression of both gluconeogenic and lipogenic genes. Under fasting conditions, FOXO1 drives the expression of gluconeogenic enzymes. In addition, FOXO1 induces the transcription of genes involved in the hepatic assembly of VLDL, reducing hepatic steatosis [106]. The genetic ablation of FOXO increases susceptibility to NAFLD and NASH in mice [105]. Specifically, the deletion of FOXO1/3 or FOXO1/3/4 genes in mouse livers leads to mild or moderate hepatic steatosis, even when mice are maintained on a regular chow diet [105]. Exposing the mice to HFD supplemented with cholesterol further exacerbates steatosis in FOXO1/3/4-deficient mice [105]. Conversely, the overexpression of a constitutively active FOXO1 reduces hepatic triglycerides [105]. On the other hand, livers of NASH patients exhibit a greater expression of FOXO1 compared to patients with simple steatosis as well as metabolically healthy patients with and without obesity [29]. More investigation into FOXO1 activity during different stages of human liver disease is needed to establish mechanisms and physiological relevance.

3.6. HNF4α

HNF4α is a member of the nuclear hormone receptor superfamily and has been shown to play an essential role in maintaining bile acid, lipid, and glucose homeostasis. HNF4α translates extracellular endocrine signals and intracellular stress and nutritional state onto transcriptional responses in the liver. HNF4α is regulated by growth hormone, glucocorticoids, thyroid hormone, insulin, transforming growth factor beta (TGFβ), estrogen, and cytokines [107]. HNF4α target genes have been identified in the liver, pancreas, and colon. In the liver, the targets include genes involved in glucose (PEPCK, glucose-6-phosphatase (G6Pase)), bile (CYP7A1), xenobiotics and drug metabolism (CYP3A4, CYP2D6, and CYP2E1) [108]. HNF4α also regulates circulating levels of cholesterol and triglycerides by inducing the transcription of genes that encode for apolipoproteins. HFD-induced oxidative stress promotes hepatic steatosis by blocking the activity of HNF4α in mice [109]. The expression of HNF4α is decreased in NASH patients [25]. Furthermore, a systematic integrative analysis of gene transcription has identified HNF4α as 'the central gene' in the NASH pathogenesis [25].

3.7. PPARδ

In addition to its activation of fatty acid oxidation, PPARδ improves glucose homeostasis and protects from insulin resistance by promoting insulin secretion in the pancreatic islet β-cells [110,111] and by increasing energy utilization [112]. Mice lacking PPARδ expression have reduced energy expenditure and are glucose-intolerant. In contrast, receptor activation by GW50516, a PPARδ-specific agonist, suppresses hepatic glucose output, improves insulin sensitivity and increases glucose disposal in mice [112]. This increase in energy disposal has been linked to increased β-oxidation in the skeletal muscle of mice following GW50516 treatment [113].

4. Inflammation

The hepatic inflammatory response is an important driving force for NASH progression as it promotes sustained hepatic fibrogenesis. Transcription factors activated in response to inflammatory stimuli mainly belong to the family of nuclear factor of the κ light chain enhancer of B cells (NF-κBs), interferon regulatory factors (IRFs), STAT, and activator protein 1 (AP-1) [114]. Other factors that have also been implicated in the transcriptional regulation of the inflammatory response include apoptosis antagonizing transcription factor (AATF, synonym: che-1), SHP, Runt-related transcription factor 2 (Runx2), and C/EBPβ. In addition to inflammation-specific regulators, transcriptional regulators of lipid homeostasis PPARα, PPARγ, CAR, and LXR also affect the hepatic inflammatory state (Table 1).

4.1. NF-κB

NF-κB is a protein complex that controls cytokine production and cell survival, and as such, it plays a key role in the immune response to infection. NF-κB is also critical for the development of inflammation in various metabolic disorders such as T2DM [115] and is highly activated in both mice and patients with NASH [30,116]. The pharmacological inhibition of NF-κB signaling protects MCD-fed mice from the pathogenesis of NASH with significant reductions in hepatocellular injury and hepatic inflammation. Furthermore, the stage of inflammation and fibrosis in livers of NASH patients correlates with the expression of the p65 subunit of NF-κB [117].

4.2. IRFs

IRFs are a family of transcription factors that regulate the transcription of interferons and consist of nine members. Most IRFs are involved in innate immunity and defense against pathogens. IRF family members impose variable impacts on inflammation in the pathogenesis of NAFLD. Studies using mice with the deletion of IRF7 expression indicated that IRF7 promotes weight gain, hepatic fat deposition, and insulin resistance in the setting of HFD [118]. In contrast, a similar study using IRF9-deficient mice demonstrated that IRF9 promotes insulin sensitivity and attenuates inflammation and hepatic steatosis [119]. Interestingly, IRF9 was shown to interact with PPARα and activate its target genes [119].

4.3. STAT

STAT family members with inflammatory biological functions (STAT1 and STAT3) have been associated with NAFLD and NASH. The oxidative hepatic environment in obesity inhibits the STAT1 and STAT3 phosphatase, T cell protein tyro-sine phosphatase (TCPTP), which results in increased STAT1 and STAT3 signaling. This in turn increases the risk of developing NASH and HCC in the setting of excessive nutrition [32]. Furthermore, the inactivation of TCPTP, coupled with increased STAT1 and STAT3 signaling, are easily detectable events in the livers of humans with NASH [32].

4.4. AP1

AP1 activation requires the synthesis of c-Jun and c-Fos proteins and c-Jun phosphorylation by c-Jun N-terminal kinase (JNK) for the full transactivation of target genes. Obese patients with NASH exhibit an enhanced hepatic expression of AP1 targets [30]. JNK activation and the extent of c-Jun nuclear localization correlates very well with the pathogenesis and progression of NASH in humans and mouse models [33]. Activated c-Jun promotes nuclear accumulation of JNK, which provides a positive feedback loop to further enhance AP1 transcriptional activity and exacerbate NASH progression [120,121].

4.5. AATF

AATF mediates cell proliferation and survival [122–124]. Its expression in the liver increases with simple steatosis [44]. Indicative of a role in inflammation, AATF expression increases in response to tumor necrosis factor α (TNFα)-mediated activation of SREBP1 in cultured cells. In turn, AATF induces the expression of the inflammatory cytokine monocyte chemotactic protein 1 (MCP1) by activating STAT3. Hepatic AATF expression does not increase any further with disease progression to NASH [44], suggesting that it plays a role in exacerbating simple steatosis toward the pathogenesis of inflammatory stages of steatohepatitis. However, its contribution to the progression of NASH to advanced stages remains unclear.

4.6. SHP

SHP is technically not a transcription factor, since it lacks a DNA binding domain but is still classified as such due to its sequence homology to other nuclear receptor families. The principal role of SHP is the repression of other nuclear receptors by binding and forming a dysfunctional heterodimer. SHP is a critical repressor of various genes involved in glucose and lipid metabolism and bile acid synthesis [125]. Several factors indicate a role in inflammation: first, SHP inhibits inflammatory responses that are triggered by the Toll-like receptor (TLR) [126] as well as the NLR family pyrin domain containing 3 (NLRP3) inflammasome, which consists of a multimeric protein complex that triggers inflammatory cell death and the release of pro-inflammatory cytokines interleukin (IL)-1β and IL-18 [127]. In addition, SHP suppresses inflammation by inhibiting transcription of the chemokine CCL2 whose biological function is to recruit macrophages and promote inflammation [34]. The SHP-mediated mitigation of inflammatory responses could play a protective role in NASH. SHP expression is drastically decreased in the livers of a mouse model of NASH and in the livers of

NASH patients compared healthy or steatotic livers [34]. The rescue of SHP expression in the livers of mice prevents the progression of NAFLD to NASH [34]. Mechanistically, the reduction of SHP expression in NASH was linked to inhibitory binding of c-Jun to the SHP promoter, suggesting that the JNK/SHP/NF-κB/CCL2 axis is a promising target for NASH prevention and treatment.

4.7. Runx2

Runx2 plays an important role in atherosclerosis. It has been indicated that atherosclerosis shares a similar histopathology with NASH with respect to macrophage infiltration. Indeed, experiments in mouse primary HSCs have elucidated a mechanism whereby Runx2 within HSCs promotes macrophage infiltration by increasing the transcription of MCP1 [36].

4.8. C/EBPβ

C/EBPβ was originally identified as nuclear factor interleukin-6 (NFIL6) because of its inducibility by IL-6 and its important role in the activation of acute inflammatory response genes in human hepatoma cells [128]. The livers of mice lacking C/EBPβ express reduced markers of inflammation and endoplasmic reticulum (ER) stress and exhibit decreased steatosis following an MCD diet. By contrast, C/EBPβ overexpression increases the hepatic prevalence of PPARγ, ER stress, NF-κB activation, and steatosis [27].

4.9. PPARα

In addition to its role in the regulation of metabolism, PPARα also exhibits anti-inflammatory effects through its regulation of NF-κB [129]. The treatment of non-steatotic mice with the PPARα agonist WY-14643 decreases the hepatic inflammatory gene expression profile, suggesting a direct anti-inflammatory effect of PPARα independent of changes in liver triglycerides [130].

4.10. PPARγ

Hepatic PPARγ does not only regulate hepatocyte metabolism but also plays an important regulatory role in liver-resident macrophages (Kupffer cells), where it acts as an inhibitor of macrophage activation and cytokine production. This regulation is mediated through the PPARγ1-mediated inhibition of AP-1, STAT, and NF-κB, which are the major regulators of macrophage activation and TNFα synthesis [131]. Mice with Kupffer cell-specific loss of PPARγ expression exhibit increased hepatic expression of inflammatory cytokines TNFα and IL1β and fibrosis in response to CCl$_4$-induced liver injury [132]. Conversely, PPARγ induction by rosiglitazone decreases the number of hepatic Kupffer cells, attenuating the inflammatory response as well as steatosis in a diet-induced mouse model of NAFLD [133].

4.11. CAR

CAR activation can potentially be used to delay or reduce the progression of NAFLD due to its dual anti-steatotic and anti-inflammatory effects. In the MCD mouse model of NASH, the administration of the CAR agonist 2,2′-[1,4-phenylenebis(oxy)]bis[3,5-dichloro]-pyridine (TCPOBOP) reduces inflammation and hepatocellular apoptosis by reducing the accumulation of Kupffer cells and enhancing the hepatic clearance of pro-inflammatory leukotriene B4 [134]. On the other hand, CAR knockout mice exhibit improved lipid peroxidation and hepatic fibrosis after exposure to the MCD diet [135]. Therefore, the precise role of CAR in the pathophysiology of NASH requires additional studies.

4.12. LXR

Although LXR promotes inflammation, its impact on obesity and steatosis is inconsistent. Mouse models with the deletion of LXR expression have indicated that LXR decreases inflammation by inhibiting the transcription of TNFα, IL-6, and IL-1β but increases steatosis [136]. On the other hand, the treatment of mice with the LXR antagonist SR9238 generates both anti-steatotic [137] and anti-fibrotic effects [138] with a dramatic reduction in steatosis, inflammation, and collagen disposition in the livers of mice. Overall, all studies indicate that LXR could be a valuable target for the treatment and prevention of NASH.

5. Metabolic Stress

The pathogenesis of NAFLD does not only depend on energy metabolism and inflammation but has also been mechanistically linked to increased cellular stress. Upon excessive nutrition, the ER cannot meet high metabolic demands and initiates the unfolded protein response (UPR) by activating three transmembrane factors located on the ER membrane: protein kinase R-like ER kinase (PERK), inositol-requiring enzyme 1α (IRE1α), and activating transcription factor 6 (ATF6). PERK activates eukaryotic translation initiation factor 2α (eIF2α), which in turn activates ATF4. Meanwhile, IRE1α splices the mRNA of X box-binding protein 1 (Xbp1) to its active isoform Xbp1s. ATF4, ATF6, and Xbp1 together initiate transcriptional events to resolve ER stress. However, excessive reactive oxygen species (ROS) and ER stress due to excessive lipid accumulation in the liver can lead to inflammation and hepatocyte death [139]. For instance, increased CYP2E1 expression promotes ROS production and the progression of NAFLD. In contrast, stress-induced activation of nuclear erythroid 2-related factor 2 (NRF2) protects against oxidative stress and the pathogenesis of NAFLD [140]. Furthermore, unresolved ER stress results in the activation of apoptotic transcription factor CCAAT/enhancer binding protein (CHOP). The prolonged activation of IRE1α also leads to the activation of the inflammatory transcription factors c-Jun and NF-κB. Thus, the transcription factors involved in stress-induced responses may contribute to the development of NASH (Table 1).

5.1. Xbp1

High caloric stress leads to the splicing and nuclear localization of Xbp1, which in turn transcribes factors that improve protein folding as well as lipogenesis [38]. However, obesity-induced chronic stress limits the nuclear localization of Xbp1 and aggravates ER stress and insulin resistance [141]. The rescue of Xbp1 activity in HFD-fed or *ob/ob* mice improves glucose homeostasis and reduces hepatic steatosis, which is associated with reductions in the expression of lipogenic genes [142]. Whether the improvement of hepatic steatosis in these mouse models is a direct outcome of transcriptional regulation by Xbp1 or a secondary consequence of resolved metabolic stress and improved insulin sensitivity remains unclear. Nonetheless, the lipogenic role of Xbp1 is demonstrated using a mouse model with a liver-specific ablation of Xbp1 following WD, whereby the loss of Xbp1 is associated with reduced steatosis but enhanced liver injury and fibrosis with the upregulation of type-I collagen α1 (Colα1), TGFβ1, CHOP, and p-JNK [38,143].

5.2. ATF4

In NASH patients, the mRNA expression of ATF4 and CHOP and protein expression of CHOP are significantly elevated compared to liver samples from patients with simple steatosis [40]. ATF4 depletion protects mice from high fructose-induced hepatic steatosis by reducing lipogenesis through the reduced hepatic expression of PPARγ, SREBP1c, ACC, and FASN [144].

5.3. ATF6

Hepatic ATF6 knockdown or overexpression of its dominant-negative form by adenovirus in WD-fed mice exacerbates insulin resistance and hepatic steatosis with reduced transcriptional activity of the PPARα/RXR complex. Conversely, overexpression of the cleaved active from of ATF6 protects mice from hepatic steatosis and promotes hepatic FA oxidation. Experiments in hepatocytes have shown that ATF6 promotes hepatic FA oxidation by enhancing PPARα transcriptional activity through direct interaction and activates its downstream targets such as carnitine palmitoyltransferase 1 alpha

(CPT1α) and medium-chain acyl-CoA dehydrogenase (MCAD) [145]. Activated ATF6 also interacts with SREBP2 and inhibits SREBP2 target genes in hepatocytes [146].

5.4. NRF2

NRF2 is the primary driver of gene expression via the antioxidative response elements (ARE). In response to oxidative damage such as lipid peroxidation and DNA damage, NRF2 increases the transcription of antioxidative factors, including [140,147] NRF2, which suppresses inflammation by preventing the increased transcription of pro-inflammatory cytokines [140]. Specifically, NRF2 interferes with the lipopolysaccharide-induced transcriptional upregulation of IL-6 and IL-1β. Accumulating evidence supports a protective role of NRF2 in NASH [148]. In rats and mice with diet-induced NASH, NRF2 activation improves glucose homeostasis and inhibits hepatic steatosis, inflammation, and fibrosis by decreasing lipid synthesis and upregulating β-oxidation and lipoprotein assembly [35,149]. In contrast, the loss of NRF2 exacerbates hepatic steatosis and accelerates the development of NASH in mice fed an HFD or MCD [150,151]. Mechanistically, the oxidative stress due to the deletion of NRF2 in these mice activates NF-κB and leads to the upregulation of the inflammatory cytokines IL-6 and TNFα.

5.5. CYP2E1

Although it is not a transcription factor, it is important to include CYP2E1, which becomes activated following insulin resistance and lipotoxicity [152] and promotes ROS production in the setting of NAFLD [153]. CYP2E1 plays key metabolic roles in gluconeogenesis and fatty acid metabolism. It controls the formation of lactate or glucose from the ketone body acetone [154]. Furthermore, CYP2E1 carries out the omega hydroxylation of fatty acids, increasing lipotoxicity and inflammation [155], which represent major pathophysiological mechanisms in NAFLD progression [156]. The role of CYP2E1 in liver injury was first identified following the alcohol-induced induction of CYP2E1 protein. However, clear differences exist between alcoholic liver disease (ALD)- and NAFLD-induced activation of CYP2E1: while alcohol consumption only stabilizes the CYP2E1 protein without changes in mRNA expression, excessive nutrition increases both protein stability and mRNA abundance [157]. Although the transcriptional regulation of CYP2E1 has been linked to the activities of HNF1α [158], HNF4α [108], SP1 [159], and C/EBP [154], the mechanisms by which obesity and NAFLD exacerbate CYP2E1 activity requires additional studies [153].

6. Fibrosis

Fibrosis is the strongest predictor of adverse clinical outcomes for NASH. Fibrogenesis during liver injury is initiated by the activation of HSCs in the liver [160,161]. Established inducers of fibrogenesis and HSC activation include adipocyte enhancer binding protein 1 (AEBP1), AATF, yes-associated protein (YAP), and transforming growth factor beta-(TGFβ)-mediated activation of transcription factors against decapentaplegic homolog (SMAD). In addition to these fibrosis-specific regulators, the main transcriptional regulators of lipid homeostasis (including PPARα and PPARγ) and inflammation (RUNX2 and c-Jun) have also been reported to dictate the fibrotic stage in NASH (Table 1).

6.1. TGFβ/SMAD axis

TGFβ is secreted from activated HSC and is a potent inducer of fibrogenesis. Its pro-fibrogenic effect is mainly mediated by the TGFβ receptor (TGFβR)-dependent activation of the SMAD family in HSC: the phosphorylated SMAD2/3 complex binds to SMAD4 and translocates to the nucleus to promote the transcription of fibrogenic genes including Co1α1, Co3α1, smooth muscle alpha 2 actin (αSMA), and TGFβ as well as the production of tissue inhibitor of metalloproteinases (TIMPs) [162], which promote fibrosis by inhibiting matrix degradation [163]. In contrast, Smad7 inhibits the regulation of the TGFβ signaling by recruiting ubiquitin E3 ligases that promote the degradation of TGFβR1 and by recruiting the protein phosphatase PP1C, which inactivates TGFβR1 [164]. The livers of NASH patients as well as a mouse model of NASH exhibit increased nuclear localization of the

SMAD2/3/4 complex and the reduced expression of SMAD7, which all together contribute to increased TGFβ, Colα1, and αSMA [42]. The regulation of SMAD2/3 has also highlighted the role of additional transcription factors in mediating TGFβ-mediated fibrogenesis: the interactions of the transcriptional coactivators CREB binding protein (CBP) and p300 with SMAD2/3 promotes histone acetylation and increased transcriptional activity [165]. Supporting the pathophysiological relevance of this axis, the AMPK-mediated degradation of p300 results in the inhibition of TGFβ/SMAD3-mediated fibrogenesis in HSC [166]. Finally, the transcription factor v-ets avian erythroblastosis virus E26 oncogene homolog 1 (ETS1), which is elevated in a NASH mouse model, enhances TGFβ/SMAD signaling by directly binding to SMAD3 and preventing its ubiquitination and degradation [167].

6.2. AEBP1

AEBP1 plays a role in adipogenesis [168,169], myofibroblast differentiation [170], and macrophage cholesterol homeostasis [171]. AEBP1 was identified as a key transcription factor during the transition from simple steatosis to NASH using a co-regulatory network approach, which assessed AEBP1 expression in NASH fibrosis versus other NAFLD histological classes using pairwise comparisons [172]. In support of this database analysis, AEBP1 expression increases in the setting of NASH compared to simple steatosis in the livers of $ApoE^{+/-}$ mice. A recent clinical study demonstrated that AEBP1 is specifically expressed in HSC and at a greater extent in the livers of patients with NASH [43]. The ablation of AEBP1 only in the HSC of mice protects against high fat and high cholesterol diet-induced fibrosis. Mechanistically, AEBP1 activates Wnt signaling by specifically binding frizzled-8 and low-density lipoprotein-related receptor 6, which blocks the PPARγ-dependent inhibition of activated HSC. Another study confirmed that hepatic AEBP1 is directly associated with the degree of steatosis, lobular inflammation, and fibrosis in NASH patients [168]. This study also found that AEBP1 upregulates the expression of genes identified as part of an algorithm-predicted AEBP1-associated NASH co-regulatory network [168]. These target genes include the regulators of fibrosis (*AKR1B10*, *CCDC80*, *DPT*, *EFEMP1*, *ITGBL1*, *LAMC3*, *MOXD1*, *SPP1*, and *STMN2*), ECM production and maintenance (*COL4A2* and *MARCO*), and myofibroblast transition (*ACTA2*, *COL1A1*, *COL1A2*, *SERPINE1* and *PLAU*). Taken together, these findings strongly implicate AEBP1 in the diagnosis and treatment of NASH.

6.3. YAP

The Hippo pathway and its effector YAP are particularly important for controlling liver size by regulating proliferation and growth [173]. The expression of YAP is barely detectable in healthy livers of humans and mice but becomes activated in the setting of NASH [45]. YAP is expressed in hepatocytes and activates the expression of proteins that promote fibrosis (ColL1α1, TIMP1, TGFβ2) and inflammation (TNFα, IL-1β), which stimulate the expansion of myofibroblasts and the recruitment of immune cells, exacerbating liver fibrosis [174]. YAP is also activated in Kupffer cells by the lipopolysaccharides (LPS)/TLR4 signaling pathway, where it promotes the development of NASH by enhancing the production of pro-inflammatory cytokines [175]. Further gain and loss of function experiments have shown that the activation of the YAP/transcriptional co-activator with PDZ-binding motif (TAZ) axis leads to the expression of a key matricellular chemokine (CYR61), which stimulates and recruits extrahepatic macrophages to promote liver fibrosis.

6.4. PPARα

In addition to beneficial effects on steatosis and inflammation, PPARα agonist treatment also reverses fibrosis by targeting PPARα in HSC, which decreases the expression of fibrogenic factors including Col1α1 and TIMPs and reduces the number of activated HSC. The protective effect of PPARα was further demonstrated by treating fibrotic APOE$_2$KI811A mice with the PPARα agonist fenofibrate, which protected mice from NASH by reducing both steatosis and hepatic macrophage accumulation [10]. By contrast, mice with a genetic ablation of PPARα display increased susceptibility to NASH [130,176].

6.5. PPARγ

In humans, growth factors activate HSC that display decreased PPARγ expression during the progression of NAFLD to NASH [160]. On the other hand, livers with simple steatosis exhibit increased PPARγ expression. The treatment of rats with NASH with the PPARγ agonist pioglitazone prevents hepatic fibrosis and reduces the expression of TIMPs [177]. Indicating that the inhibition of PPARγ in HSC is responsible for the increased transcription of TIMPs, the overexpression of PPARγ reduces the expression of TIMP1, TIMP2, and alpha smooth muscle actin (αSMA) and reverses hepatic fibrosis. By contrast, the HSC-specific ablation of PPARγ aggravates CCl₄-induced liver fibrosis and increases αSMA expression [132]. Collectively, these findings clearly link decreased PPARγ activity in HSC to hepatic fibrosis. Accordingly, pioglitazone ameliorates only moderate pericentrilobular fibrosis in rats with no effect on severe bridging fibrosis, which is most likely due to the reduced PPARγ availability for pioglitazone to target under the advanced stages of the disease [178]. On the other hand, the effect of TZDs on fibrosis in humans have been less clear. Unlike in rats, a meta-analysis of TZD effects from eight randomized trials ($n = 516$) on NASH-associated liver fibrosis found pioglitazone to significantly improve fibrosis, particularly in the advanced fibrosis stage with bridging fibrosis and cirrhosis compared to NASH with mild perisinusoidal/periportal fibrosis [179]. This effect could have been independent of PPARγ, as TZDs can bind alternative targets such as the mitochondrial pyruvate carrier [179]. In fact, the inhibition of the mitochondrial pyruvate carrier by a next-generation TZD (MSDC0602) was found to reverse hepatic fibrosis in mice, supporting the mitochondria pyruvate carrier as a relevant treatment target [180,181]. Nonetheless, the relevance of targeting PPARγ for the treatment of advanced fibrosis in humans remains unclear.

6.6. RUNX2

Studies have shown that Runx2 acts as a fibrogenic or tumorigenic transcription factor in hepatic fibrosis or hepatocellular carcinoma [182,183]. Runx2 is expressed in the non-parenchymal cells of the liver but not in the hepatocytes. In a mouse model of NAFLD/NASH, Runx2 becomes upregulated in the HSCs during the development of NAFLD [163].

6.7. c-Jun

The impact of c-Jun on fibrogenesis depends on the liver cell type. The deletion of c-Jun only in hepatocytes reduces steatosis but increases fibrosis, whereas its deletion in both hepatocytes and non-parenchymal cells protects against MCD-induced fibrosis in mice [142]. This was linked to reductions in the pro-inflammatory cytokine osteopontin (Opn, also known as SPP1), which is an established marker of a regenerative response called the ductular reaction (DR), which is an essential driver of fibrogenesis. Additional investigations using $Opn^{-/-}$ mice established that c-Jun expression in NPLC promotes NASH-related DR and subsequent fibrosis by upregulating Opn expression [39,184].

7. Microbiome Dysbiosis

The contribution of obesity-induced changes in the gut microbiome to the pathogenesis and progression of NAFLD [185] was initially established using germ-free mice and fecal transplant from lean [186] and diet-induced obese mice [187]. Furthermore, the inoculation of germ-free mice with the gut microbiota of obese humans [188] and NASH patients [189] leads to the onset of hepatic steatosis and NASH, respectively. These findings formed the base or microbiota-based therapies for NAFLD such as pre- and probiotics and fecal microbiota transplantation [190–192].

The gut microbiota can influence the progression of NAFLD through several pathways, which has been reviewed extensively elsewhere [193]. Briefly, these pathways include changes in gut permeability, low-grade inflammation and immune balance, the modulation of dietary choline and bile acid metabolism, and the production of endogenous substrates [186]. In this review, we highlight that the microbiota, through the production of endogenous substrates, may alter the transcriptional profile of the liver. Major metabolites that are linked to alterations in the gut microbiota include bile acids [194–196], short-chain fatty acids (SCFA) [197] and lipopolysaccharides (LPS) [189]. These metabolites can play an important role in NAFLD progression by mediating the gut–liver axis [198]. Products derived from bile acid metabolism act on FXR to decrease hepatic triglyceride levels and improve glucose metabolism [90]. Specifically, the HFD-induced remodeling of the gut microbiota increases the production of bile salt hydrolase (BSH), which is a bacterial enzyme that hydrolyzes and inactivates tauro-β-muricholic acid (T-β-MCA) [199]. T-β-MCA inhibits intestinal FXR signaling, which suppresses ceramide synthesis [200]. Therefore, microbiome dysbiosis results in increased FXR signaling and ceramide production, which in turn promotes SREBP1c activity and steatosis in the liver [201].

SCFAs have been shown to increase the AMPK activity in liver and muscle tissue [202]. The activation of AMPK triggers PGC-1α expression, which controls the transcriptional activity of PPARα, PPARγ, PPARδ, LXR, and FXR, which are important transcriptional regulators of cholesterol, lipid, and glucose metabolism [203]. LPS has been shown to activate NF-κB in cultured hepatocytes [204], which plays a major role in the development of inflammation during NAFLD progression [91] and is highly activated in both mice and patients with NASH. Furthermore, LPS can induce MAP kinase kinase-3 (MKK3) activation, which in turn stimulates C/EBPβ and C/EBPδ binding elements to promote the transcription of CYP2E1 and induce oxidative stress [154].

8. Prediction of Transcriptional Regulators by Database Analyses

8.1. Prognostic Biomarkers for Human NAFLD and NASH

Many transcriptomic studies have been conducted to elucidate novel biomarkers for the different stages of NAFLD, including steatosis, ballooning, and fibrosis. To elucidate the transcriptional changes that are associated with human NAFLD, we procured publicly available human NAFLD/NASH transcriptome data from the Gene Expression Omnibus (GEO) and subjected them to Ingenuity Pathway Analysis for the prediction of changes in upstream factors (Table 2). Predictions were based on two GEO datasets with strong power analysis (Table 2) as well as a previously published Ingenuity Pathway Analysis (IPA)-based prediction analysis [7,205,206]. The activation of PPARγ was the only consistent prediction for simple steatosis, whereas the onset of fibrosis was associated with changes in a larger number of transcription factors, which were consistent in at least half of the datasets. These included the activation of inflammation (NF-κB, RELA, JUN, IRF1, IRF3, STAT1, SP1), glucose production (FOXO1), and lipogenesis (SREBP1), as well as the inhibition of PPARα, PPARγ, and RXRα. The activation of C/EBPβ, CTNNB1, and SMAD3 and the inhibition of HNF4α and SMAD7 were also associated with NASH and NASH-induced HCC, suggesting that these factors might contribute to the pathogenesis of advanced stage fibrosis.

Table 2. Ingenuity Pathway Analysis (IPA) prediction of upstream mechanistic networks that are commonly regulated in the livers of humans and mice with NAFLD.

Regulation in Human Fibrosis	Transcription Factor/Regulator	Human							Mouse Model							
		Steatosis		Fibrosis				HCC	Steatosis			NASH				
		[c] Non-fibrotic NAFLD vs. Healthy	[e] Steatotic vs. Healthy	[a] Fibrotic vs. Healthy	[b] Fibrotic vs. Non-Fibrotic NAFLD	[d] NASH vs. Healthy	[f] External IPA NASH	[g] External IPA HCC	[h] HFD	[i] WD	[j] MCD	[k] NASH Diet	[l] NASH Diet + CCl₄	[n] CCl₄	[m] WD + CCl₄	[o] STAM
Consistent Activation (2 ≥ datasets)	FOXO1 *		▨	■						▨	■	■	■	■	■	
	IRF1 *		▨	■		■					■	■		■	■	
	IRF3 *		▨	■		■					■	■				
	JUN *	■	▨	■	■		■	■				■		■		
	NFκB *	■	▨	■	■		■	■				■			■	
	RELA *	■	▨	■	■		■	■				■	■	■	■	
	SP1 *			■			■					■		■		
	SREBP1 *											■	■	■	■	
	STAT1 *	■	▨		■	■						■	■	■	■	■
	C/EBPβ †		▨		■		■	■		▨		■	■	■	■	■
	CTNNB1 †						■	■							■	
	SMAD3 †											■				
Activation (1 dataset)	CREB			■										■		
	EGR1			■												
	ESR2															
	IRF7															
	LXR												▨			
	NFAT			■				■						■		
	NRF2					■		■								
	RARα				■						■				■	
	RUNX2				■						■					
	SPI1					■								■	■	
	STAT2					■									■	

Table 2. *Cont.*

The shaded cells in the original table encode regulation (red = activation, blue = inhibition) and cannot be read as text values; marks are transcribed as ■ for a shaded/filled cell and left empty where blank.

Regulation in Human Fibrosis	Transcription Factor/Regulator	[c] Non-fibrotic NAFLD vs. Healthy	[e] Steatotic vs. Healthy	[a] Fibrotic vs. Healthy	[b] Fibrotic vs. Non-Fibrotic NAFLD	[d] NASH vs. Healthy	[f] External IPA NASH	[g] External IPA HCC	HFD [h]	WD [i]	MCD [j]	NASH Diet [k]	NASH Diet + CCl4 [l]	CCl4 [n]	WD + CCl4 [m]	STAM [o]
		Human — Steatosis		**Human — Fibrosis**				**HCC**	**Mouse — Steatosis**		**Mouse — NASH**					
Consistent Inhibition (2 ≥ datasets)	PPARα *	■		■	■		■		■		■	■	■			■
	PPARγ *	■							■		■	■	■			
	RXRα *	■		■			■		■	■					■	
	HNF4α †						■	■								
	SMAD7 †															
Inhibition (1 dataset)	AHR				■				■							
	HDAC1				■											
	HNF1α															
	NR1h			■									■	■		
	NR3C1															
	NR5A2				■										■	
	RBL1															
	STAT5a													■		
	THRβ									■						
Inconsistent Regulation	STAT3		■	■				■					■			
	MYC						■	■							■	
	p53		■	■										■		
	IRF8		■			■						■		■		
	ESR1		■	■							■					

Human GEO Accession GSE130970 was divided into three independent IPA comparative analyses: [a] Advanced fibrotic (fibrosis score > 3, $n = 16$) versus healthy ($n = 8$), [b] Fibrotic versus non-fibrotic NAFLD (NAS > 3, $n = 11$), and [c] non-fibrotic NAFLD versus healthy. Human GEO Accession GSE89632 was similarly analyzed in three independent analyses comparing transcriptomic changes among human livers with [d] NASH ($n = 19$) vs. healthy ($n = 24$), NASH vs. simple steatosis ($n = 20$) and [e] simple steatosis vs. healthy. The conclusions of a previously published upstream regulators analysis for [f] NASH and [g] NASH-associated HCC are included as well. The mouse models of steatosis using [h] HFD (GSE93132) and [i] Western diet (GSE99010) as well as mouse models of NASH using [j] MCD diet (GSE93132), [k] NASH diet (GSE52748), [l] NASH diet coupled with CCl4 treatment (GSE129525), [m] CCl4 treatment alone (GSE99010) and [n] Western diet coupled with CCl4 treatment (GSE99010). The observations from the [o] STAM NASH model are included as well. Transcriptomic changes of 2-fold or more were included in the IPA. The table includes the mechanistic network of the transcription factors with a prediction Z score of greater than 2 for activation (red) or less than −2 for inhibition (blue). Datasets for mouse hepatocellular carcinoma (HCC) models using extended CCl4 treatment for 24 weeks were excluded from the IPA prediction. The analysis of human livers with NASH vs. simple steatosis from GSE89632 dataset did not yield any prediction for significant changes in upstream activity and was excluded from the table. Abbreviations: forkhead protein O (FoxO), interferon regulatory factor (IRF), nuclear factor of the κ light chain enhancer of B cells (NF-κB), v-rel avian reticuloendotheliosis viral oncogene homolog A (RELA), Specific Protein 1 (SP1), sterol regulatory element binding protein (SREBP), signal transducer and activator of transcription (STAT), CCAAT/enhancer binding protein (C/EBP), Catenin Beta 1 (CTNNB1), transcription factors against decapentaplegic homolog (SMAD), cyclic AMP-responsive element-binding protein (CREB), early growth response 1 (EGR1), estrogen receptor (ESR), liver X receptor (LXR), nuclear factor of activated T-cells (NFAT), nuclear factor. * Consistent regulation in 2 or more human NASH datasets. † Consistent regulation in human NASH and HCC.

8.2. Altered Transcription Factors in Mouse Models of NAFLD and NASH

The same strategy was applied to predict the changes in the activity of transcription factors in mouse models of NAFLD/NASH. We performed IPA upstream activity prediction analysis for publicly available liver transcriptome data from mouse models of steatosis that were established by feeding high caloric diets [18,207] as well as mouse models of NASH that were established by feeding an MCD diet [207], NASH diet, or a combination of high caloric diets coupled with CCl$_4$ treatment [18,208]. Additionally, we included the observations of a previously published STZ-induced NASH and HCC model (STAM) [7]. Transgenic mouse models that involve genetic manipulations were excluded, since our comparative analysis was not aimed at delineating the transcriptional consequences of rare gene variants in humans and mice. As anticipated, the activation of most consistent pathways in humans (Table 2) were also confirmed in most mouse models. However, in contrast to the downregulation of PPARα, PPARγ, and RXRα in human livers with NASH, these pathways were upregulated in most mouse models of NASH (Table 2). The activity regulation of PPARα, PPARγ, and RXRα in mouse models of NASH was instead more representative of their activity in human livers with simple steatosis (Table 2).

IPA analysis of the mouse models also identified pathways that were not predicted to be affected among human NASH datasets. Among these, the activation of SMAD2, SMAD4, YAP1, NOTCH1, EP300, p63, and the inhibition of nuclear receptor corepressor (NCOR) has been previously linked to human NASH by independent studies (Table 3) [42,166,173,209–212]. Therefore, most mouse models mimic the transcriptional signature of human NASH for these transcription factors. However, the consistent inhibition of SREBP2 and the activation of fos proto-oncogene (FOS) and PGC1α in mouse NASH models mimicked human steatosis but were absent in the setting of human fibrosis (Table 3) [102,213,214]. Furthermore, increased FOS mRNA in fibrotic versus non-fibrotic NAFLD patients was in line with increased EGR1 activity, which promotes FOS expression, as previously published (Table 2). However, IPA did not predict FOS activation, as this would be anticipated to inhibit NF-κB and SP1 and activate CEBBP, which was in contrast with the regulation in fibrotic livers (Table 2). Other frequently altered transcriptional mechanisms in mouse NASH models, which were not previously associated with human NASH, included PPARδ, HIF1α, MED1, NCOA1, NCOA2, SMARCA4, FOXO3, HDAC2, STAT5b, and STAT6 (Table 4). Individual transcriptomic datasets from mouse livers also predicted the regulation of unique pathways for each dataset, which were not predicted to be regulated in other mouse models (Table 4). Since IPA prediction of upstream factors in human NASH also failed to identify changes in the activity of these sets of transcription factors in Tables 3 and 4, studying their relevance in the pathogenesis of NASH in humans would be beneficial prior to investigating their roles in pre-clinical rodent models of NASH. It is worth mentioning that the activation of ChREBP and C/EBPα were only confirmed in the mouse models using MCD and WD coupled with CCl$_4$, respectively, but they were not detected in human fibrosis datasets. Another category of altered transcription factors belonged to those that were altered in a single human dataset but not in any of the mouse models (Table 5). Although the activity regulation of these factors could be relevant in the pathogenesis of NASH, corroborating evidence is lacking.

To determine how the transcriptional activity of popular NASH mouse models faired against human NASH, we implemented a scoring strategy ranging from +2 to −2 for each transcription factor: +2 for the confirmation of a transcriptional activity in a mouse model, which was observed in more than one human NASH dataset (i.e., NF-κB); −2 for the reversal of a transcriptional activity, which was observed in more than one human NASH dataset (i.e., PPARγ); +1 for the confirmation of a transcriptional activity, which was observed only in one human NASH dataset (i.e., SMAD7); −1 for the reversal of a transcriptional activity, which was observed only in one human NASH dataset (i.e., THRβ for CCl_4 model); -1 when multiple confirmations for a transcriptional activity among human datasets remained unchanged in a mouse model (i.e., NF-κB for NASH diet + CCl_4 model); 0 for a lack of transcriptional activity in a mouse model, which was also observed in some of the human NASH datasets (i.e., THRb for all models except CCl_4); and 0 when a transcriptional activity was predicted to be inconsistently regulated among different human NASH datasets regardless of the state of the activity of that transcription factor within the mouse models (i.e., STAT3). From a possible maximum score of +47 for all the common transcription factors (Table 2), the NASH diet, MCD diet, NASH diet + CCl_4, CCl_4 alone, and WD + CCl_4 netted total scores of 23, 27, −10, 12 and 7, respectively, suggesting that the NASH diet and MCD diet exhibit transcriptional activity profiles that are more representative of human NASH, whereas the models that involved CCl_4 treatment did not. We excluded the STAM mouse model due to the low number of predicted matches.

Table 3. IPA prediction of upstream regulators that were detected in the livers of mouse models of NASH but not in human NASH cohorts.

	[j] MCD	[k] NASH Diet	[l] NASH Diet + CCl₄	[n] CCl₄	[m] WD + CCl₄	Association with Human Fibrosis
SMAD4						NASH
SMAD2						NASH
YAP1						NASH
NOTCH1						NASH
EP300						NASH
NCOR						NASH
p63						NASH, steatosis
SREBP2						Steatosis
CAR						Steatosis
FOS						Steatosis, insulin resistance
PGC1α						Steatosis, insulin resistance
PPARδ						N/A
HIF1α						N/A
MED1						N/A
NCOA1						N/A
SMARCA4						N/A
NCOA2						N/A
FOXO3						N/A
HDAC2						N/A
STAT5b						N/A
STAT6						N/A

Mouse models of NASH using [j] MCD diet (GSE93132), [k] NASH diet (GSE52748), [l] NASH diet coupled with CCl_4 treatment (GSE129525), [m] CCl_4 treatment alone (GSE99010) and [n] Western diet coupled with CCl_4 treatment (GSE99010). Abbreviations: transcription factors against decapentaplegic homolog (SMAD), yes-associated protein (YAP), notch receptor 1 (NOTCH1), Histone Acetyltransferase P300 (EP300), nuclear receptor corepressor (NCOR), sterol regulatory element binding protein (SREBP), constitutive androstane receptor (CAR), fos proto-oncogene (FOS), PPARγ coactivator 1 alpha (PGC1α), peroxisome proliferator-activated receptor (PPAR), hypoxia inducible factor 1α (HIF1α), mediator complex subunit 1 (MED1), nuclear receptor coactivator (NCOA), SWI/SNF related, matrix associated, actin dependent regulator of chromatin subfamily A member 4 (SMARCA4), forkhead protein O (FoxO), histone deacetylase (HDAC), signal transducer and activator of transcription (STAT).

Table 4. IPA prediction of upstream mechanistic networks that are unique to each mouse model.

	[j] MCD	[k] NASH Diet	[l] NASH Diet + CCl$_4$	[n] CCl$_4$	[m] WD + CCl$_4$
AR		■			
ARNTL			■		
CDKN2A		■			
C/EBPα					■
ChREBP	■				
CIITA				■	
E2F	■				
FOXO4					■
HNF1α		■			
HSF1				■	
IRF9				■	
KLF4					■
MAX					■
MYB					■
PGR			■		
RARB					■
RB1	■				
RORA					■
SNAI					■
SP3	■				
STAT4	■				
TCF7L2					■
THRα				■	■
VDR					■
WT1					■
Ybx1					■
ZNFn1a1			■		

Mouse models of NASH using [j] MCD diet (GSE93132), [k] NASH diet (GSE52748), [l] NASH diet coupled with CCl$_4$ treatment (GSE129525), [m] CCl$_4$ treatment alone (GSE99010) and [n] Western diet coupled with CCl$_4$ treatment (GSE99010). Abbreviations: androgen receptor (AR), aryl hydrocarbon receptor nuclear translocator like (ARNTL), cyclin dependent kinase inhibitor 2A (CDKN2A), CCAAT/enhancer binding protein (C/EBP), class ii major histocompatibility complex transactivator (CIITA), forkhead protein O (FoxO), hepatocyte nuclear factor (HNF), heat shock transcription factor 1 (HSF1), interferon regulatory factor (IRF), kruppel like factor 4 (KLF4), MYC associated factor X (MAX), myb proto-oncogene (MYB), progesterone receptor (PGR), retinoic acid receptor beta (RARB), retinoblastoma transcriptional corepressor 1 (RB1), retinoic acid receptor-related orphan receptor alpha (RORA), snail family transcriptional repressor (SNAI), specificity protein 3 (SP3), signal transducer and activator of transcription (STAT), transcription factor 7 like 2 (TCF7L2), thyroid hormone receptor α (THRα), vitamin D receptor (VDR), Wilms' tumor protein (WT1), Y box-binding protein 1 (Ybx1), IKAROS family zinc finger 1 (ZNFn1a1).

Table 5. IPA prediction of upstream mechanistic networks that are unique to each human NASH cohort.

	[a] Fibrotic vs. Healthy	[b] Fibrotic vs. Non-Fibrotic NAFLD	[d] NASH vs. Healthy	[f] External IPA NASH
CCND1		■		
CCNE1		■		
HMGB1	■			
IRF2			■	
IRF5	■			
KLF2	■			
NRIP1				■
SOX2				■

Human GEO Accession GSE130970 was divided into three independent IPA comparative analyses: [a] Advanced fibrotic (fibrosis score > 3, n = 16) versus healthy (n = 8), [b] Fibrotic versus non-fibrotic NAFLD (NAS > 3, n = 11), and [d] non-fibrotic NAFLD versus healthy. [f] Previously reported IPA of NASH (Kakehashi et al.). Abbreviations: cyclin D1 (CCND1), cyclin E1 (CCNE1), high mobility group box 1 (HMGB1), interferon regulatory factor (IRF), kruppel like factor 2 (KLF2), nuclear receptor interacting protein 1 (NRIP1), sex determining region Y box transcription factor 2 (SOX2).

9. Conclusions

Maladaptive responses to obesity results in the activation of inflammatory and fibrogenic pathways in the liver. Here, we reviewed the transcription factors, the activity of which have been commonly associated with obesity-induced NAFLD and NASH. The development of NAFLD and NASH strongly correlates with the dysregulation of transcriptional regulators that play a role in lipid metabolism, inflammation, metabolic stress, and fibrosis. Interestingly, the review of gluconeogenic transcription factors indicated a protective function against steatosis and NASH, since their loss often resulted in disease. The field of main regulators will continue to increase with heightened focus on delineating new pathways in the pathogenesis of NAFLD, as each of the areas discussed in this review are still being actively researched and adding to our understanding of the transcriptional regulation of NAFLD.

Our review also indicates that none of the diet-based rodent models replicate all the features of the human pathophysiology. Our observations suggested that the FCP diet and MCD diet exhibit transcriptional activity profiles that are more representative of human NASH, whereas the models that involved chemical induction, such as CCl_4 treatment, did not. The generation of novel experimental models that more accurately reproduce human pathophysiology, including mice with humanized livers [215], will be central to the discovery of tractable targets for the management of NAFLD.

Author Contributions: Conceptualized the outline of the review: S.S.; performed literature search: S.S., J.Q. and B.A.E.; wrote and edited the manuscript: S.S., J.Q. and B.A.E.; conceptualized the outline: B.A.E., directed and validated the review: B.A.E.; analyzed publicly available datasets: B.A.E. All authors have read and agreed to the published version of the manuscript.

References

1. Machado, M.V.; Cortez-Pinto, H. Non-alcoholic fatty liver disease: What the clinician needs to know. *World J. Gastroenterol.* **2014**, *20*, 12956–12980. [CrossRef] [PubMed]
2. Younossi, Z.; Anstee, Q.M.; Marietti, M.; Hardy, T.; Henry, L.; Eslam, M.; George, J.; Bugianesi, E. Global burden of NAFLD and NASH: Trends, predictions, risk factors and prevention. *Nat. Rev. Gastroenterol. Hepatol.* **2017**, *15*, 11–20. [CrossRef]
3. Iwaisako, K.; Brenner, D.A.; Kisseleva, T. What's new in liver fibrosis? The origin of myofibroblasts in liver fibrosis. *J. Gastroenterol. Hepatol.* **2012**, *27*, 65–68. [CrossRef] [PubMed]
4. Benedict, M.; Zhang, X. Non-alcoholic fatty liver disease: An expanded review. *World J. Hepatol.* **2017**, *9*, 715–732. [CrossRef] [PubMed]
5. Oseini, A.M.; Sanyal, A.J. Therapies in non-alcoholic steatohepatitis (NASH). *Liver Int.* **2017**, *37*, 97–103. [CrossRef] [PubMed]
6. Paschos, P.; Paletas, K. Non alcoholic fatty liver disease and metabolic syndrome. *Hippokratia* **2009**, *13*, 9–19.
7. Kakehashi, A.; Stefanov, V.E.; Ishii, N.; Okuno, T.; Fujii, H.; Kawai, K.; Kawada, N.; Wanibuchi, H. Proteome Characteristics of Non-Alcoholic Steatohepatitis Liver Tissue and Associated Hepatocellular Carcinomas. *Int. J. Mol. Sci.* **2017**, *18*, 434. [CrossRef]
8. Buzzetti, E.; Pinzani, M.; Tsochatzis, E.A. The multiple-hit pathogenesis of non-alcoholic fatty liver disease (NAFLD). *Metabolism* **2016**, *65*, 1038–1048. [CrossRef]
9. Zaret, K.S.; Carroll, J.S. Pioneer transcription factors: Establishing competence for gene expression. *Genes Dev.* **2011**, *25*, 2227–2241. [CrossRef]
10. Shiri-Sverdlov, R.; Wouters, K.A.M.; Van Gorp, P.; Gijbels, M.J.; Noël, B.; Buffat, L.; Staels, B.; Maeda, N.; Van Bilsen, M.; Hofker, M.H. Early diet-induced non-alcoholic steatohepatitis in APOE2 knock-in mice and its prevention by fibrates. *J. Hepatol.* **2006**, *44*, 732–741. [CrossRef]
11. Horie, Y.; Suzuki, A.; Kataoka, E.; Sasaki, T.; Hamada, K.; Sasaki, J.; Mizuno, K.; Hasegawa, G.; Kishimoto, H.; Iizuka, M.; et al. Hepatocyte-specific Pten deficiency results in steatohepatitis and hepatocellular carcinomas. *J. Clin. Investig.* **2004**, *113*, 1774–1783. [CrossRef] [PubMed]
12. Nakagawa, H.; Umemura, A.; Taniguchi, K.; Font-Burgada, J.; Dhar, D.; Ogata, H.; Zhong, Z.; Valasek, M.A.; Seki, E.; Hidalgo, J.; et al. ER stress cooperates with hypernutrition to trigger TNF-dependent spontaneous HCC development. *Cancer Cell* **2014**, *26*, 331–343. [CrossRef] [PubMed]

13. Ito, M.; Suzuki, J.; Tsujioka, S.; Sasaki, M.; Gomori, A.; Shirakura, T.; Hirose, H.; Ito, M.; Ishihara, A.; Iwaasa, H.; et al. Longitudinal analysis of murine steatohepatitis model induced by chronic exposure to high-fat diet. *Hepatol. Res.* **2007**, *37*, 50–57. [CrossRef] [PubMed]

14. Stephenson, K.; Kennedy, L.; Hargrove, L.; Demieville, J.; Thomson, J.; Alpini, G.; Francis, H.L. Updates on Dietary Models of Nonalcoholic Fatty Liver Disease: Current Studies and Insights. *Gene Expr.* **2018**, *18*, 5–17. [CrossRef]

15. Nakae, D.; Mizumoto, Y.; Andoh, N.; Tamura, K.; Horiguchi, K.; Endoh, T.; Kobayashi, E.; Tsujiuchi, T.; Denda, A.; Lombardi, B.; et al. Comparative Changes in the Liver of Female Fischer-344 Rats after Short-Term Feeding of a Semipurified or a Semisynthetic L-Amino Acid-Defined Choline-Deficient Diet. *Toxicol. Pathol.* **1995**, *23*, 583–590. [CrossRef]

16. Mamikutty, N.; Thent, Z.; Suhaimi, F. Fructose-Drinking Water Induced Nonalcoholic Fatty Liver Disease and Ultrastructural Alteration of Hepatocyte Mitochondria in Male Wistar Rat. *BioMed Res. Int.* **2015**, *2015*, 1–7. [CrossRef]

17. Fujii, M.; Shibazaki, Y.; Wakamatsu, K.; Honda, Y.; Kawauchi, Y.; Suzuki, K.; Arumugam, S.; Watanabe, K.; Ichida, T.; Asakura, H.; et al. A murine model for non-alcoholic steatohepatitis showing evidence of association between diabetes and hepatocellular carcinoma. *Med. Mol. Morphol.* **2013**, *46*, 141–152. [CrossRef]

18. Tsuchida, T.; Lee, Y.A.; Fujiwara, N.; Ybanez, M.; Allen, B.; Martins, S.; Fiel, M.I.; Goossens, N.; Chou, H.-I.; Hoshida, Y.; et al. A simple diet- and chemical-induced murine NASH model with rapid progression of steatohepatitis, fibrosis and liver cancer. *J. Hepatol.* **2018**, *69*, 385–395. [CrossRef]

19. Sinton, M.; Hay, D.C.; Drake, A.J. Metabolic control of gene transcription in non-alcoholic fatty liver disease: The role of the epigenome. *Clin. Epigenet.* **2019**, *11*, 104. [CrossRef]

20. Montagner, A.; Polizzi, A.; Fouché, E.; Ducheix, S.; Lippi, Y.; Lasserre, F.; Barquissau, V.; Régnier, M.; Lukowicz, C.; Benhamed, F.; et al. Liver PPARα is crucial for whole-body fatty acid homeostasis and is protective against NAFLD. *Gut* **2016**, *65*, 1202–1214. [CrossRef]

21. Ponugoti, B.; Kemper, J.K.; Fang, S. Functional Interaction of Hepatic Nuclear Factor-4 and Peroxisome Proliferator-Activated Receptor- Gamma Coactivator 1 alpha in CYP7A1 Regulation Is Inhibited by a Key Lipogenic Activator, Sterol Regulatory Element-Binding Protein-1c. *Mol. Endocrinol.* **2007**, *21*, 2698–2712. [CrossRef] [PubMed]

22. Benhamed, F.; Denechaud, P.-D.; Lemoine, M.; Robichon, C.; Moldes, M.; Bertrand-Michel, J.; Ratziu, V.; Serfaty, L.; Housset, C.; Capeau, J.; et al. The lipogenic transcription factor ChREBP dissociates hepatic steatosis from insulin resistance in mice and humans. *J. Clin. Investig.* **2012**, *122*, 2176–2194. [CrossRef] [PubMed]

23. Tanaka, N.; Aoyama, T.; Kimura, S.; Gonzalez, F.J. Targeting nuclear receptors for the treatment of fatty liver disease. *Pharmacol. Ther.* **2017**, *179*, 142–157. [CrossRef] [PubMed]

24. Ahn, S.B.; Jang, K.; Jun, D.W.; Lee, B.H.; Shin, K.J. Expression of Liver X Receptor Correlates with Intrahepatic Inflammation and Fibrosis in Patients with Nonalcoholic Fatty Liver Disease. *Dig. Dis. Sci.* **2014**, *59*, 2975–2982. [CrossRef] [PubMed]

25. Baciu, C.; Pasini, E.; Angeli, M.; Schwenger, K.; Afrin, J.; Humar, A.; Fischer, S.; Patel, K.; Allard, J.; Bhat, M. Systematic integrative analysis of gene expression identifies HNF4A as the central gene in pathogenesis of non-alcoholic steatohepatitis. *PLoS ONE* **2017**, *12*, e0189223. [CrossRef]

26. Kaltenecker, D.; Themanns, M.; Mueller, K.M.; Spirk, K.; Suske, T.; Merkel, O.; Kenner, L.; Luís, A.; Kozlov, A.; Haybaeck, J.; et al. Hepatic growth hormone-JAK2-STAT5 signalling: Metabolic function, non-alcoholic fatty liver disease and hepatocellular carcinoma progression. *Cytokine* **2019**, *124*, 154569. [CrossRef]

27. Rahman, S.M.; Janssen, R.C.; Jiang, H.; Qadri, I.; MacLean, K.N.; Friedman, J.E.; Schroeder-Gloeckler, J.M. CCAAT/enhancing binding protein β deletion in mice attenuates inflammation, endoplasmic reticulum stress, and lipid accumulation in diet-induced nonalcoholic steatohepatitis. *Hepatology* **2007**, *45*, 1108–1117. [CrossRef]

28. Piccinin, E.; Villani, G.; Moschetta, A. Metabolic aspects in NAFLD, NASH and hepatocellular carcinoma: The role of PGC1 coactivators. *Nat. Rev. Gastroenterol. Hepatol.* **2018**, *16*, 160–174. [CrossRef]

29. Valenti, L.; Rametta, R.; Dongiovanni, P.; Maggioni, M.; Fracanzani, A.L.; Zappa, M.; Lattuada, E.; Roviaro, G.; Fargion, S. Increased Expression and Activity of the Transcription Factor FOXO1 in Nonalcoholic Steatohepatitis. *Diabetes* **2008**, *57*, 1355–1362. [CrossRef]

30. Videla, L.; Tapia, G.; Rodrigo, R.; Pettinelli, P.; Haim, D.; Santibáñez, C.; Araya, A.V.; Smok, G.; Csendes, A.; Gutiérrez, L.; et al. Liver NF-κB and AP-1 DNA Binding in Obese Patients. *Obesity* **2009**, *17*, 973–979. [CrossRef]

31. Severa, M.; Islam, S.A.; Waggoner, S.N.; Jiang, Z.; Kim, N.D.; Ryan, G.; Kurt-Jones, E.; Charo, I.; Caffrey, D.R.; Boyartchuk, V.L.; et al. The transcriptional repressor BLIMP1 curbs host defenses by suppressing expression of the chemokine CCL8. *J. Immunol.* **2014**, *192*, 2291–2304. [CrossRef] [PubMed]

32. Grohmann, M.; Wiede, F.; Dodd, G.T.; Gurzov, E.N.; Ooi, G.J.; Butt, T.; Rasmiena, A.A.; Kaur, S.; Gulati, T.; Goh, P.K.; et al. Obesity Drives STAT-1-Dependent NASH and STAT-3-Dependent HCC. *Cell* **2018**, *175*, 1289.e20–1306.e20. [CrossRef] [PubMed]

33. Dorn, C.; Engelmann, J.C.; Saugspier, M.; Koch, A.; Hartmann, A.; Müller-Nurasyid, M.; Spang, R.; Bosserhoff, A.K.; Hellerbrand, C. Increased expression of c-Jun in nonalcoholic fatty liver disease. *Lab. Investig.* **2014**, *94*, 394–408. [CrossRef] [PubMed]

34. Zou, A.; Magee, N.; Deng, F.; Lehn, S.; Zhong, C.; Zhang, Y. Hepatocyte nuclear receptor SHP suppresses inflammation and fibrosis in a mouse model of nonalcoholic steatohepatitis. *J. Biol. Chem.* **2018**, *293*, 8656–8671. [CrossRef]

35. Shimozono, R.; Asaoka, Y.; Yoshizawa, Y.; Aoki, T.; Noda, H.; Yamada, M.; Kaino, M.; Mochizuki, H. Nrf2 Activators Attenuate the Progression of Nonalcoholic Steatohepatitis–Related Fibrosis in a Dietary Rat Model. *Mol. Pharmacol.* **2013**, *84*, 62–70. [CrossRef]

36. Zhong, L.; Huang, L.; Xue, Q.; Liu, C.; Xu, K.; Shen, W.; Deng, L. Cell-specific elevation of Runx2 promotes hepatic infiltration of macrophages by upregulating MCP-1 in high-fat diet-induced mice NAFLD. *J. Cell. Biochem.* **2019**, *120*, 11761–11774. [CrossRef]

37. Lebeaupin, C.; Vallee, D.; Rousseau, D.; Patouraux, S.; Bonnafous, S.; Adam, G.; Luciano, F.; Luci, C.; Anty, R.; Iannelli, A.; et al. Bax inhibitor-1 protects from nonalcoholic steatohepatitis by limiting inositol-requiring enzyme 1 alpha signaling in mice. *Hepatology* **2018**, *68*, 515–532. [CrossRef]

38. Lee, A.-H.; Scapa, E.F.; Cohen, D.E.; Glimcher, L.H. Regulation of Hepatic Lipogenesis by the Transcription Factor XBP1. *Science* **2008**, *320*, 1492–1496. [CrossRef]

39. Cazanave, S.; Podtelezhnikov, A.; Jensen, K.; Seneshaw, M.; Kumar, D.P.; Min, H.-K.; Santhekadur, P.K.; Banini, B.; Mauro, A.G.; Oseini, A.M.; et al. The Transcriptomic Signature of Disease Development and Progression of Nonalcoholic Fatty Liver Disease. *Sci. Rep.* **2017**, *7*, 17193. [CrossRef]

40. Gonzalez-Rodriguez, A.; Mayoral, R.; Agra, N.; Valdecantos, M.P.; Pardo, V.; E Miquilena-Colina, M.; Vargas-Castrillón, J.; Iacono, O.L.; Corazzari, M.; Fimia, G.M.; et al. Impaired autophagic flux is associated with increased endoplasmic reticulum stress during the development of NAFLD. *Cell Death Dis.* **2014**, *5*, e1179. [CrossRef]

41. Lee, S.; Kim, S.; Hwang, S.; Cherrington, N.J.; Ryu, D.-Y. Dysregulated expression of proteins associated with ER stress, autophagy and apoptosis in tissues from nonalcoholic fatty liver disease. *Oncotarget* **2017**, *8*, 63370–63381. [CrossRef] [PubMed]

42. Dattaroy, D.; Pourhoseini, S.; Das, S.; Alhasson, F.; Seth, R.; Nagarkatti, M.; Michelotti, G.A.; Diehl, A.M.; Chatterjee, S. Micro-RNA 21 inhibition of SMAD7 enhances fibrogenesis via leptin-mediated NADPH oxidase in experimental and human nonalcoholic steatohepatitis. *Am. J. Physiol. Liver Physiol.* **2014**, *308*, G298–G312. [CrossRef] [PubMed]

43. Teratani, T.; Tomita, K.; Suzuki, T.; Furuhashi, H.; Irie, R.; Nishikawa, M.; Yamamoto, J.; Hibi, T.; Miura, S.; Minamino, T.; et al. Aortic carboxypeptidase-like protein, a WNT ligand, exacerbates nonalcoholic steatohepatitis. *J. Clin. Investig.* **2018**, *128*, 1581–1596. [CrossRef] [PubMed]

44. Kumar, D.P.; Santhekadur, P.K.; Seneshaw, M.; Mirshahi, F.; Tuculescu, C.U.; Sanyal, A.J. A Regulatory Role of Apoptosis Antagonizing Transcription Factor in the Pathogenesis of Nonalcoholic Fatty Liver Disease and Hepatocellular Carcinoma. *Hepatology* **2019**, *69*, 1520–1534. [CrossRef]

45. Patel, S.H.; Camargo, F.D.; Yimlamai, D. Hippo Signaling in the Liver Regulates Organ Size, Cell Fate, and Carcinogenesis. *Gastroenterology* **2016**, *152*, 533–545. [CrossRef] [PubMed]

46. Souza-Mello, V. Peroxisome proliferator-activated receptors as targets to treat non-alcoholic fatty liver disease. *World J. Hepatol.* **2015**, *7*, 1012–1019. [CrossRef]

47. Ip, E.; Farrell, G.; Robertson, G.; Hall, P.; Kirsch, R.; Leclercq, I. Central role of PPARα-dependent hepatic lipid turnover in dietary steatohepatitis in mice. *Hepatology* **2003**, *38*, 123–132. [CrossRef]

48. Musso, G.; Gambino, R.; Cassader, M.; Pagano, G. A meta-analysis of randomized trials for the treatment of nonalcoholic fatty liver disease. *Hepatology* **2010**, *52*, 79–104. [CrossRef]

49. Lee, Y.K.; Park, J.E.; Lee, M.; Hardwick, J.P. Hepatic lipid homeostasis by peroxisome proliferator-activated receptor gamma 2✩. *Liver Res.* **2018**, *2*, 209–215. [CrossRef]

50. Greenstein, A.W.; Majumdar, N.; Yang, P.; Subbaiah, P.V.; Kineman, R.D.; Cordoba-Chacon, J. Hepatocyte-specific, PPARγ-regulated mechanisms to promote steatosis in adult mice. *J. Endocrinol.* **2016**, *232*, 107–121. [CrossRef]

51. Medina-Gómez, G.; Gray, S.L.; Yetukuri, L.; Shimomura, K.; Virtue, S.; Campbell, M.; Curtis, R.K.; Jimenez-Liñan, M.; Blount, M.; Yeo, G.S.H.; et al. PPAR gamma 2 Prevents Lipotoxicity by Controlling Adipose Tissue Expandability and Peripheral Lipid Metabolism. *PLoS Genet.* **2007**, *3*, e64. [CrossRef] [PubMed]

52. Morán-Salvador, E.; López-Parra, M.; García-Alonso, V.; Titos, E.; Martínez-Clemente, M.; González-Périz, A.; López-Vicario, C.; Barak, Y.; Arroyo, V.; Claria, J. Role for PPARγ in obesity-induced hepatic steatosis as determined by hepatocyte- and macrophage-specific conditional knockouts. *FASEB J.* **2011**, *25*, 2538–2550. [CrossRef] [PubMed]

53. Matsusue, K.; Haluzík, M.; Lambert, G.; Yim, S.-H.; Gavrilova, O.; Ward, J.M.; Brewer, B.; Reitman, M.L.; Gonzalez, F.J. Liver-specific disruption of PPARγ in leptin-deficient mice improves fatty liver but aggravates diabetic phenotypes. *J. Clin. Investig.* **2003**, *111*, 737–747. [CrossRef]

54. Pettinelli, P.; Videla, L. Up-Regulation of PPAR-γ mRNA Expression in the Liver of Obese Patients: An Additional Reinforcing Lipogenic Mechanism to SREBP-1c Induction. *J. Clin. Endocrinol. Metab.* **2011**, *96*, 1424–1430. [CrossRef] [PubMed]

55. Pan, X.; Wang, P.; Luo, J.; Wang, Z.; Song, Y.; Ye, J.; Hou, X. Adipogenic changes of hepatocytes in a high-fat diet-induced fatty liver mice model and non-alcoholic fatty liver disease patients. *Endocrine* **2014**, *48*, 834–847. [CrossRef] [PubMed]

56. Ratziu, V.; Charlotte, F.; Bernhardt, C.; Giral, P.; Halbron, M.; Lenaour, G.; Hartmann-Heurtier, A.; Bruckert, E.; Poynard, T.; LIDO Study Group. Long-term efficacy of rosiglitazone in nonalcoholic steatohepatitis: Results of the fatty liver improvement by rosiglitazone therapy (FLIRT 2) extension trial. *Hepatology* **2009**, *51*, 445–453. [CrossRef]

57. Ratziu, V.; Giral, P.; Jacqueminet, S.; Charlotte, F.; Hartemann–Heurtier, A.; Serfaty, L.; Podevin, P.; Lacorte, J.; Bernhardt, C.; Bruckert, E.; et al. Rosiglitazone for Nonalcoholic Steatohepatitis: One-Year Results of the Randomized Placebo-Controlled Fatty Liver Improvement With Rosiglitazone Therapy (FLIRT) Trial. *Gastroenterology* **2008**, *135*, 100–110. [CrossRef]

58. Cusi, K.; Orsak, B.; Bril, F.; Lomonaco, R.; Hecht, J.; Ortiz-Lopez, C.; Tio, F.; Hardies, J.; Darland, C.; Musi, N.; et al. Long-Term Pioglitazone Treatment for Patients With Nonalcoholic Steatohepatitis and Prediabetes or Type 2 Diabetes Mellitus. *Ann. Intern. Med.* **2016**, *165*, 305. [CrossRef]

59. Feige, J.N.; Gelman, L.; Tudor, C.; Engelborghs, Y.; Wahli, W.; Desvergne, B. Fluorescence Imaging Reveals the Nuclear Behavior of Peroxisome Proliferator-activated Receptor/Retinoid X Receptor Heterodimers in the Absence and Presence of Ligand. *J. Biol. Chem.* **2005**, *280*, 17880–17890. [CrossRef]

60. Kliewer, S.A.; Forman, B.M.; Blumberg, B.; Ong, E.S.; Borgmeyer, U.; Mangelsdorf, D.J.; Umesono, K.; Evans, R.M. Differential expression and activation of a family of murine peroxisome proliferator-activated receptors. *Proc. Natl. Acad. Sci. USA* **1994**, *91*, 7355–7359. [CrossRef]

61. Bays, H.E.; Schwartz, S.; Littlejohn, T.; Kerzner, B.; Krauss, R.M.; Karpf, D.B.; Choi, Y.-J.; Wang, X.; Naim, S.; Roberts, B.K. MBX-8025, A Novel Peroxisome Proliferator Receptor-? Agonist: Lipid and Other Metabolic Effects in Dyslipidemic Overweight Patients Treated with and without Atorvastatin. *J. Clin. Endocrinol. Metab.* **2011**, *96*, 2889–2897. [CrossRef] [PubMed]

62. Riserus, U.; Sprecher, D.; Johnson, T.; Olson, E.; Hirschberg, S.; Liu, A.; Fang, Z.; Hegde, P.; Richards, D.; Sarov-Blat, L.; et al. Activation of Peroxisome Proliferator-Activated Receptor (PPAR) Promotes Reversal of Multiple Metabolic Abnormalities, Reduces Oxidative Stress, and Increases Fatty Acid Oxidation in Moderately Obese Men. *Diabetes* **2007**, *57*, 332–339. [CrossRef] [PubMed]

63. Shimano, H. SREBPs: Physiology and pathophysiology of the SREBP family. *FEBS J.* **2008**, *276*, 616–621. [CrossRef] [PubMed]

64. Fatehi-Hassanabad, Z.; Chan, C.B. Transcriptional regulation of lipid metabolism by fatty acids: A key determinant of pancreatic β-cell function. *Nutr. Metab.* **2005**, *2*, 1. [CrossRef] [PubMed]

65. Walker, A.K.; Yang, F.; Jiang, K.; Ji, J.-Y.; Watts, J.L.; Purushotham, A.; Boss, O.; Hirsch, M.L.; Ribich, S.; Smith, J.J.; et al. Conserved role of SIRT1 orthologs in fasting-dependent inhibition of the lipid/cholesterol regulator SREBP. *Genes Dev.* **2010**, *24*, 1403–1417. [CrossRef]

66. Bruschi, F.V.; Tardelli, M.; Claudel, T.; Trauner, M. PNPLA3 expression and its impact on the liver: Current perspectives. *Hepatic Med.* **2017**, *9*, 55–66. [CrossRef] [PubMed]

67. Cohen, J.C.; Horton, J.D.; Hobbs, H.H. Human Fatty Liver Disease: Old Questions and New Insights. *Science* **2011**, *332*, 1519–1523. [CrossRef]

68. Dongiovanni, P.; Donati, B.; Fares, R.; Lombardi, R.; Mancina, R.M.; Romeo, S.; Valenti, L. PNPLA3 I148M polymorphism and progressive liver disease. *World J. Gastroenterol.* **2013**, *19*, 6969–6978. [CrossRef]

69. Sookoian, S.; Pirola, C.J. Meta-analysis of the influence of I148M variant of patatin-like phospholipase domain containing 3 gene (PNPLA3) on the susceptibility and histological severity of nonalcoholic fatty liver disease. *Hepatology* **2011**, *53*, 1883–1894. [CrossRef]

70. Kohjima, M.; Higuchi, N.; Kato, M.; Kotoh, K.; Yoshimoto, T.; Fujino, T.; Yada, M.; Yada, R.; Harada, N.; Enjoji, M.; et al. SREBP-1c, regulated by the insulin and AMPK signaling pathways, plays a role in nonalcoholic fatty liver disease. *Int. J. Mol. Med.* **2008**, *21*, 507–511. [CrossRef]

71. Horton, J.D.; Goldstein, J.L.; Brown, M.S. SREBPs: Activators of the complete program of cholesterol and fatty acid synthesis in the liver. *J. Clin. Investig.* **2002**, *109*, 1125–1131. [CrossRef]

72. Kim, J.Y.; Garcia-Carbonell, R.; Yamachika, S.; Zhao, P.; Dhar, D.; Loomba, R.; Kaufman, R.J.; Saltiel, A.R.; Karin, M. ER Stress Drives Lipogenesis and Steatohepatitis via Caspase-2 Activation of S1P. *Cell* **2018**, *175*, 133–145.e15. [CrossRef] [PubMed]

73. Caballero, F.; Fernandez, A.; De Lacy, A.M.; Fernándezcheca, J.C.; Caballería, J.; García-Ruiz, C. Enhanced free cholesterol, SREBP-2 and StAR expression in human NASH. *J. Hepatol.* **2009**, *50*, 789–796. [CrossRef] [PubMed]

74. Ueda, A.; Hamadeh, H.K.; Webb, H.K.; Yamamoto, Y.; Sueyoshi, T.; Afshari, C.A.; Lehmann, J.M.; Negishi, M. Diverse roles of the nuclear orphan receptor CAR in regulating hepatic genes in response to phenobarbital. *Mol. Pharmacol.* **2002**, *61*, 1–6. [CrossRef] [PubMed]

75. Gao, J.; He, J.; Zhai, Y.; Wada, T.; Xie, W. The Constitutive Androstane Receptor Is an Anti-obesity Nuclear Receptor That Improves Insulin Sensitivity*. *J. Biol. Chem.* **2009**, *284*, 25984–25992. [CrossRef]

76. Dong, B.; Saha, P.K.; Huang, W.; Chen, W.; Abu-Elheiga, L.; Wakil, S.J.; Stevens, R.D.; Ilkayeva, O.; Newgard, C.B.; Chan, L.; et al. Activation of nuclear receptor CAR ameliorates diabetes and fatty liver disease. *Proc. Natl. Acad. Sci. USA* **2009**, *106*, 18831–18836. [CrossRef] [PubMed]

77. Patel, M.B.; Oza, N.A.; Anand, I.S.; Deshpande, S.S.; Patel, C.N. Liver X Receptor: A Novel Therapeutic Target. *Indian J. Pharm. Sci.* **2008**, *70*, 135–144. [CrossRef]

78. Han, C.Y. Update on FXR Biology: Promising Therapeutic Target? *Int. J. Mol. Sci.* **2018**, *19*, 2069. [CrossRef]

79. Park, J.-G.; Xu, X.; Cho, S.; Hur, K.Y.; Lee, M.-S.; Kersten, S.; Lee, A.-H. CREBH-FGF21 axis improves hepatic steatosis by suppressing adipose tissue lipolysis. *Sci. Rep.* **2016**, *6*, 27938. [CrossRef]

80. Nakagawa, Y.; Shimano, H. CREBH Regulates Systemic Glucose and Lipid Metabolism. *Int. J. Mol. Sci.* **2018**, *19*, 1396. [CrossRef]

81. Lee, M.-W.; Chanda, D.; Yang, J.; Oh, H.; Kim, S.S.; Yoon, Y.-S.; Hong, S.; Park, K.; Lee, I.-K.; Choi, C.S.; et al. Regulation of Hepatic Gluconeogenesis by an ER-Bound Transcription Factor, CREBH. *Cell Metab.* **2010**, *11*, 331–339. [CrossRef]

82. Danno, H.; Ishii, K.-A.; Nakagawa, Y.; Mikami, M.; Yamamoto, T.; Yabe, S.; Furusawa, M.; Kumadaki, S.; Watanabe, K.; Shimizu, H.; et al. The liver-enriched transcription factor CREBH is nutritionally regulated and activated by fatty acids and PPARα. *Biochem. Biophys. Res. Commun.* **2010**, *391*, 1222–1227. [CrossRef] [PubMed]

83. Xu, X.; Park, J.-G.; So, J.-S.; Hur, K.Y.; Lee, A.-H. Transcriptional regulation of apolipoprotein A-IV by the transcription factor CREBH. *J. Lipid Res.* **2014**, *55*, 850–859. [CrossRef] [PubMed]

84. Cheng, N.; Xu, X.; Simon, T.; Boudyguina, E.; Deng, Z.; Verhague, M.; Lee, A.-H.; Shelness, G.S.; Weinberg, R.B.; Parks, J.S. Very Low Density Lipoprotein Assembly Is Required for cAMP-responsive Element-binding Protein H Processing and Hepatic Apolipoprotein A-IV Expression. *J. Biol. Chem.* **2016**, *291*, 23793–23803. [CrossRef] [PubMed]

85. Lee, J.H.; Giannikopoulos, P.; Duncan, S.A.; Wang, J.; Johansen, C.T.; Brown, J.D.; Plutzky, J.; Hegele, R.A.; Glimcher, L.H.; Lee, A.-H. The transcription factor cyclic AMP–responsive element–binding protein H regulates triglyceride metabolism. *Nat. Med.* **2011**, *17*, 812–815. [CrossRef] [PubMed]

86. Zhang, C.; Wang, G.; Zheng, Z.; Maddipati, K.R.; Zhang, X.; Dyson, G.; Williams, P.; Duncan, S.A.; Kaufman, R.J.; Zhang, K. Endoplasmic reticulum-tethered transcription factor cAMP responsive element-binding protein, hepatocyte specific, regulates hepatic lipogenesis, fatty acid oxidation, and lipolysis upon metabolic stress in mice. *Hepatology* **2012**, *55*, 1070–1082. [CrossRef] [PubMed]

87. Satoh, A.; Han, S.-I.; Araki, M.; Nakagawa, Y.; Ohno, H.; Mizunoe, Y.; Kumagai, K.; Murayama, Y.; Osaki, Y.; Iwasaki, H.; et al. CREBH Improves Diet-Induced Obesity, Insulin Resistance, and Metabolic Disturbances by FGF21-Dependent and FGF21-Independent Mechanisms. *iScience* **2020**, *23*, 100930. [CrossRef] [PubMed]

88. Zhang, Y.; Kast-Woelbern, H.R.; Edwards, P.A. Natural Structural Variants of the Nuclear Receptor Farnesoid X Receptor Affect Transcriptional Activation. *J. Biol. Chem.* **2002**, *278*, 104–110. [CrossRef]

89. Xi, Y.; Li, H. Role of farnesoid X receptor in hepatic steatosis in nonalcoholic fatty liver disease. *Biomed. Pharmacother.* **2020**, *121*, 109609. [CrossRef]

90. Kalaany, N.Y.; Mangelsdorf, D.J. LXRS AND FXR: The Yin and Yang of Cholesterol and Fat Metabolism. *Annu. Rev. Physiol.* **2006**, *68*, 159–191. [CrossRef]

91. Jiao, Y.; Lu, Y.; Li, X.-Y. Farnesoid X receptor: A master regulator of hepatic triglyceride and glucose homeostasis. *Acta Pharmacol. Sin.* **2014**, *36*, 44–50. [CrossRef] [PubMed]

92. Barclay, J.; Nelson, C.N.; Ishikawa, M.; Murray, L.A.; Kerr, L.M.; McPhee, T.R.; Powell, E.E.; Waters, M.J. GH-Dependent STAT5 Signaling Plays an Important Role in Hepatic Lipid Metabolism. *Endocrinology* **2011**, *152*, 181–192. [CrossRef] [PubMed]

93. Baik, M.; Nam, Y.S.; Piao, M.; Kang, H.J.; Park, S.J.; Lee, J.-H. Liver-specific deletion of the signal transducer and activator of transcription 5 gene aggravates fatty liver in response to a high-fat diet in mice. *J. Nutr. Biochem.* **2016**, *29*, 56–63. [CrossRef] [PubMed]

94. Ko, C.-Y.; Chang, W.-C.; Wang, J.-M. Biological roles of CCAAT/Enhancer-binding protein delta during inflammation. *J. Biomed. Sci.* **2015**, *22*, 6. [CrossRef] [PubMed]

95. Matsusue, K.; Gavrilova, O.; Lambert, G.; Brewer, H.B.; Ward, J.M.; Inoue, Y.; Leroith, D.; Gonzalez, F.J. Hepatic CCAAT/Enhancer Binding Protein α Mediates Induction of Lipogenesis and Regulation of Glucose Homeostasis in Leptin-Deficient Mice. *Mol. Endocrinol.* **2004**, *18*, 2751–2764. [CrossRef] [PubMed]

96. Yoon, J.C.; Puigserver, P.; Chen, G.; Donovan, J.; Wu, Z.; Rhee, J.; Adelmant, G.; Stafford, J.M.; Kahn, C.R.; Granner, D.K.; et al. Control of hepatic gluconeogenesis through the transcriptional coactivator PGC-1. *Nature* **2001**, *413*, 131–138. [CrossRef] [PubMed]

97. Yu, Y.; Maguire, T.G.; Alwine, J.C. ChREBP, a glucose-responsive transcriptional factor, enhances glucose metabolism to support biosynthesis in human cytomegalovirus-infected cells. *Proc. Natl. Acad. Sci. USA* **2014**, *111*, 1951–1956. [CrossRef]

98. Kim, M.-S.; Krawczyk, S.A.; Doridot, L.; Fowler, A.J.; Wang, J.X.; Trauger, S.A.; Noh, H.-L.; Kang, H.J.; Meissen, J.K.; Blatnik, M.; et al. ChREBP regulates fructose-induced glucose production independently of insulin signaling. *J. Clin. Investig.* **2016**, *126*, 4372–4386. [CrossRef]

99. Herman, M.A.; Peroni, O.D.; Villoria, J.; Schön, M.R.; Abumrad, N.A.; Blüher, M.; Klein, S.; Kahn, B.B. A novel ChREBP isoform in adipose tissue regulates systemic glucose metabolism. *Nature* **2012**, *484*, 333–338. [CrossRef]

100. Xu, X.; So, J.-S.; Park, J.-G.; Lee, A.-H. Transcriptional control of hepatic lipid metabolism by SREBP and ChREBP. *Semin. Liver Dis.* **2013**, *33*, 301–311. [CrossRef]

101. Austin, S.; St-Pierre, J. PGC1 and mitochondrial metabolism—Emerging concepts and relevance in ageing and neurodegenerative disorders. *J. Cell Sci.* **2012**, *125*, 4963–4971. [CrossRef] [PubMed]

102. Aharoni-Simon, M.; Hann-Obercyger, M.; Pen, S.; Madar, Z.; Tirosh, O. Fatty liver is associated with impaired activity of PPARγ-coactivator 1α (PGC1α) and mitochondrial biogenesis in mice. *Lab. Investig.* **2011**, *91*, 1018–1028. [CrossRef] [PubMed]

103. Erion, D.M.; Ignatova, I.D.; Yonemitsu, S.; Nagai, Y.; Chatterjee, P.; Weismann, D.; Hsiao, J.J.; Zhang, D.; Iwasaki, T.; Stark, R.; et al. Prevention of Hepatic Steatosis and Hepatic Insulin Resistance by Knockdown of cAMP Response Element-Binding Protein. *Cell Metab.* **2009**, *10*, 499–506. [CrossRef] [PubMed]

104. Carter, M.E.; Brunet, A. FOXO transcription factors. *Curr. Biol.* **2007**, *17*, R113–R114. [CrossRef]

105. Dong, X.C. FOXO transcription factors in non-alcoholic fatty liver disease☆. *Liver Res.* **2017**, *1*, 168–173. [CrossRef]

106. Sparks, J.; Dong, H.H. FoxO1 and hepatic lipid metabolism. *Curr. Opin. Lipidol.* **2009**, *20*, 217–226. [CrossRef]

107. Lu, H. Crosstalk of HNF4α with extracellular and intracellular signaling pathways in the regulation of hepatic metabolism of drugs and lipids. *Acta Pharm. Sin. B* **2016**, *6*, 393–408. [CrossRef]

108. Liu, H.; Lou, G.; Li, C.; Wang, X.; Cederbaum, A.I.; Gan, L.; Xie, B. HBx Inhibits CYP2E1 Gene Expression via Downregulating HNF4α in Human Hepatoma Cells. *PLoS ONE* **2014**, *9*, e107913. [CrossRef]

109. Yu, D.; Chen, G.; Pan, M.; Zhang, J.; He, W.; Liu, Y.; Nian, X.; Sheng, L.; Xu, B. High fat diet-induced oxidative stress blocks hepatocyte nuclear factor 4α and leads to hepatic steatosis in mice. *J. Cell. Physiol.* **2018**, *233*, 4770–4782. [CrossRef]

110. Ravnskjaer, K.; Frigerio, F.; Boergesen, M.; Nielsen, T.; Maechler, P.; Mandrup, S. PPARδ is a fatty acid sensor that enhances mitochondrial oxidation in insulin-secreting cells and protects against fatty acid-induced dysfunction. *J. Lipid Res.* **2009**, *51*, 1370–1379. [CrossRef]

111. Iglesias, J.; Barg, S.; Vallois, D.; Lahiri, S.; Roger, C.; Yessoufou, A.; Pradevand, S.; McDonald, A.; Bonal, C.; Reimann, F.; et al. PPARβ/δ affects pancreatic β cell mass and insulin secretion in mice. *J. Clin. Investig.* **2012**, *122*, 4105–4117. [CrossRef] [PubMed]

112. Lee, C.-H.; Olson, P.; Hevener, A.; Mehl, I.; Chong, L.-W.; Olefsky, J.M.; Gonzalez, F.J.; Ham, J.; Kang, H.; Peters, J.M.; et al. PPARδ regulates glucose metabolism and insulin sensitivity. *Proc. Natl. Acad. Sci. USA* **2006**, *103*, 3444–3449. [CrossRef] [PubMed]

113. Tanaka, T.; Yamamoto, J.; Iwasaki, S.; Asaba, H.; Hamura, H.; Ikeda, Y.; Watanabe, M.; Magoori, K.; Ioka, R.X.; Tachibana, K.; et al. Activation of peroxisome proliferator-activated receptor δ induces fatty acid β-oxidation in skeletal muscle and attenuates metabolic syndrome. *Proc. Natl. Acad. Sci. USA* **2003**, *100*, 15924–15929. [CrossRef] [PubMed]

114. Smale, S.T.; Natoli, G. Transcriptional Control of Inflammatory Responses. *Cold Spring Harb. Perspect. Biol.* **2014**, *6*, a016261. [CrossRef]

115. Karin, M.; Yamamoto, Y.; Wang, Q.M. The IKK NF-κB system: A treasure trove for drug development. *Nat. Rev. Drug Discov.* **2004**, *3*, 17–26. [CrossRef]

116. Pena, A.D.; Leclercq, I.; Field, J.; George, J.; Jones, B.; Farrell, G. NF-κB Activation, Rather Than TNF, Mediates Hepatic Inflammation in a Murine Dietary Model of Steatohepatitis. *Gastroenterology* **2005**, *129*, 1663–1674. [CrossRef]

117. Ribeiro, P.S.; Cortez-Pinto, H.; Solá, S.; Castro, R.E.; Ramalho, R.; Baptista, A.; Moura, M.C.; Camilo, M.E.; Rodrigues, C.M.P.; Baptista, A. Hepatocyte Apoptosis, Expression of Death Receptors, and Activation of NF-κB in the Liver of Nonalcoholic and Alcoholic Steatohepatitis Patients. *Am. J. Gastroenterol.* **2004**, *99*, 1708–1717. [CrossRef]

118. Wang, X.-A.; Zhang, R.; Zhang, S.; Deng, S.; Jiang, D.; Zhong, J.; Yang, L.; Wang, T.; Hong, S.; Guo, S.; et al. Interferon regulatory factor 7 deficiency prevents diet-induced obesity and insulin resistance. *Am. J. Physiol. Metab.* **2013**, *305*, E485–E495. [CrossRef]

119. Iyer, S.; Upadhyay, P.K.; Majumdar, S.S.; Nagarajan, P. Animal Models Correlating Immune Cells for the Development of NAFLD/NASH. *J. Clin. Exp. Hepatol.* **2015**, *5*, 239–245. [CrossRef]

120. Ferreira, D.M.S.; Castro, R.E.; Machado, M.V.; Evangelista, T.; Silvestre, A.; Costa, A.; Coutinho, J.; Carepa, F.; Cortez-Pinto, H.; Rodrigues, C.M.P. Apoptosis and insulin resistance in liver and peripheral tissues of morbidly obese patients is associated with different stages of non-alcoholic fatty liver disease. *Diabetology* **2011**, *54*, 1788–1798. [CrossRef]

121. Schreck, I.; Al-Rawi, M.; Mingot, J.-M.; Scholl, C.; Diefenbacher, M.E.; O'Donnell, P.; Bohmann, D.; Weiss, C. c-Jun localizes to the nucleus independent of its phosphorylation by and interaction with JNK and vice versa promotes nuclear accumulation of JNK. *Biochem. Biophys. Res. Commun.* **2011**, *407*, 735–740. [CrossRef] [PubMed]

122. Bruno, T.; Iezzi, S.; De Nicola, F.; Di Padova, M.; DeSantis, A.; Scarsella, M.; Di Certo, M.G.; Leonetti, C.; Floridi, A.; Passananti, C.; et al. Che-1 activates XIAP expression in response to DNA damage. *Cell Death Differ.* **2007**, *15*, 515–520. [CrossRef]

123. DeSantis, A.; Bruno, T.; Catena, V.; De Nicola, F.; Goeman, F.; Iezzi, S.; Sorino, C.; Ponzoni, M.; Bossi, G.; Federico, V.; et al. Che-1-induced inhibition of mTOR pathway enables stress-induced autophagy. *EMBO J.* **2015**, *34*, 1214–1230. [CrossRef] [PubMed]

124. DeSantis, A.; Bruno, T.; Catena, V.; De Nicola, F.; Goeman, F.; Iezzi, S.; Sorino, C.; Gentileschi, M.P.; Germoni, S.; Monteleone, V.; et al. Che-1 modulates the decision between cell cycle arrest and apoptosis by its binding to p53. *Cell Death Dis.* **2015**, *6*, e1764. [CrossRef] [PubMed]

125. Zhang, K.; Wang, S.; Malhotra, J.; Hassler, J.R.; Back, S.H.; Wang, G.; Chang, L.; Xu, W.; Miao, H.; Leonardi, R.; et al. The unfolded protein response transducer IRE1α prevents ER stress-induced hepatic steatosis. *EMBO J.* **2011**, *30*, 1357–1375. [CrossRef] [PubMed]

126. Yuk, J.-M.; Shin, N.-M.; Lee, H.-M.; Kim, J.-J.; Kim, S.-W.; Jin, H.S.; Yang, C.-S.; Park, K.A.; Chanda, D.; Kim, N.-K.; et al. The orphan nuclear receptor SHP acts as a negative regulator in inflammatory signaling triggered by Toll-like receptors. *Nat. Immunol.* **2011**, *12*, 742–751. [CrossRef]

127. Yang, C.-S.; Kim, J.-J.; Kim, T.S.; Jo, E.-K.; Kim, S.Y.; Lee, H.-M.; Shin, N.-M.; Nguyen, L.T.; Lee, M.-S.; Jin, H.S.; et al. Small heterodimer partner interacts with NLRP3 and negatively regulates activation of the NLRP3 inflammasome. *Nat. Commun.* **2015**, *6*, 6115. [CrossRef] [PubMed]

128. Poli, V. The Role of C/EBP Isoforms in the Control of Inflammatory and Native Immunity Functions. *J. Biol. Chem.* **1998**, *273*, 29279–29282. [CrossRef]

129. Berghe, W.V.; Vermeulen, L.; Delerive, P.; De Bosscher, K.; Staels, B.; Haegeman, G. A Paradigm for Gene Regulation: Inflammation, NF-κB and PPAR. *Adv. Exp. Med. Biol.* **2003**, *544*, 181–196. [CrossRef]

130. Stienstra, R.; Mandard, S.; Patsouris, D.; Maass, C.; Kersten, S.; Muller, M. Peroxisome Proliferator-Activated Receptor α Protects against Obesity-Induced Hepatic Inflammation. *Endocrinology* **2007**, *148*, 2753–2763. [CrossRef]

131. Ricote, M.; Li, A.C.; Willson, T.M.; Kelly, C.J.; Glass, C.K. The peroxisome proliferator-activated receptor-γ is a negative regulator of macrophage activation. *Nature* **1998**, *391*, 79–82. [CrossRef] [PubMed]

132. Morán-Salvador, E.; Titos, E.; Rius, B.; González-Périz, A.; García-Alonso, V.; López-Vicario, C.; Miquel, R.; Barak, Y.; Arroyo, V.; Claria, J. Cell-specific PPARγ deficiency establishes anti-inflammatory and anti-fibrogenic properties for this nuclear receptor in non-parenchymal liver cells. *J. Hepatol.* **2013**, *59*, 1045–1053. [CrossRef]

133. Luo, W.; Xu, Q.; Wang, Q.; Wu, H.; Hua, J. Effect of modulation of PPAR-γ activity on Kupffer cells M1/M2 polarization in the development of non-alcoholic fatty liver disease. *Sci. Rep.* **2017**, *7*, 44612. [CrossRef] [PubMed]

134. Baskin-Bey, E.S.; Anan, A.; Isomoto, H.; Bronk, S.F.; Gores, G.J. Constitutive androstane receptor agonist, TCPOBOP, attenuates steatohepatitis in the methionine choline-deficient diet-fed mouse. *World J. Gastroenterol.* **2007**, *13*, 5635–5641. [CrossRef] [PubMed]

135. Yamazaki, Y.; Kakizaki, S.; Horiguchi, N.; Sohara, N.; Sato, K.; Takagi, H.; Mori, M.; Negishi, M. The role of the nuclear receptor constitutive androstane receptor in the pathogenesis of non-alcoholic steatohepatitis. *Gut* **2006**, *56*, 565–574. [CrossRef] [PubMed]

136. Venteclef, N.; Jakobsson, T.; Ehrlund, A.; Damdimopoulos, A.; Mikkonen, L.; Ellis, E.; Nilsson, L.-M.; Parini, P.; Jänne, O.A.; Gustafsson, J.-Å.; et al. GPS2-dependent corepressor/SUMO pathways govern anti-inflammatory actions of LRH-1 and LXRβ in the hepatic acute phase response. *Genes Dev.* **2010**, *24*, 381–395. [CrossRef]

137. Griffett, K.; Solt, L.A.; Elgendy, B.; Kamenecka, T.M.; Burris, T.P. A Liver-Selective LXR Inverse Agonist That Suppresses Hepatic Steatosis. *ACS Chem. Biol.* **2012**, *8*, 559–567. [CrossRef]

138. Griffett, K.; Welch, R.D.; Flaveny, C.A.; Kolar, G.R.; Neuschwander-Tetri, B.A.; Burris, T.P. The LXR inverse agonist SR9238 suppresses fibrosis in a model of non-alcoholic steatohepatitis. *Mol. Metab.* **2015**, *4*, 353–357. [CrossRef]

139. Kim, K.H.; Lee, M.-S. Pathogenesis of Nonalcoholic Steatohepatitis and Hormone-Based Therapeutic Approaches. *Front. Endocrinol.* **2018**, *9*, 485. [CrossRef]

140. Xu, D.; Xu, M.; Jeong, S.; Qian, Y.; Wu, H.; Xia, Q.; Kong, X. The Role of Nrf2 in Liver Disease: Novel Molecular Mechanisms and Therapeutic Approaches. *Front. Pharmacol.* **2019**, *9*, 9. [CrossRef]

141. Lee, J.; Sun, C.; Zhou, Y.; Lee, J.; Gökalp, D.; Herrema, H.; Park, S.W.; Davis, R.J.; Ozcan, U. p38 MAPK-mediated regulation of Xbp1s is crucial for glucose homeostasis. *Nat. Med.* **2011**, *17*, 1251–1260. [CrossRef] [PubMed]

142. Herrema, H.; Zhou, Y.; Zhang, D.; Lee, J.; Hernandez, M.A.S.; Shulman, G.I.; Ozcan, U. XBP1s Is an Anti-lipogenic Protein. *J. Biol. Chem.* **2016**, *291*, 17394–17404. [CrossRef] [PubMed]

143. Liu, X.; Henkel, A.S.; Lecuyer, B.E.; Schipma, M.J.; Anderson, K.A.; Green, R.M. Hepatocyte X-box binding protein 1 deficiency increases liver injury in mice fed a high-fat/sugar diet. *Am. J. Physiol. Liver Physiol.* **2015**, *309*, G965–G974. [CrossRef] [PubMed]

144. Xiao, G.; Zhang, T.; Yu, S.; Lee, S.; Calabuig-Navarro, V.; Yamauchi, J.; Ringquist, S.; Dong, H.H. ATF4 Protein Deficiency Protects against High Fructose-induced Hypertriglyceridemia in Mice*. *J. Biol. Chem.* **2013**, *288*, 25350–25361. [CrossRef]

145. Chen, X.; Zhang, F.; Gong, Q.; Cui, A.; Zhuo, S.; Hu, Z.; Han, Y.; Gao, J.; Sun, Y.; Liu, Z.; et al. Hepatic ATF6 Increases Fatty Acid Oxidation to Attenuate Hepatic Steatosis in Mice through Peroxisome Proliferator-Activated Receptor Alpha. *Diabetes* **2016**, *65*, 1904–1915. [CrossRef]

146. Zeng, L.; Lu, M.; Mori, K.; Luo, S.; Lee, A.S.; Zhu, Y.; Shyy, J.Y.-J. ATF6 modulates SREBP2-mediated lipogenesis. *EMBO J.* **2004**, *23*, 950–958. [CrossRef]

147. Tang, W.; Jiang, Y.-F.; Ponnusamy, M.; Diallo, M. Role of Nrf2 in chronic liver disease. *World J. Gastroenterol.* **2014**, *20*, 13079–13087. [CrossRef]

148. Gupte, A.A.; Lyon, C.J.; Hsueh, W.A. Nuclear Factor (Erythroid-Derived 2)-Like-2 Factor (Nrf2), a Key Regulator of the Antioxidant Response to Protect Against Atherosclerosis and Nonalcoholic Steatohepatitis. *Curr. Diabetes Rep.* **2013**, *13*, 362–371. [CrossRef]

149. Sharma, R.S.; Harrison, D.J.; Kisielewski, D.; Cassidy, D.M.; McNeilly, A.D.; Gallagher, J.R.; Walsh, S.V.; Honda, T.; McCrimmon, R.J.; Dinkova-Kostova, A.T.; et al. Experimental Nonalcoholic Steatohepatitis and Liver Fibrosis Are Ameliorated by Pharmacologic Activation of Nrf2 (NF-E2 p45-Related Factor 2). *Cell. Mol. Gastroenterol. Hepatol.* **2017**, *5*, 367–398. [CrossRef]

150. Chowdhry, S.; Nazmy, M.H.; Meakin, P.J.; Dinkova-Kostova, A.T.; Walsh, S.V.; Tsujita, T.; Dillon, J.; Ashford, M.L.; Hayes, J. Loss of Nrf2 markedly exacerbates nonalcoholic steatohepatitis. *Free Radic. Biol. Med.* **2010**, *48*, 357–371. [CrossRef]

151. Liu, Z.; Dou, W.; Ni, Z.; Wen, Q.; Zhang, R.; Qin, M.; Wang, X.; Tang, H.; Cao, Y.; Wang, J.; et al. Deletion of Nrf2 leads to hepatic insulin resistance via the activation of NF-κB in mice fed a high-fat diet. *Mol. Med. Rep.* **2016**, *14*, 1323–1331. [CrossRef] [PubMed]

152. Woodcroft, K.J.; Hafner, M.S.; Novak, R.F. Insulin signaling in the transcriptional and posttranscriptional regulation of CYP2E1 expression. *Hepatology* **2002**, *35*, 263–273. [CrossRef] [PubMed]

153. Leung, T.-M.; Nieto, N. CYP2E1 and oxidant stress in alcoholic and non-alcoholic fatty liver disease. *J. Hepatol.* **2013**, *58*, 395–398. [CrossRef] [PubMed]

154. Kelicen, P.; Tindberg, N. Lipopolysaccharide Induces CYP2E1 in Astrocytes through MAP Kinase Kinase-3 and C/EBPbeta and -Delta. *J. Biol. Chem.* **2003**, *279*, 15734–15742. [CrossRef]

155. Daly, A.K. Relevance of CYP2E1 to Non-alcoholic Fatty Liver Disease. *Membr. Biog.* **2013**, *67*, 165–175. [CrossRef]

156. Svegliati-Baroni, G.; Pierantonelli, I.; Torquato, P.; Marinelli, R.; Ferreri, C.; Chatgilialoglu, C.; Bartolini, D.; Galli, F. Lipidomic biomarkers and mechanisms of lipotoxicity in non-alcoholic fatty liver disease. *Free Radic. Biol. Med.* **2019**, *144*, 293–309. [CrossRef]

157. Aubert, J.; Begriche, K.; Knockaert, L.; Robin, M.; Fromenty, B. Increased expression of cytochrome P450 2E1 in nonalcoholic fatty liver disease: Mechanisms and pathophysiological role. *Clin. Res. Hepatol. Gastroenterol.* **2011**, *35*, 630–637. [CrossRef]

158. Liu, S.-Y.; Gonzalez, F.J. Role of the Liver-Enriched Transcription Factor HNF-1α in Expression of theCYP2E1Gene. *DNA Cell Biol.* **1995**, *14*, 285–293. [CrossRef]

159. Jin, M.; Ande, A.; Kumar, A.; Kumar, S. Regulation of cytochrome P450 2e1 expression by ethanol: Role of oxidative stress-mediated pkc/jnk/sp1 pathway. *Cell Death Dis.* **2013**, *4*, e554. [CrossRef]

160. Tsuchida, T.; Friedman, S.L. Mechanisms of hepatic stellate cell activation. *Nat. Rev. Gastroenterol. Hepatol.* **2017**, *14*, 397–411. [CrossRef]

161. Koyama, Y.; Xu, J.; Liu, X.; Brenner, D.A. New Developments on the Treatment of Liver Fibrosis. *Dig. Dis.* **2016**, *34*, 589–596. [CrossRef]

162. Meng, X.-M.; Nikolic-Paterson, D.J.; Lan, H.-Y. TGF-β: The master regulator of fibrosis. *Nat. Rev. Nephrol.* **2016**, *12*, 325–338. [CrossRef] [PubMed]

163. Wobser, H.; Dorn, C.; Weiss, T.S.; Amann, T.; Bollheimer, C.; Büttner, R.; Schölmerich, J.; Hellerbrand, C. Lipid accumulation in hepatocytes induces fibrogenic activation of hepatic stellate cells. *Cell Res.* **2009**, *19*, 996–1005. [CrossRef] [PubMed]

164. Xu, P.; Liu, J.; Derynck, R. Post-translational regulation of TGF-β receptor and Smad signaling. *FEBS Lett.* **2012**, *586*, 1871–1884. [CrossRef]

165. Inoue, Y.; Itoh, Y.; Abe, K.; Okamoto, T.; Daitoku, H.; Fukamizu, A.; Onozaki, K.; Hayashi, H. Smad3 is acetylated by p300/CBP to regulate its transactivation activity. *Oncogene* **2006**, *26*, 500–508. [CrossRef] [PubMed]

166. Lim, J.-Y.; Oh, M.-A.; Kim, W.H.; Sohn, H.-Y.; Park, S.I. AMP-activated protein kinase inhibits TGF-?-induced fibrogenic responses of hepatic stellate cells by targeting transcriptional coactivator p300. *J. Cell. Physiol.* **2011**, *227*, 1081–1089. [CrossRef] [PubMed]

167. Liu, E.; Liu, Z.; Zhou, Y.; Chen, M.; Wang, L.; Li, J. MicroRNA-142-3p inhibits trophoblast cell migration and invasion by disrupting the TGF-β1/Smad3 signaling pathway. *Mol. Med. Rep.* **2019**, *19*, 3775–3782. [CrossRef]

168. Gerhard, G.S.; Hanson, A.; Wilhelmsen, D.; Piras, I.S.; Still, C.D.; Chu, X.; Petrick, A.T.; Distefano, J.K. AEBP1 expression increases with severity of fibrosis in NASH and is regulated by glucose, palmitate, and miR-372-3p. *PLoS ONE* **2019**, *14*, e0219764. [CrossRef]

169. Kim, S.-W.; Muise, A.M.; Lyons, P.J.; Ro, H.-S. Regulation of Adipogenesis by a Transcriptional Repressor That Modulates MAPK Activation. *J. Biol. Chem.* **2001**, *276*, 10199–10206. [CrossRef]

170. Jager, M.; Lee, M.-J.; Li, C.; Farmer, S.R.; Fried, S.K.; Layne, M.D. Aortic carboxypeptidase-like protein enhances adipose tissue stromal progenitor differentiation into myofibroblasts and is upregulated in fibrotic white adipose tissue. *PLoS ONE* **2018**, *13*, e0197777. [CrossRef]

171. Majdalawieh, A.; Zhang, L.; Fuki, I.V.; Rader, D.J.; Ro, H.-S. Adipocyte enhancer-binding protein 1 is a potential novel atherogenic factor involved in macrophage cholesterol homeostasis and inflammation. *Proc. Natl. Acad. Sci. USA* **2006**, *103*, 2346–2351. [CrossRef] [PubMed]

172. Lou, Y.; Chen, Y.-D.; Sun, F.-R.; Shi, J.-P.; Song, Y.; Yang, J. Potential Regulators Driving the Transition in Nonalcoholic Fatty Liver Disease: A Stage-Based View. *Cell. Physiol. Biochem.* **2017**, *41*, 239–251. [CrossRef] [PubMed]

173. Camargo, F.D.; Gokhale, S.; Johnnidis, J.B.; Fu, N.; Bell, G.W.; Jaenisch, R.; Brummelkamp, T.R. YAP1 Increases Organ Size and Expands Undifferentiated Progenitor Cells. *Curr. Biol.* **2007**, *17*, 2054–2060. [CrossRef] [PubMed]

174. Mooring, M.; Fowl, B.H.; Lum, S.Z.C.; Liu, Y.; Yao, K.; Softic, S.; Kirchner, R.; Bernstein, A.; Singhi, A.D.; Jay, D.G.; et al. Hepatocyte Stress Increases Expression of YAP and TAZ in Hepatocytes to Promote Parenchymal Inflammation and Fibrosis. *Hepatology* **2019**. [CrossRef]

175. Song, K.; Kwon, H.; Han, C.; Chen, W.; Zhang, J.; Ma, W.; Dash, S.; Gandhi, C.R.; Wu, T. YAP in Kupffer cells enhances the production of pro-inflammatory cytokines and promotes the development of non-alcoholic steatohepatitis. *Hepatology* **2019**. [CrossRef] [PubMed]

176. Abdelmegeed, M.A.; Yoo, S.-H.; Henderson, L.E.; Gonzalez, F.J.; Woodcroft, K.J.; Song, B.-J. PPARalpha expression protects male mice from high fat-induced nonalcoholic fatty liver. *J. Nutr.* **2011**, *141*, 603–610. [CrossRef]

177. Kawaguchi, K.; Sakaida, I.; Tsuchiya, M.; Omori, K.; Takami, T.; Okita, K. Pioglitazone prevents hepatic steatosis, fibrosis, and enzyme-altered lesions in rat liver cirrhosis induced by a choline-deficient l-amino acid-defined diet. *Biochem. Biophys. Res. Commun.* **2004**, *315*, 187–195. [CrossRef]

178. Leclercq, I.A.; Sempoux, C.; Stärkel, P.; Horsmans, Y. Limited therapeutic efficacy of pioglitazone on progression of hepatic fibrosis in rats. *Gut* **2006**, *55*, 1020–1029. [CrossRef]

179. Colca, J.R.; McDonald, W.G.; Cavey, G.S.; Cole, S.L.; Holewa, D.D.; Brightwell-Conrad, A.S.; Wolfe, C.L.; Wheeler, J.S.; Coulter, K.R.; Kilkuskie, P.M.; et al. Identification of a Mitochondrial Target of Thiazolidinedione Insulin Sensitizers (mTOT)—Relationship to Newly Identified Mitochondrial Pyruvate Carrier Proteins. *PLoS ONE* **2013**, *8*, e61551. [CrossRef]

180. McCommis, K.S.; Hodges, W.T.; Brunt, E.M.; Nalbantoglu, I.; McDonald, W.G.; Holley, C.; Fujiwara, H.; Schaffer, J.E.; Colca, J.; Finck, B.N. Targeting the mitochondrial pyruvate carrier attenuates fibrosis in a mouse model of nonalcoholic steatohepatitis. *Hepatology* **2017**, *65*, 1543–1556. [CrossRef]

181. Skat-Rørdam, J.; Ipsen, D.H.; Lykkesfeldt, J.; Tveden-Nyborg, P. A role of peroxisome proliferator-activated receptor γ in non-alcoholic fatty liver disease. *Basic Clin. Pharmacol. Toxicol.* **2019**, *124*, 528–537. [CrossRef] [PubMed]

182. Hattori, S.; Dhar, D.K.; Hara, N.; Tonomoto, Y.; Onoda, T.; Ono, T.; Yamanoi, A.; Tachibana, M.; Tsuchiya, M.; Nagasue, N. FR-167653, a selective p38 MAPK inhibitor, exerts salutary effect on liver cirrhosis through downregulation of Runx2. *Lab. Investig.* **2007**, *87*, 591–601. [CrossRef]

183. Cao, Z.; Sun, B.; Zhao, X.; Zhang, Y.; Gu, Q.; Liang, X.; Dong, X.; Zhao, N. The Expression and Functional Significance of Runx2 in Hepatocellular Carcinoma: Its Role in Vasculogenic Mimicry and Epithelial–Mesenchymal Transition. *Int. J. Mol. Sci.* **2017**, *18*, 500. [CrossRef] [PubMed]

184. Sahai, A.; Malladi, P.; Melin-Aldana, H.; Green, R.M.; Whitington, P.F. Upregulation of osteopontin expression is involved in the development of nonalcoholic steatohepatitis in a dietary murine model. *Am. J. Physiol. Liver Physiol.* **2004**, *287*, G264–G273. [CrossRef]

185. Kolodziejczyk, A.A.; Zheng, D.; Shibolet, O.; Elinav, E. The role of the microbiome in NAFLD and NASH. *EMBO Mol. Med.* **2018**, *11*, e9302. [CrossRef] [PubMed]

186. Bäckhed, F.; Ding, H.; Wang, T.; Hooper, L.V.; Koh, G.Y.; Nagy, A.; Semenkovich, C.F.; Gordon, J.I. The gut microbiota as an environmental factor that regulates fat storage. *Proc. Natl. Acad. Sci. USA* **2004**, *101*, 15718–15723. [CrossRef] [PubMed]

187. Zeng, H.; Liu, J.; Jackson, M.I.; Zhao, F.-Q.; Yan, L.; Combs, G.F. Fatty liver accompanies an increase in lactobacillus species in the hind gut of C57BL/6 mice fed a high-fat diet. *J. Nutr.* **2013**, *143*, 627–631. [CrossRef] [PubMed]

188. Wang, R.; Li, H.; Yang, X.; Xue, X.; Deng, L.; Shen, J.; Zhang, M.; Zhao, L.; Zhang, C. Genetically Obese Human Gut Microbiota Induces Liver Steatosis in Germ-Free Mice Fed on Normal Diet. *Front. Microbiol.* **2018**, *9*. [CrossRef]

189. Chiu, C.-C.; Ching, Y.-H.; Li, Y.-P.; Liu, J.-Y.; Huang, Y.-T.; Huang, Y.-W.; Yang, S.-S.; Huang, W.-C.; Chuang, H.-L. Nonalcoholic Fatty Liver Disease Is Exacerbated in High-Fat Diet-Fed Gnotobiotic Mice by Colonization with the Gut Microbiota from Patients with Nonalcoholic Steatohepatitis. *Nutrients* **2017**, *9*, 1220. [CrossRef]

190. Lambert, J.E.; Parnell, J.A.; Eksteen, B.; Raman, M.; Bomhof, M.R.; Rioux, K.P.; Madsen, K.L.; Reimer, R.A. Gut microbiota manipulation with prebiotics in patients with non-alcoholic fatty liver disease: A randomized controlled trial protocol. *BMC Gastroenterol.* **2015**, *15*, 169. [CrossRef]

191. Perumpail, B.J.; Li, A.A.; John, N.; Sallam, S.; Shah, N.D.; Kwong, W.; Cholankeril, G.; Kim, D.; Ahmed, A. The Therapeutic Implications of the Gut Microbiome and Probiotics in Patients with NAFLD. *Diseases* **2019**, *7*, 27. [CrossRef]

192. Cheng, Y.-W.; Phelps, E.; Ganapini, V.; Khan, N.; Ouyang, F.; Xu, H.; Khanna, S.; Tariq, R.; Friedman-Moraco, R.J.; Woodworth, M.H.; et al. Fecal microbiota transplantation for the treatment of recurrent and severe Clostridium difficileinfection in solid organ transplant recipients: A multicenter experience. *Arab. Archaeol. Epigr.* **2018**, *19*, 501–511. [CrossRef]

193. Aron-Wisnewsky, J.; Gaborit, B.; Dutour, A.; Clément, K. Gut microbiota and non-alcoholic fatty liver disease: New insights. *Clin. Microbiol. Infect.* **2013**, *19*, 338–348. [CrossRef] [PubMed]

194. Arab, J.P.; Karpen, S.J.; Dawson, P.A.; Arrese, M.; Trauner, M. Bile acids and nonalcoholic fatty liver disease: Molecular insights and therapeutic perspectives. *Hepatology* **2016**, *65*, 350–362. [CrossRef] [PubMed]

195. Cruz-Ramón, V.; Chinchilla-López, P.; Ramírez-Pérez, O.; Méndez-Sánchez, N. Bile Acids in Nonalcoholic Fatty Liver Disease: New Concepts and Therapeutic Advances. *Ann. Hepatol.* **2017**, *16*, S58–S67. [CrossRef]

196. Chiang, J.Y. Bile acid metabolism and signaling in liver disease and therapy. *Liver Res.* **2017**, *1*, 3–9. [CrossRef]

197. Leung, C.; Rivera, L.; Furness, J.B.; Angus, P.W. The role of the gut microbiota in NAFLD. *Nat. Rev. Gastroenterol. Hepatol.* **2016**, *13*, 412–425. [CrossRef]

198. Wang, L.; Wan, Y.-J.Y. The role of gut microbiota in liver disease development and treatment. *Liver Res.* **2019**, *3*, 3–18. [CrossRef]

199. Jones, B.V.; Begley, M.; Hill, C.; Gahan, C.G.; Marchesi, J.R. Functional and comparative metagenomic analysis of bile salt hydrolase activity in the human gut microbiome. *Proc. Natl. Acad. Sci. USA* **2008**, *105*, 13580–13585. [CrossRef]

200. Xie, C.; Jiang, C.; Shi, J.; Gao, X.; Sun, D.; Sun, L.; Wang, T.; Takahashi, S.; Anitha, M.; Krausz, K.W.; et al. An Intestinal Farnesoid X Receptor–Ceramide Signaling Axis Modulates Hepatic Gluconeogenesis in Mice. *Diabetes* **2016**, *66*, 613–626. [CrossRef]

201. Jiang, C.; Xie, C.; Li, F.; Zhang, L.; Nichols, R.G.; Krausz, K.W.; Cai, J.; Qi, Y.; Fang, Z.-Z.; Takahashi, S.; et al. Intestinal farnesoid X receptor signaling promotes nonalcoholic fatty liver disease. *J. Clin. Investig.* **2014**, *125*, 386–402. [CrossRef] [PubMed]

202. Gao, Z.; Yin, J.; Zhang, J.; Ward, R.E.; Martin, R.J.; Lefevre, M.; Cefalu, W.T.; Ye, J. Butyrate Improves Insulin Sensitivity and Increases Energy Expenditure in Mice. *Diabetes* **2009**, *58*, 1509–1517. [CrossRef] [PubMed]

203. Besten, G.D.; Van Eunen, K.; Groen, A.K.; Venema, K.; Reijngoud, D.-J.; Bakker, B.M. The role of short-chain fatty acids in the interplay between diet, gut microbiota, and host energy metabolism. *J. Lipid Res.* **2013**, *54*, 2325–2340. [CrossRef] [PubMed]

204. Liu, S.; Gallo, D.J.; Green, A.M.; Williams, D.L.; Gong, X.; Shapiro, R.A.; Gambotto, A.A.; Humphris-Narayanan, E.; Vodovotz, Y.; Billiar, T.R. Role of Toll-Like Receptors in Changes in Gene Expression and NF-κB Activation in Mouse Hepatocytes Stimulated with Lipopolysaccharide. *Infect. Immun.* **2002**, *70*, 3433–3442. [CrossRef] [PubMed]

205. Hoang, S.A.; Oseini, A.; Feaver, R.E.; Cole, B.K.; Asgharpour, A.; Vincent, R.; Siddiqui, M.S.; Lawson, M.J.; Day, N.; Taylor, J.; et al. Gene Expression Predicts Histological Severity and Reveals Distinct Molecular Profiles of Nonalcoholic Fatty Liver Disease. *Sci. Rep.* **2019**, *9*, 12541. [CrossRef] [PubMed]

206. Arendt, B.M.; Comelli, E.M.; Ma, D.W.; Lou, W.; Teterina, A.; Kim, T.; Fung, S.K.; Wong, D.K.; McGilvray, I.D.; Fischer, S.E.; et al. Altered hepatic gene expression in nonalcoholic fatty liver disease is associated with lower hepatic n-3 and n-6 polyunsaturated fatty acids. *Hepatology* **2015**, *61*, 1565–1578. [CrossRef]

207. Cichocki, J.A.; Furuya, S.; Konganti, K.; Luo, Y.-S.; McDonald, T.J.; Iwata, Y.; Chiu, W.A.; Threadgill, D.W.; Pogribny, I.P.; Rusyn, I. Impact of Nonalcoholic Fatty Liver Disease on Toxicokinetics of Tetrachloroethylene in Mice. *J. Pharmacol. Exp. Ther.* **2017**, *361*, 17–28. [CrossRef]

208. Maeso-Diaz, R.; Boyer-Diaz, Z.; Lozano, J.J.; Ortega-Ribera, M.; Peralta, C.; Bosch, J.; Gracia-Sancho, J. New rat model of advanced nash mimicking pathophysiological features and transcriptomic signature of the human disease. *Cells* **2019**, *8*, 1062. [CrossRef]

209. Qin, G.; Wang, G.Z.; Guo, D.D.; Bai, R.-X.; Wang, M.; Du, S.Y. Deletion of *Smad4* reduces hepatic inflammation and fibrogenesis during nonalcoholic steatohepatitis progression. *J. Dig. Dis.* **2018**, *19*, 301–313. [CrossRef]

210. Valenti, L.; Mendoza, R.M.; Rametta, R.; Maggioni, M.; Kitajewski, C.; Shawber, C.J.; Pajvani, U.B. Hepatic notch signaling correlates with insulin resistance and nonalcoholic fatty liver disease. *Diabetes* **2013**, *62*, 4052–4062. [CrossRef]

211. Liang, N.; Damdimopoulos, A.; Goni, S.; Huang, Z.; Vedin, L.L.; Jakobsson, T.; Giudici, M.; Ahmed, O.; Pedrelli, M.; Barilla, S.; et al. Hepatocyte-specific loss of GPS2 in mice reduces non-alcoholic steatohepatitis via activation of PPARα. *Nat. Commun.* **2019**, *10*, 1684. [CrossRef] [PubMed]

212. Porteiro, B.; Fondevila, M.F.; Delgado, T.C.; Iglesias, C.; Imbernon, M.; Iruzubieta, P.; Crespo, J.; Zabala-Letona, A.; Ferno, J.; Gonzalez-Teran, B.; et al. Hepatic p63 regulates steatosis via IKKβ/ER stress. *Nat. Commun.* **2017**, *8*, 15111. [CrossRef] [PubMed]

213. Li, Z.; Yu, P.; Wu, J.; Tao, F.; Zhou, J. Transcriptional regulation of early growth response gene-1 (EGR1) is associated with progression of nonalcoholic fatty liver disease (NAFLD) in patients with insulin resistance. *Med. Sci. Monit.* **2019**, *25*, 2293–3004. [CrossRef] [PubMed]

214. Cheng, C.; Deng, X.; Xu, K. Increased expression of sterol regulatory element binding protein-2 alleviates autophagic dysfunction in NAFLD. *Int. J. Mol. Med.* **2018**, *41*, 1877–1886. [CrossRef]

215. Kabbani, M.; Michailidis, E.; Steensels, S.; Zou, C.H.; Zeck, B.; Inna, R.L.; Fulmer, C.G.; Quirk, C.; Ashbrook, A.W.; Belkaya, S.; et al. PNPLA3-148M Overexpression in primary human hepatocytes exacerbates steatosis in tissue culture and chimeric mouse models of NAFLD. *Hepatology* **2019**, *70*, 1325A–1326A.

4

Metabolomic and Lipidomic Biomarkers for Premalignant Liver Disease Diagnosis and Therapy

Diren Beyoğlu and Jeffrey R. Idle *

Arthur G. Zupko's Division of Systems Pharmacology and Pharmacogenomics, Arnold & Marie Schwartz College of Pharmacy and Health Sciences, Long Island University, 75 Dekalb Avenue, Brooklyn, NY 11201, USA; diren.beyoglu@liu.edu

* Correspondence: jeff.idle@liu.edu

Abstract: In recent years, there has been a plethora of attempts to discover biomarkers that are more reliable than α-fetoprotein for the early prediction and prognosis of hepatocellular carcinoma (HCC). Efforts have involved such fields as genomics, transcriptomics, epigenetics, microRNA, exosomes, proteomics, glycoproteomics, and metabolomics. HCC arises against a background of inflammation, steatosis, and cirrhosis, due mainly to hepatic insults caused by alcohol abuse, hepatitis B and C virus infection, adiposity, and diabetes. Metabolomics offers an opportunity, without recourse to liver biopsy, to discover biomarkers for premalignant liver disease, thereby alerting the potential of impending HCC. We have reviewed metabolomic studies in alcoholic liver disease (ALD), cholestasis, fibrosis, cirrhosis, nonalcoholic fatty liver (NAFL), and nonalcoholic steatohepatitis (NASH). Specificity was our major criterion in proposing clinical evaluation of indole-3-lactic acid, phenyllactic acid, N-lauroylglycine, decatrienoate, N-acetyltaurine for ALD, urinary sulfated bile acids for cholestasis, cervonoyl ethanolamide for fibrosis, 16α-hydroxyestrone for cirrhosis, and the pattern of acyl carnitines for NAFL and NASH. These examples derive from a large body of published metabolomic observations in various liver diseases in adults, adolescents, and children, together with animal models. Many other options have been tabulated. Metabolomic biomarkers for premalignant liver disease may help reduce the incidence of HCC.

Keywords: metabolomics; lipidomics; biomarker; premalignant; alcoholic liver disease; cholestasis; fibrosis; cirrhosis; NAFL; NASH

---

1. The Need for Biomarkers of Premalignant Liver Disease

Hepatocellular carcinoma (HCC) and intrahepatic cholangiocarcinoma (ICC) are the commonest types of primary liver cancer, and their combined incidence ranks among the highest cancer rates in the world [1]. HCC in particular is a major health problem, with an annual death rate in excess of 500,000 worldwide [2]. HCC in the United States, which comprises 75% of all primary liver cancers [3], has been attributed primarily to a number of infectious and lifestyle causes. The principal attributable factors among these are alcohol (32.0% in males, 30.7% in females), adiposity (26.6% in males, 15.6% in females), hepatitis C virus (HCV) infection (17.5% overall), smoking (9.0% in males, 8.0% in females), diabetes (6.9% in males, 5.5% in females), and hepatitis B virus (HBV) infection (5.3% overall). In contrast, in China, HBV (53.8% overall) is the principal cause, with adiposity a relatively minor contributor (7.2% in males, 4.2% in females) [4]. These causative factors produce insults to the liver that include inflammation, steatosis, and fibrosis, all of which can progress through various stages, in particular cirrhosis, that can eventually lead to HCC. In recent years, there have been multiple attempts to develop predictive biomarkers of HCC, but many of these have involved the study of HCC cases themselves. Understanding the progression from hepatic insult through premalignant stages to HCC would seem to be the most fruitful means of predicting the development of HCC in susceptible individuals. In this review, we examine the investigations into key premalignant stages of HCC and ICC that have employed metabolomics both in patients and in animal models. In particular, we have focused on the metabolomics of alcoholic liver disease (ALD), cholestasis, fibrosis, cirrhosis, nonalcoholic fatty liver (steatosis, NAFL), and nonalcoholic steatohepatitis (NASH). In each case, we evaluated whether the experimental data provide sufficient grounds, especially in terms of specificity, to warrant further development of clinical biomarkers of hepatic premalignancy. Additionally, we considered only metabolites that were upregulated as potential biomarkers for the aforementioned premalignant liver diseases. The references cited in this review were culled from PubMed searches with keywords metabolomics OR metabonomics AND the various disease entities, such as alcoholic liver disease. Some references also arose from the bibliographies cited by publications found in these initial searches.

2. Hepatic Metabolism

The human body comprises around 34 trillion cells of which ca. 240 billion (0.7%) make up the approximately 1.5 kg of healthy liver, the largest solid organ and the biggest gland in the body. Of the roughly 20,000 human protein-coding genes, 60% are transcribed in the liver, many of which are not expressed in any other tissue [5]. Studies in mice using single cell transcriptomics revealed that about half of all hepatocyte genes were expressed in a zonal manner, supporting the concept that different liver regions have diverse metabolic functions. This was interpreted as being due to variable microenvironments attributable to gradients of oxygen, nutrients, and hormones [6]. Metabolic reactions that are specific to the liver include de novo synthesis and secretion of the primary bile acids glycocholate, taurocholate, glycochenodeoxycholate, and taurochenodeoxycholate, together with ornithine degradation. Overall, the liver is the most metabolically-active tissue, followed by adipose tissue and skeletal muscle [5]. Parenchymal hepatocytes comprise up to 85% of the liver volume, with sinusoidal endothelial cells, perisinusoidal stellate cells and phagocytic Kupffer cells, with intrahepatic lymphocytes making up the rest. Strong evidence suggests that different hepatic cell types possess variable gene expression profiles [6–8]. The liver is therefore highly heterogeneous in both gene expression and metabolic function. Assignment of metabolic function to discrete hepatic regions based upon in vivo observations alone is extremely challenging, since metabolic phenotypes vary between cell types and also across the liver. The role of in vitro studies in this regard will be increasingly important as aids to the interpretation of in vivo metabolic phenotyping. For example, laser capture microdissection has been employed as an adjunct to genomic, transcriptomic, and proteomic analyses of liver diseases [9], but so far, rarely for metabolic profiling of liver tissue.

3. Metabolomics—The What, the How, and the Why

It is two decades since Jeremy Nicholson and colleagues introduced the concept of metabonomics, with the promise of biomarker discovery from changes in metabolite profiles that result from constitutional differences such as disease or genetics or from exogenous challenges due to drug administration or exposure to toxicants [10]. The initial protocols based upon high-resolution proton nuclear magnetic resonance spectroscopy (^{1}H NMR) of body fluids have been supplemented by an array of additional technologies, based mostly on mass spectrometry (MS), which have infiltrated virtually every branch of biology and medicine. The literature currently stands at virtually 30,000 PubMed citations with almost 6000 in 2019 alone. The identification and quantitation of all metabolites in a given organism or biofluid was at first seen as a realistic goal [11]. However, as the biochemical complexity and analytical shortcomings came more into focus, global metabolite quantitation was abandoned, and more realistic definitions emerged, such as, "metabolomics studies the low molecular weight metabolites [e.g., <1.5 kDa] found in cells and organisms, usually through the analysis of plasma/serum, urine or cell culture medium using mainly MS or NMR technologies" [12]. There has also been some confusion regarding the use of the terms "metabolomics" and "metabonomics." Although it has been stated that the difference in terms is not a technical one, and that the terminologies are often used interchangeably [13], almost without exception, metabonomics published reports were conducted using NMR rather than MS. Other commonly-used phrases include untargeted and targeted metabolic phenotyping. Untargeted metabolomics is commonly conducted by first separating the biological analytes that have a large range of physicochemical properties using ultraperformance liquid chromatography (UPLC) with either reversed phase (RP) and/or hydrophobic interaction chromatography (HILIC) columns [14]. Interfaced by electrospray ionization (ESI) in either positive (ESI+) and/or negative (ESI-) mode, the UPLC eluate is analyzed by quadrupole time-of-flight mass spectrometry (QTOFMS). This may yield in excess of 5000 ions in each ionization mode, which should not be interpreted as 5000 biological constituents, as many of these features correspond to adducts, dimers, multiply charged species, and fragment ions formed in the electrosprayer. In targeted metabolomics, specific metabolites, for example amino acids or acyl carnitines, are quantitated using stable isotope labeled standards [15]. This is frequently conducted using tandem mass spectrometry, often with a triple quadrupole mass spectrometer (TQMS), rather than a QTOFMS. Another common technology used in metabolomics is gas chromatography-mass spectrometry (GC-MS). This has the benefit of a high confidence in metabolite identification, albeit for a small number of metabolites and a lower throughput than UPLC-QTOFMS. The technologies available for metabolomic analysis have recently been reviewed in detail [16].

In a typical metabolomics experiment, two or more groups of samples are investigated. These could be biofluids from a patient group and age- and sex-matched healthy controls, genetically-modified mice and their wild-type (WT) controls, and persons or experimental animals that have been administered a drug, specific diet, or with some other lifestyle variable (e.g. smoking or particular occupation), compared with a suitable control group. Analysis of the biofluids, usually urine and/or serum/plasma, by MS- or NMR-based methods produces a data table that must first be preprocessed (normalization, scaling, peak picking) prior to multivariate data analysis (MDA). It is first prudent to conduct unsupervised MDA, for example, with principal components analysis (PCA), which reveals the internal structure of the dataset, the principal components of variance, and the existence of any outliers. A number of presentations of the data are common, including the scores plot (with one data point for each sample) and the loadings plot, which for MS methods show the ions responsible for the distribution of samples in the scores plot. If each sample group analyzed clusters and separates from the other group(s), then this leads to supervised analyses such as partial least squares-discriminant analysis (PLS-DA) and orthogonal PLS-DA (OPLS-DA). Unless at least a partial separation of scores was observed in the PCA analysis, there is a danger that the data could be overmodeled using these supervised analyses. The literature is replete with examples of this. The generated loadings plots can be used with various software packages that assist in the identification of metabolites that differ significantly between the test groups. The reader is directed to specific reviews in this area [17–19].

Various estimates of distinct human metabolomes have been reported that were derived using multiple analytical platforms to gain maximum metabolite coverage. The human cerebrospinal fluid metabolome (308 metabolites) [20], the human serum metabolome (4229 "highly probable" metabolites) [21], the human urine metabolome (2651 "confirmed" metabolites) [22], and the human fecal metabolome (>6000 identified metabolites) [23] have all been described. The culmination of these efforts is the human metabolome database (HMDB 4.0) that comprises 114,100 total metabolites that encompass "the complete collection of small molecules found in the human body including peptides, lipids, amino acids, nucleic acids, carbohydrates, organic acids, biogenic amines, vitamins, minerals, food additives, drugs, cosmetics, contaminants, pollutants, and just about any other chemical that humans ingest, metabolize, catabolize or come into contact with" [24]. This still may be the tip of the iceberg. It has been estimated that humans are probably exposed to some 1–3 million discrete chemicals in their lifetimes [11] of which >25,000 have already been described in the diet [25].

The lipidome refers to the total number of lipid species present in a cell, tissue, organ, organism, or biofluid such as plasma. Although there is overlap with the human metabolome, the human lipidome is expected to be highly complex due in great part to the varying chain lengths and degrees of unsaturation, together with structural isomerism. As of January 2018, there were more than 40,000 lipid structures listed in the LIPID MAPS database [26]. Our conservative estimate is that the human lipidome is made up of at least 100,000 discrete lipid entities.

Based on the foregoing evidence, it is likely that a human metabolome that includes the lipidome may have some 200,000 members. As stated above, there are thought to be ~20,000 protein coding human genes, although the exact number is yet to be determined. The total number of cellular proteins (proteome) may be 16,000–17,000, similar to the total number of mRNA transcripts (transcriptome) obtained by untargeted RNA sequencing (RNA-seq) [27]. In addition, the existence of a human core proteome of 10,000–12,000 ubiquitously expressed proteins has been postulated, whose primary function is the general control and maintenance of cells [28]. Many of these are enzymes, and therefore contribute to the human metabolome, either through the metabolism of a single specific metabolite or pair of metabolites, such as lactate dehydrogenase or in a pleiotropic fashion, such as the thousands of potential metabolites produced by the human cytochromes P450 [29]. Nevertheless, it has been estimated that there are 1–2 million "protein entities" that are expressed in a cell at a given time as a result of posttranslational modifications (PTMs), such as acetylation, phosphorylation, and glycosylation [30]. To study mechanisms of liver disease through the lens of untargeted proteomics would be an extremely demanding task. However, targeted proteomics in the form of specific protein biomarkers in plasma or serum has a long history. This is because of the availability of commercial antibodies against virtually every protein and this forms the basis of convenient quantitative immunoassays such as ELISA.

The expression of phenotypes, including metabolic phenotypes, from a genomic sequence that is transcribed, spliced, and translated to protein with potential post-translational modifications, is analogous to the information flow involved when listening to a music compact disk or some other digital music format. In the former case, the genome is analogous to the compact disk itself, which without the apparatus for converting it to sound, is simply a digital storage system (Figure 1). This is why the metabolic phenotype is more revealing of the status of a cell, tissue, or organism than a genetic sequence, because it more resembles the musical experience rather than analyzing the so-called pits and lands (Figure 1) on a CD.

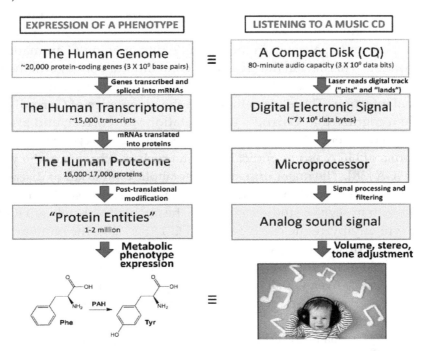

Figure 1. The flow of genetic information vs. digital music data flow.

In terms of generating new knowledge regarding the liver, metabolomics has for some years offered this opportunity. Because the liver is the seat of much of the body's metabolic processes, the systemic measurement of metabolites that originate in the liver should provide clear signposts to liver wellbeing or disease. This alone justifies the inclusion of metabolomic protocols in the study of hepatic pathogenesis. As we will demonstrate below, a plethora of such studies has already been reported, but the picture is still not in focus. We will seek to highlight the potential biomarkers that can be determined through metabolomics and that point most directly to disease mechanisms. We will discuss below the shortcomings of the current trend of identifying metabolomic biomarkers as risk factors for liver disease.

4. Biomarkers—The Good, the Bad, and the Ugly

A biomarker has been characterized as "a defined characteristic that is measured as an indicator of normal biological processes, pathogenic processes, or responses to an exposure or intervention, including therapeutic interventions." It has also been emphasized that biomarkers can be medical measurements, including physiological measurements, blood tests, molecular analyses of biopsies, genetic or metabolic data, and measurements from images [31]. Blood pressure and blood glucose are commonly determined biomarkers of both pathogenic processes and therapeutic interventions. Neither of these biomarkers point to mechanisms of either disease or therapeutic response. Measurement of the pressure of various parts of the arterial circulation was initiated in the mid-18th century by the English clergyman Stephen Hales [32]. The testing of the color, smell, and taste of urine as indicators of disease goes back at least as far as the ancient Greeks, with diagnostic 'urine charts' dating from the Middle Ages [13]. Determination of blood glucose developed relatively recently and as a substitute to urine taste as a diagnostic biomarker for diabetes [33].

The first metabolic biomarkers that indicated disease mechanisms are contained in the remarkable work of Sir Archibald Garrod (1857–1936) who coined the phrases "inborn errors of metabolism" [34] and "chemical individuality" [35] in the early part of the 20th century. Garrod contended that four diseases, i.e., alkaptonuria, albinism, cystinuria, and pentosuria, were Mendelian autosomal recessive traits, therefore pointing to genetic mechanisms for each. Moreover, he recognized that increased urinary homogentisic acid (HGA; known then as "alkapton acid") in newborn babies with alkaptonuria that stained their diapers black could be further increased by the oral administration of tyrosine or a diet rich in proteins containing aromatic amino acids such as tyrosine and phenylalanine [36]. This led Garrod to propose an impairment in the aromatic ring opening of aromatic amino acids as the mechanism of alkaptonuria. This flew in the face of the contemporaneous "germ theory of disease" that focused on external rather than inborn causes of disease, and maintained that alkaptonuria resulted from a gastrointestinal infection. These ideas hindered the acceptance of Garrod's concepts for many years [37]. Today, we recognize that Garrod's interpretation was correct, and also that mutations in the *HGO* gene causing a deficiency in hepatic homogentisate 1,2-dioxygenase (EC 1.13.11.5) activity result in an accumulation of HGA and its clinical sequelae such as ochronosis, the yellowish staining of connective tissue by HGA [38]. The major impact of a metabolic biomarker of disease (HGA) is that the mechanism when unmasked can lead to potential therapies of the disease. In the case of alkaptonuria, nitisinone has been shown in several studies to reduce the circulating levels of HGA. Nitisinone is an inhibitor of 4-hydroxyphenylpyruvate dioxygenase (EC 1.13.11.27), the enzyme responsible for the formation of HGA. A daily dose of 2 mg slowed progression of alkaptonuria and arrested ocular and ear ochronosis [39]. This old example of alkaptonuria is a clear-cut prototype for a metabolic biomarker of disease that originates in the liver, which has led to both an understanding of the disease mechanism and its potential treatment. Sadly, many recent examples of liver disease metabolic biomarkers have not lived up to this paradigm.

Alpha-fetoprotein (AFP) was reported in 1956 to be in human fetal serum but not in the serum of healthy adults. The production of AFP by fetal liver largely ceases before birth [40]. The discovery a few years later of AFP in animal models with hepatocellular carcinoma (HCC) [41] led to clinical investigations that associated AFP with HCC. It has been stated that ~70% HCC secrete AFP [42] and up to 40% of HCC patients may not show elevated serum AFP [43]. This suboptimal sensitivity is coupled with specificity issues in relation to premalignant liver diseases such as hepatitis and cirrhosis, together with ovarian and testicular malignancies. Therefore, the clinical interpretation of serum AFP with respect to HCC requires care. Nevertheless, serum AFP is widely used as both a diagnostic and prognostic biomarker for HCC [42–44]. In these regards, it is recognized that it should be replaced with more specific and sensitive biomarkers [43,44]. Neither European nor American guidelines for HCC screening include serum AFP concentration [45].

Although osteopontin (OPN), a protein normally expressed in kidney and bone, has a high sensitivity for the detection of HCC, its elevation can be linked to more than 30 types of cancer [45] and to many other diseases, including diseases of the liver [46]. Its employment as a HCC risk biomarker is clearly inappropriate. We will examine below whether metabolomics can disclose liver disease biomarkers with high sensitivity and especially with high specificity.

Of the biomarkers for liver disease discussed above, the determination of metabolite HGA to diagnose the rare inborn error of metabolism alkaptonuria is by far the most sensitive and specific. Studies in experimental animals in the 1950s suggested that homogentisate 1,2-dioxygenase was expressed in liver, to a lesser extent in kidney, and with little enzyme activity reported for heart, skeletal muscle, brain, intestine, spleen, and blood [47]. Contemporary biochemical and molecular methodologies have recently revealed that homogentisate 1,2-dioxygenase is expressed in human and mouse brain, explaining the various observations of brain pigmentation found in cases of alkaptonuria [48]. Both AFP and OPN are compromised by insufficient specificity, which would require them to be used in combination with other biomarkers for liver disease risk.

5. Biomarkers of Premalignant Liver Disease

5.1. Alcoholic Liver Disease (ALD)

Excessive alcohol consumption is a global healthcare problem that accounts for almost 1% of all global deaths and 50% of all liver cirrhosis-attributable deaths [49]. The spectrum of hepatic lesions includes steatosis, alcoholic steatohepatitis (ASH), alcoholic hepatitis, fibrosis, cirrhosis, and HCC. Alcohol is a principal cause of end-stage liver disease, for which the only curative treatment is transplantation [50]. The insult on the liver by alcohol is closely related to the fact that the liver is the site of most of the metabolism of alcohol. Alcohol dehydrogenase (ADH; EC 1.1.1.1) converts ethanol to acetaldehyde with the generation of NADH reducing equivalents. Subsequent metabolism by acetaldehyde dehydrogenase (ALDH; EC 1.2.1.3) generates further equivalents of NADH. The elevated ratio of $NADH/NAD^+$ due to excess alcohol consumption is responsible for many of the biochemical consequences in the liver. For example, lactic acidosis, hyperuricemia, enhanced lipogenesis, and depressed fatty acid β-oxidation have long been known to be driven by excess hepatic NADH [51]. However, the influence of ethanol exposure on lipid metabolism is considerably more complicated than redox inhibition of fatty acid β-oxidation [52].

Much of the understanding of the mechanisms of liver disease have been generated using animal models. In pioneering studies, rats fed a 5% ethanol diet (36% total calories) had a plasma glycerolipid profile that mirrored the serum ethanol profile. Relative to paired rats fed a sucrose diet, the ethanol-fed rats displayed a 3-fold increase in total hepatic lipids and an 8-fold greater hepatic triglyceride content [53]. This early work led to the establishment of the Lieber-Decarli experimental alcohol diet [54], which is still widely employed [55]. Binge ethanol administration to mice (5 g/kg in three divided doses over 36 h) has also been used [56], in which case, hepatic S-adenosylmethionine (SAM), cysteine, and glutathione were decreased, while hypotaurine and taurine levels were elevated. These findings were interpreted as being due to both oxidative injury and a rapid elevation in cysteine dioxygenase (EC 1.13.11.20) activity, responsible for the production of hypotaurine and taurine. These markers could be attenuated by the co-administration of betaine, thought to be due to the regulation by betaine of hepatic levels of SAM and GSH [56]. Changes in hepatic lipid profiles occurred after chronic feeding of Yucatan micropigs (20–40 kg) with a 40% ethanol folate-deficient diet. In alcoholic pigs, hepatic triglycerides were elevated with increased desaturation of fatty acids (16:0 to 16:1n7 and 18:0 to 18:1n9) by stearoyl-CoA desaturase (SCD; EC 1.14.19.1) and decreased fatty acid elongation pathway (ELOVL5; EC 2.3.1.199) and phosphatidylethanolamine N-methyltransferase (PEMT; EC 2.1.1.17) activity. This latter enzyme attenuation led to a shift from phosphatidylethanolamines to phosphatidylcholines in the liver [57].

The above studies of the effect of alcohol administration were highly targeted, and therefore, limited in their description of the hepatic metabolic phenotype induced by alcohol. They were also limited by the vastly different protocols of ethanol administration. A study in mice was conducted using the Lieber-Decarli diet treated wild-type (WT) and $Ppara$-null mice (PPARα is a nuclear receptor that regulates much of lipid metabolism including fatty acid β-oxidation) [58]. Six months' chronic alcohol exposure led to increased hepatic triglyceride accumulation in the $Ppara$-null mice. Urines collected from 2 to 6 months were analyzed using an untargeted metabolomic protocol by UPLC-ESI-QTOFMS, and showed differential elevated metabolite profiles for the WT and null mice. In WT mice, the principal elevated urinary metabolites resulting from alcohol administration were ethyl sulfate and ethyl-β-D-glucuronide, secondary metabolites of ethanol, together with 4-hydroxyphenylacetic acid and its sulfate conjugate. These were also found for the null mice and, in addition, elevated urinary excretion of indole-3-lactic acid was found only in the $Ppara$-null mice, which was mechanistically related to the administration of ethanol in these animals. In a subsequent and more detailed investigation [59] that used WT and $Ppara$-null mice with two different strain backgrounds, indole-3-lactic acid and phenyllactic acid were reported as ALD biomarkers, with their formation arising from their corresponding pyruvic acids having been driven by the NADH hepatic overload due to ethanol consumption (Figure 2). The mechanism-based biomarkers also shed light on the development of steatosis, driven by the deficit in NAD^+ and the hepatic increase in NADH. The redox inhibition of fatty acid β-oxidation is an initial step of triglyceride and lipid droplet accumulation in the liver [52]. Metabolomic investigations in rats fed the Lieber-DeCarli liquid diet for 2 and 3 months have been conducted using high-field ^{1}H and ^{31}P NMR. These studies reported a two-fold increase in plasma triglycerides and a halving of plasma free fatty acids, mirroring smaller but statistically significant changes in the liver. Both total and free cholesterol were increased two-fold in the liver [60]. Metabolomics has identified specific lipids in serum that were associated with alcohol-induced liver diseases, specifically, N-lauroylglycine identified cirrhosis with 100% sensitivity and 90% specificity, while decatrienoic acid could evaluate liver disease severity with 100% sensitivity and specificity [61].

N-Acetyltaurine (NAT) has been reported to be a biomarker of alcohol exposure in mice, arising from metabolism of ethanol to acetaldehyde via ADH and CYP2E1 (EC 1.14.13.n7), and further by ALDH to acetate [62]. NAT is not specific to alcohol exposure, since it has been described as a biomarker of gamma-irradiation in both rats [63] and rhesus monkeys [64]. NAT urinary excretion has been reported in healthy human subjects who drank alcohol (0.66 to 0.84 g/kg) [65]. In blood, NAT concentration as a biomarker of alcohol exposure was of limited value [66]. To date, NAT has not been evaluated with respect to liver disease.

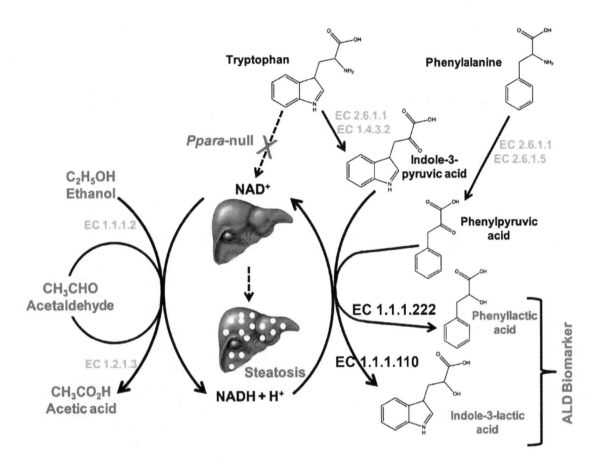

Figure 2. Generation of mechanism-based biomarkers of ALD (adapted from Manna et al., 2011 [59] with permission).

Chronic alcohol exposure in both experimental animals and humans leads to functional perturbations in the intestinal microbiota as determined by metabolomic investigations of intestinal metabolites. A wide range of altered intestinal microbiota metabolites has been reported, including decreased amino acids, changes in steroid, lipid, carnitine, and bile acid metabolism. Short-chain fatty acids (SCFAs) that are produced by bacterial fermentation were lowered by alcohol administration to rats, with the exception of acetate, which is an end-product of ethanol metabolism [67,68]. Additionally, saturated long-chain fatty acid (LCFA) biosynthesis by the microbiota is reduced by ethanol administration. These attenuated LCFA metabolites have been shown to contribute to alcohol-associated dysbiosis, influencing ALD [69]. Microbial metabolites combined with reduced levels of *Lactobacillus* trigger intestinal inflammation and liver disease following alcohol administration highlighting the role of gut microbiome-liver cross talk in ALD [49]. Studies that identified metabolomic and lipidomic biomarkers of alcoholic liver disease are listed in Table 1.

Table 1. Metabolomic and lipidomic biomarkers of alcoholic liver disease.

Species	Alcohol Dose	Pathology	Metabolites Reported	Ref.
Rat	20% or 36% of total calories; 24 days	Hepatomegaly Fatty infiltration	Plasma triglycerides↑ Plasma phospholipids↑ Hepatic triglycerides↑ 8-fold	[53]
Rat	5% alcohol Lieber-DeCarli diet; 2-3 months	Fatty infiltration Mild inflammatory infiltrate; 3 months Mild oxidative stress, 3 months	Liver triglycerides↑ Liver cholesterol↑ Liver phospholipids and lysophospholipids↓	[60]
Rat	6 g/kg alcohol + high-fat diet	Regional laminar necrosis and edema around central vein. Inflammatory cell infiltrate.	Total of 37 core ALD biomarkers identified. Pathways perturbed included TCA cycle, carbohydrate and amino acid metabolism.	[70]
Mouse	5 g/kg every 12 h X 3	Serum ALT↑ Hepatic CYP2E1↑	Malondialdehyde↑ Methionine↑ Hypotaurine↑ Taurine↑ SAM↓ GSH↓	[56]
Mouse 129 Sv WT and *Ppara*-null	4% alcohol Lieber-DeCarli diet; 2–6 months	Little change after 1 month	Ethylsulfate↑ Ethyl-β-D-glucuronide↑ 4-hydroxyphenylacetic acid (4HPAA)↑ 4HPAA sulfate↑ in both WT and null. Indole-3-lactic acid↑ in null only.	[58]
Mouse 129 Sv and C57BL/6 WT and *Ppara*-null	4% alcohol Lieber-DeCarli diet; 1 month	Steatosis in B6 null mice	Indole-3-lactic acid↑ and phenyllactic acid↑ in alcohol-treated *Ppara*-null mouse, both 129 Sv and C57BL/6	[59]
Mouse WT and *Cyp2e1*-null	2.2%, 4.5%, 5.4% Lieber-DeCarli semi-solid diet; 21 days	CYP2E1↑ in WT Microvesicular and macrovesicular steatosis around central vein; WT>null	Hepatic and serum triglycerides↑ in WT only. Urinary *N*-acetyltaurine, 4HPAA sulfate, ethylsulfate, ethyl-β-D-glucuronide↑	[62]
Mouse	4.896 g/kg; 7 days	ALT↑ AST↑ Focal hepatic necrosis Inflammatory infiltrate	Serum Malondialdehyde↑ GSH↓ GSSG↑ Methylglyoxal↑	[71]
Mouse	5% alcohol Lieber-DeCarli diet; 8 weeks	Mild steatohepatitis No fibrosis	Correlation between urinary and fecal metabolites. Many fecal and urinary metabolites altered. Amino acid metabolism perturbed. Indole-3-lactic acid↑	[72]
Mouse *Cramp*-null and WT	5% alcohol Lieber-DeCarli diet; 24 days	Not clearly stated	In alcohol-fed WT, fecal taurine, α-aminoisobutyric acid, nicotinic acid, serine, SCFAs↓ In alcohol-fed null mice, only nicotinic acid↑	[73]

Table 1. *Cont.*

Species	Alcohol Dose	Pathology	Metabolites Reported	Ref.
Micropig	40% total calories Folate-depleted diet	Not determined	Hepatic triglycerides↑ SCD pathway↑ ELOVL5 pathway↑ PEMT pathway↓ Phospholipid export↓	[57]
Human	100–300 g/day; 10 days 118 g/day; 11 days, 141 g/day; 8 days	Fatty infiltration	Plasma triglycerides↑	[53]
Human	30 ALD patients (mean daily alcohol consumption 109.7 g/day) vs. 10 healthy controls	Cirrhosis (80%) Decompensated cirrhosis (DC; 23%)	*N*-Lauroylglycine↑ in cirrhosis. Decatrienoic acid associated with disease severity.	[61]
Human	30 Alcohol use disorder (AUD), 13 alcoholic hepatitis (AH) and 16 nonalcoholic controls	ALT↑ (AUD = AH) AST↑ (AH>>AUD)	Seven serum oxylipins and nine fecal oxylipins↑ Results related to inflammation and platelet aggregation. Inflammatory ω-6 PUFA oxylipins counteracted by ω-3 bioactive lipid mediators.	[74]
Human	64 AH patients, 26 DC patients without AH	AST and GGT↑ (AH > DC). Other serum markers and MELD score AH = DC	Metabolomic signature of AH claimed but not disclosed.	[75]

5.2. Cholestasis

Cholestasis is the impaired formation or secretion of bile into the small intestine, and can be classified as intrahepatic or extrahepatic, together with obstructive or nonobstructive. There are many causes of the various manifestations of cholestasis including gallstones, malignancy, and defective bile acid synthesis and secretion [76]. Metabolomics has been employed to attempt to distinguish between the different mechanisms of cholestasis. In the first such study, rat models of inhibited biliary secretion (intrahepatic) and obstructed bile flow (extrahepatic) were employed, and urine was analyzed by ¹H NMR. It was concluded that bile acids, valine, and methyl malonate were possible cholestatic biomarkers [77]. These biomarkers did not appear to be specific to cholestatic injury. Another early approach was to use metabolomics to understand the metabolic consequences of perturbed bile acid (BA) homeostasis, as occurs in cholestasis. The farnesoid X receptor (FXR) is a nuclear receptor that regulates genes involved in BA synthesis, metabolism, and transport. *Fxr*-null and WT mice dosed with the FXR ligands CA or LCA generated metabolites indicative of intrahepatic cholestasis. These included the sulfate and β-D-glucuronic acid conjugates of *p*-cresol [78], a fermentation product of tyrosine produced by *Clostridium difficile* in the gut [79], thereby providing further evidence of gut microbiota-liver crosstalk. Other metabolites related to cholestasis included corticosterone and CA metabolites, with the latter being produced by induced CYP3A11 [78]. Furthermore, in LCA-induced experimental intrahepatic cholestasis in mice, TGFβ-SMAD3 signaling mediated the alterations in phospholipid and BA metabolism [80]. In a rat model for cholestasis, mass spectrometry-based targeted metabolomics revealed elevations in urinary taurine and hypotaurine (5- to 9-fold). The largest increases between cholestatic and control rats were for CA, LCA, deoxycholic acid, and ursodeoxycholic acid (10- to 23-fold, respectively) [81]. Four independent rat studies that employed the experimental cholestatic compound α-naphthylisothiocyanate (ANIT) reported that both free and conjugated primary BAs were significantly elevated above controls by ANIT administration [82–85]. It has been demonstrated that several traditional Chinese medicine (TCM) remedies for treating jaundice can reverse the metabolomic fingerprint of ANIT, and therefore, protect against ANIT-induced cholestasis. These treatments include paeoniflorin (from the dried root of *Paeonia lactiflora*) [83,84], rhubarb [85], Yinchenhao decoction (from the above ground parts of *Artemisia annua*) [86], chicken bile powder (containing mainly taurochenodeoxycholic acid that is deconjugated in the gut producing the primary BA that is a FXR ligand) [87], Huangqi decoction (a TCM comprising Radix Astragali and Radix Glycyrrhizae) [88], gentiopicroside (from *Gentiana rigescens* Franch. ex Hemsl.) [89], and Da-Huang-Xiao-Shi decoction [90]. In addition to TCMs, melatonin (100 mg/kg p.o.) has been administered to rats 24 h after they had received ANIT (25 mg/kg i.p.). This high dose of melatonin (relative to the 4-20 mg/kg doses used in mouse melatonin studies [91,92]) produced a modest reduction in serum liver enzymes and bilirubin with a less severe liver histology. The metabolomic changes in serum due to melatonin administration were unexceptional and, in part, derived metabolically from melatonin [93]. The mechanism of ANIT-induced cholestasis continues to be investigated using metabolomic tools. The plasma and liver biomarkers described in mice administered ANIT gave rise to the conclusion that the cholestatic liver injury might correlate significantly with hepatocyte necrosis, metabolic disorders, and an imbalance of intestinal microbiome ecology as a result of BA accumulation [94].

A metabolomic investigation has also been reported, whereby regulation of BA metabolism by the nuclear receptor PPARα and inhibition of NF-κB/STAT3 signaling protected against cholestasis induced by ANIT [95]. Furthermore, a lipidomic study of ANIT-induced intrahepatic cholestasis uncovered the role of the aryl hydrocarbon receptor (AHR) in regulating expression of choline kinase (CHK) in mice. Knockout of the *Ahr* gene significantly reversed ANIT-induced lipid metabolism via *Chka* expression, and reversed the intrahepatic cholestasis [96]. Vascular protein sorting-associated protein 33B (VPS33B) is involved in the trafficking of intracellular proteins to distinct organelles. Mutations in *VPS33B* are associated with a neonatal syndrome that includes cholestasis (OMIM 208085). Using the lipidomic and metabolomic profiles of hepatic *Vps33b*-null male mice, which displayed cholestasis with elevated serum liver enzymes and total bilirubin and total BAs, demonstrated the importance of VPS33B in BA, glycerolipid, phospholipid, and sphingolipid metabolism. In particular, the elevation of hepatic ceramides was thought to influence apoptosis and the progression of cholestasis [97].

Bile duct ligation (BDL) is a nonchemical means to produce experimental cholestasis in rats. Compared with sham operated rats, BDL rats displayed oxidative stress, with diminished serum GSH, total antioxidant capacity, and superoxide dismutase and glutathione peroxidase activities, with upregulated serum malondialdehyde. Changes in certain amino acids, lipids, Krebs cycle intermediates, and lactic acid were signs of the effects of cholestasis on energy metabolism [98]. The BDL cholestasis rat model was shown to generate similar metabolic characteristics as thioacetamide (TAA)-induced cholestasis in rats, with excessive fatty acid oxidation, insufficient glutathione regeneration, and disturbed gut microbiota. These features in both rat models could be reversed by the TCM Huang-Lian-Jie-Du-Decoction [99]. A metabolomic study recently compared three models of chemically-induced cholestasis, using ANIT, 3,5-diethoxycarbonyl-1,4-dihydrocollidine (DDC), or LCA. BAs were increased in all three models, whereas arginine was decreased. Hepatic protoporphyrin IX, a metabolic precursor of heme and cytochrome c, was increased only in the DDC model [100].

Both primary biliary cholangitis (PBC) (previously known as primary biliary cirrhosis) and primary sclerosing cholangitis (PSC) are chronic cholestatic liver diseases. PBC and PSC patients were investigated using targeted profiling of serum BAs. In PBC with cholestasis, total primary BAs (CA and chenodeoxycholic acid) were 13.5-fold higher than noncholestatic donors, in particular, their taurine conjugates (34- to 46.5-fold accumulation) [101]. A similar pattern of elevated free and conjugated primary BAs was reported in another PBC metabolomic investigation. The total secondary BAs (deoxycholic acid and LCA) were not significantly altered in PBC, nor were the 6α-hydroxylated BAs (hyocholic acid and hyodeoxycholic acid). In PSC with cholestasis, primary

BAs were more abundant and both secondary BAs, and 6α-hydroxylated BAs were significantly reduced. The authors recognized that the BA composition of bile requires determination in these two cholestatic diseases [102]. Similar findings were reported in a later study that also included some small changes in free fatty acids and markers of inflammation and oxidative stress [103]. Furthermore, BAs increased during progression of PBC with a decline in acylcarnitines, such as propionyl and butyryl carnitine [104]. The metabolic signatures of PBC and celiac disease have been compared and contrasted with healthy controls using ^{1}H NMR-based metabolomics on serum and urine. Both diseases showed distinct metabolite patterns, although relatively few metabolites, such as pyruvate, lactate, glutamate, glutamine, hippurate, and trigonelline (a metabolite of niacin also found in coffee) were described [105]. It is unclear whether the differences described were due to dietary factors. Intrahepatic cholestasis of pregnancy (ICP) has an incidence of between 0.1% (Europe) and 15.6% (South America) [106]. A urinary metabolomic study of ICP revealed several significant predictive biomarkers of ICP, including the primary BA metabolites glycocholic acid and chenodeoxycholic acid 3-sulfate [107]. In a serum targeted metabolomics ICP study, 60 BAs were detected of which most conjugated BAs were elevated in ICP. Metabolomics was also employed to monitor BAs during treatment with ursodeoxycholic acid [108]. Targeted metabolomics of urinary sulfated BAs was used to define biomarkers for the diagnosis and grading of ICP. Total sulfated BAs were remarkably increased in ICP, particularly those formed from glycine and taurine conjugated BAs. Clear clustering and separation of the PCA and OPLS-DA scores for controls, mild ICP, and severe ICP were reported, and are depicted in Figure 3. In order to better understand how ICP endangers the fetus and the links between fetal BA homeostasis and sulfation capacity, a metabolomic investigation in pregnant swine was conducted. It was found that sulfation played a pivotal role in maintaining BA homeostasis in the fetus. Furthermore, fetal mortality showed an exponential increase in relation to the total BA increase from week 60 to week 90 [109]. A controversial condition related to ICP that is asymptomatic and difficult to distinguish from ICP is asymptomatic hypercholanemia of pregnancy (AHP). A targeted metabolomics study was undertaken in order to establish a differential diagnosis of AHP. Compared to a control group, AHP had several higher urinary BAs and sulfated BAs than controls, and more that were lower in AHP than ICP. Glycocholic acid and tauro-ω-muricholic acid were a potential combination biomarker for AHP, whereas a further combination biomarker involving BA sulfates could distinguish AHP from ICP [110]. Metabolomic profiling of maternal hair was conducted to find predictive biomarkers of ICP. Despite the identification of 105 metabolites in hair, none was associated with ICP [111].

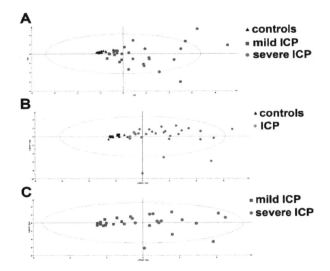

Figure 3. (**A**) PCA scores plot for controls vs. mild ICP vs. severe ICP; (**B**) OPLS-DA scores plot for controls vs. ICP; (**C**) OPLS-DA scores plot for mild ICP vs. severe ICP. Note the data clustering and separation (taken from Li et al., 2018 [112] with permission).

Cholestasis may also occur in neonates. Infantile hepatitis syndrome (IHS) and biliary atresia (BLA) are the most common in the first three months of life. Using GC-MS metabolomics on urine, it was reported that IHS could be distinguished from BLA with the biomarkers *N*-acetyl-D-mannosamine and α-aminoadipic acid [113]. A summary of studies is given in Table 2.

Table 2. Metabolomic and lipidomic biomarkers of cholestasis.

Species	Manipulation/Condition	Pathology	Analytical Methodology	Metabolites Reported	Ref.
Rat	Inhibition of bile secretion vs. bile flow obstruction	Intrahepatic cholestasis vs. extrahepatic cholestasis	¹H NMR	Bile acids↑ Bilirubin↑ vs. Bile acids↑ BCAAs↑ SCFAs↑	[77]
Mouse	*Fxr*-null vs. WT treated with FXR ligands CA and LCA	Cholestasis	UPLC-ESI-QTOFMS	*p*-Cresol sulfate and β-D-glucuronide↑ Corticosterone metabolites↑ Cholic acid metabolites↑	[78]
Rat	Eisai hyperbilirubinemic rat	Cholestasis	UPLC-TQMS	Taurine↑ Hypotaurine↑ Unconjugated primary and secondary bile acids↑	[81]
Rat	ANIT Methapyrilene Dimethylnitrosamine	Cholestasis	UPLC-TQMS GC-MS UPLC-QTOFMS	Bile acids↑ Arginine↓ Pantothenate↑ Protoporphyrin IX↑ Palmitoyl carnitine↑ Arachidonic, linoleic and oleic acids↓	[82–85]
Mouse	*Vps33b*-depleted mouse	Cholestasis	UPLC-MS	Serum bile acids↑ triglycerides↑ and sphingomyelins↑	[97]
Rat	Bile duct ligation (BDL)	Cholestasis	UPLC-QTOFMS	Phenylalanine↑ Glutamate↑ Tyrosine↑ Kynurenine↑ Lactate↑ LPC(14:0) ↑ Glycine↑ Succinate↑ MDA↑ GSH↑ Valine↓ Isoleucine↓ Citrate↓ Palmitate↓ Taurine↓ LPC(19:0)↓	[98]
Rat	TAA or BDL	Cholestasis	¹H NMR	BDL vs. TAA: 2-Hydroxybutyrate↑ BCAAs↑ Lysine↑ Arginine↑ Glycine↑ Citrate↑ 2-Oxoglutarate↑ Fumarate↑ Hippurate↑ Phenacetylglycine↑	[99]
Mouse	ANIT or DDC or LCA	Cholestasis	UPLC-QTOFMS	Phospholipids↑ Protoporphyrin IX↑ GSH↓	[100]
Human	Primary biliary cholangitis	Cholestasis	UPLC-QTOFMS	Primary bile acids↑ Phospholipids↑ Oleic and Linoleic acids↑	[101–103]
Human	Intrahepatic cholestasis of pregnancy (ICP)	Cholestasis	HPLC-QTOFMS	MG(22:5) ↑ LPE(22:5) ↑ L-Homocysteine sulfonic acid↑ Glycocholic acid↑ Chenodeoxycholic acid 3-sulfate↑	[107]
Human	Hypercholanemia of pregnancy (HCP) vs. ICP	Cholestasis	UPLC-QTOFMS	Sulfated bile acid pattern used for differential diagnosis of HCP and ICP	[110]
Human	Infantile hepatitis syndrome (IHS) vs. biliary atresia	Cholestasis	GC-MS	*N*-Acetyl-D-mannosamine and α-Aminoadipic acid used for differential diagnosis	[113]

5.3. Fibrosis and Cirrhosis

Fibrosis occurs when damage to the liver causing overactive wound healing leads to the formation of scarring or deposition of extracellular matrix proteins including collagen. This process occurs in most chronic liver diseases, and can ultimately lead to cirrhosis and liver failure. Such end-stage liver disease may require transplantation [114]. Fibrosis is staged 0 to 4 by liver biopsy using the METAVIR scoring system, F0 = no fibrosis, F1 = portal fibrosis, F2 = periportal fibrosis, F3 = bridging fibrosis, F4 = cirrhosis. Fibrosis is also graded according to the severity of the underlying disease process, activity grades A0 to A3 [115]. Fibrosis and cirrhosis are primarily caused by hepatitis or chronic alcoholism, but can also arise due to nonalcoholic fatty liver disease (NAFLD), including nonalcoholic steatohepatitis (NASH). In compensated cirrhosis, the liver is still able to perform most of its basic functions despite the scarring. Compensated cirrhosis involves Stage 1 (no varices, no ascites) and Stage 2 (varices, no ascites). In decompensated cirrhosis, excessive scarring inhibits basic liver functions and comprises Stage 3 (ascites ± varices) and Stage 4 (bleeding varices ± ascites) [116]. The 1-year survival for compensated and decompensated cirrhosis is 87.3% and 75.0% and 5-year survival is 66.5% and 45.4%, respectively [117]. As the terminal stages of liver fibrosis that can lead to HCC have a high morbidity and mortality with only transplantation as a therapeutic option, there have been extensive studies using metabolomics to define biomarkers for the underlying disease progression.

Relatively few investigations have sought biomarkers of fibrosis using metabolomics. The greatest both quantity and quality of potential biomarker data has been leveraged using mass spectrometry methodologies. Metabolic pathways associated with hepatic fibrosis, specifically, for carbohydrates, amino acids, and lipids, have been reviewed [118]. In a Japanese study that employed CE-TOFMS and LC-TOFMS, the progression of fibrosis in NAFLD was reported to be associated with increased serum concentrations of several metabolites, among them the sulfates of the three steroids etiocholanolone (a major testosterone metabolite), dehydroepiandrosterone (a precursor of androgens and estrogens) and 16α-hydroxy-dehydroepiandrosterone (a precursor of estriol). The first of these sulfates decreased in relation to fibrosis progression from F0/F1 to F4, while the last steroid sulfate increased during fibrosis progression, especially when expressed as a ratio to either of the other two sulfates [119]. Although these steroid sulfates and their ratios appeared to be biomarkers of fibrosis progression in NAFLD, the key biomarker, 16α-hydroxy-dehydroepiandrosterone sulfate, has also been reported in serum of patients with breast cancer and endometrial cancer [120]. A Brazilian study in chronic hepatitis C collected large amounts of clinical data on 69 fibrotic patients classified with fibrosis by METAVIR that was significant (≥F2; 42), nonsignificant (<F2; 27), also as advanced (≥F3; 28), nonadvanced (<F3; 41), and as cirrhosis (F4; 18) and noncirrhosis (<F4; 51). ^{1}H NMR was used to analyze serum, but not to identify metabolites. The PLS-DA 3-D scores plots showed clustering and separation for F0-F1 vs. F2-F4, F0-F2 vs. F3-F4 with partial separation of F0-F3 vs. F4, leading the authors to hypothesize that their metabolomic strategy could distinguish between significant fibrosis, advanced fibrosis, and cirrhosis [121]. Without knowledge of the altered metabolites central to the metabolomic model used, it is not possible to delineate whether the discriminatory signals arise as biomarkers for the disease process or due to confounding factors such as comorbidities or drug treatment, as commented in another similar case (see below) [122]. A ^{1}H NMR-based metabolomic study was conducted in rats injected i.p. for 8 weeks with CCl4. Seven metabolites were diminished in urine of treated rats compared with controls, namely, 2-oxoglutarate, citrate, dimethylamine, phenacetylglycine, creatinine, and hippurate. Only taurine urinary excretion was found to be significantly elevated in this rat model of fibrosis [123]. A subsequent report from this group found more metabolomic changes in their CCl4 fibrosis rat model. They proposed that the TCM *Corydalis saxicola* Bunting exhibited antifibrotic effects by regulating ALT, FXR, COX-2, metalloproteinase-1, and angiotensinogen based upon network analysis with their NMR metabolomic data [124], about which we remain skeptical. Shi-Wei-Gan-Ning-Pill (SWGNP) is a multicomponent Tibetan recipe used to treat viral hepatitis, hepatic fibrosis and steatosis, cirrhosis, and HCC. In a study in the CCl4 rat model, SWGNP was also administered at a low, medium, and high dose, equivalent to 3-, 6-, and 12-times the clinical dose, respectively. ^{1}H NMR-based metabolomics was conducted on liver extracts and serum. A total of 39 metabolites were identified in rat liver extracts and 28 in serum. Alterations in energy metabolites suggested that the liver responded to CCl4 crisis by metabolic remodeling from mitochondrial respiration to cytosolic aerobic glycolysis, increased fatty acid β-oxidation, glycogenolysis, and metabolism of ketone bodies. The medium and high doses of SWGNP significantly decreased the histological scores in the CCl4 model, together with fibrosis and

oxidative stress markers. SWGNP also reversed changes in amino acids and nucleosides caused by CCl4. The authors concluded that SWGNP could alleviate liver fibrosis caused by CCl4 [125]. Another Tibetan folk remedy has been investigated in the CCl4 rat fibrosis model, that of *Herpetospermum caudigerum* Wall. (HCW), the Himalayan Bitter Gourd, a large climbing plant that grows at an altitude of 1500 to 3600 m, whose dry ripe seeds have been used as a hepatoprotectant. In the CCl4 experiments, HCW was administered at doses of 1 and 3 g/kg. HCW produced similar effects on fibrosis markers as SWGNP, with the exception that the lower dose was more effective than the higher dose. The metabolomic effects and proposed mechanisms were very similar for HCW [126] to those of SWGNP [125]. The active principles of neither of these TCMs have been identified, except that HCW was said to comprise mainly lignans, coumarins, triterpenes, saponins, phenols, essential oils, amino acids, and trace elements [126]. The underlying antifibrotic mechanisms of these TCM remedies remain unknown, despite the clues provided by metabolomics.

Earliest serum biomarkers of liver cirrhosis (LC) were derived from chronic hepatitis B patients in China, and comprised the four primary bile salts found by UPLC-QTOFMS [127]. However, elevated glycine and taurine conjugated primary bile acids are not specific to LC (see above). A similar population studied using GC-MS identified several elevated metabolic intermediates in cirrhotic serum, including butanoic and hexanoic acid [128]. These two SCFAs are presumably products of the gut microflora (see above). Amino acid D- and L-enantiomers in serum and urine have been examined using two-dimensional gas chromatography-time-of-flight mass spectrometry (GC X GC-TOFMS) in 25 LC patients and 16 controls in Germany. No L-amino acids were significantly higher in the serum of LC patients, although several were significantly higher in controls. In contrast, D-alanine and D-proline were significantly elevated in LC serum, and D-valine, D-leucine, and D-threonine were only detected in LC serum [129]. It is attractive to consider these D-amino acids as candidate biomarkers for LC. However, only D-serine and D-aspartate are considered human tissue-derived, while the rest most likely arise from microbial sources, either in the diet or from the gut microbiota [130]. This may be further evidence of gut microbiota-liver cross-talk in liver disease. Further evidence of this crosstalk is furnished by a Chinese study that examined stool samples by UPLC-ESI-QTOFMS taken from cirrhotic patients (etiologies either HBV, HCV or alcohol; 17) and healthy controls (24). The two groups clustered and separated in both the PCA and PLS-DA scores plots. Several metabolites that were reduced in cirrhotic feces, chenodeoxycholic acid, 7-ketolithocholic acid, urobilin, and urobilinogen. A number of metabolites were more prominent in cirrhotic feces, including amino acids, and long-chain fatty acids and their carnitine esters. These findings were interpreted as due to changes in biliary function and the gut microbiota in cirrhosis leading to fat malabsorption [131]. Another Chinese study claimed that taurocholate was not merely a biomarker for cirrhosis progression, but also actively promoted this progression. Of the 12 BAs targeted using UPLC-TQMS, taurocholate increased 76-fold between LC (32) and HV (27). This was said to be due to increased synthesis. In addition, the promotion of cirrhosis progression by taurocholate was postulated to be due to stellate cell activation via the TLR4 pathway [132].

We have reported a metabolomic and lipidomic investigation of into Swiss HCC patients (20) using UPLC-ESI-QTOFMS and GC-MS, in which LC patients (7) were included together with healthy volunteers (HV; 6) and an acute myelogenous leukemia (AML) control group (22). With one exception, all the HCC patients also had LC. Interestingly, LC and HCC clustered together in both the unsupervised (PCA) and supervised (PLS-DA) scores plots, and clearly segregated from the HV and AML clusters. This suggests that the greatest insult to liver metabolism resulted from LC rather than HCC. No elevated biomarkers specific to LC were described, although several were found for HCC (see below) [133]. The investigation by GC-MS of urine from HCV-positive untreated Egyptian patients with LC (40) and HCC (55), together with HV (45) essentially confirmed the findings of metabolomic similarity between LC and HCC patients. With the exception of AFP, serum biochemistry was similar for the LC and HCC. Several urinary metabolites were elevated above HV for both LC and HCC in a similar fashion, including serine, glycine, threonine, and citrate [134]. Although not stated, the HCC patients almost certainly also had LC, underlining the difficulties of distinguishing between HCC and LC in studies of this kind for an HCV population. In a Chinese study of LC (20), healthy controls (20) and HCC (59) using UPLC-ESI-QTOFMS, three ions corresponding to canavaninosuccinate (CVS) were virtually absent in LC serum relative to the other groups [135]. CVS is a derivative of aspartate formed from ureidohomoserine; aspartate is further converted to creatine [136]. The extinction of CVS in LC serum is an appealing biomarker for LC, except that it is also massively reduced in plasma of chronic kidney disease patients relative to controls, correlating strongly with the glomerular filtration rate [137]. A US study compared patients with high both liver and kidney disease severity (ascites present, GFR ≤ 60; n = 34) with those with low liver and kidney disease (ascites absent, GFR ≥ 60; n = 69) severity. Using UPLC-ESI-TQMS, 34/1028 plasma metabolites were significantly increased in the severe hepatorenal dysfunction group. The greatest change (2.39) was for 4-acetamidobutanoate, the acetylated metabolite of GABA and a product of arginine and proline metabolism (http://www.hmdb.ca/metabolites/HMDB0003681). Pathway enrichment analysis identified glucuronidation and methylation, together with ascorbate and aldarate metabolism, that were linked to hepatorenal dysfunction [138]. Another study in China used both NMR and UPLC-ESI-QTOFMS to analyze serum from LC (42), HCC (43) and HV (18). Several phospholipids and fatty acids together with bilirubin were elevated in LC vs. HV [139], findings similar to those which we had previously reported in Swiss patients [133]. A UK study that employed both NMR and UPLC-ESI-QTOFMS of plasma from 248 subjects examined the differences between surviving and nonsurviving patients with decompensated cirrhosis. NMR profiles of nonsurvivors had increased plasma lactate, tyrosine, methionine and phenylalanine. UPLC-ESI-QTOFMS showed that lysophosphatidylcholines (LPC) and phosphatidylcholines (PC) were downregulated in nonsurvivors. LPC concentrations negatively correlated with the circulating markers of cell death, M30 and M65. Therefore, metabolomic phenotyping ("metabotyping") was said to accurately predict mortality in decompensated cirrhosis, due to LPC and amino acid metabolism dysregulation that reflected hepatocyte cell death [140]. Using LC-MS, a Chinese group profiled 43 steroids in the urine of HV (21), LC (21), and HCC (28) relative to urinary creatinine. The PCA scores plot showed some overlap between these three groups. Many steroids in LC displayed lower urinary excretion than HV controls, including pregnanediol, corticosterone, androsterone, etiocholanolone, dehydroepiandrosterone, and testosterone. In contrast, LC urinary excretion of 16α-hydroxyestrone was markedly elevated above HV controls. These findings are consistent with what has been described as a "feminization" phenotype in LC [141]. It is worth noting that these investigators treated the urines with sulfatase and β-glucuronidase prior to steroid analysis to determine total (free plus conjugated) steroids; therefore, their results are difficult to compare with those cited above where sulfated steroids were quantitated [120]. Using GC-MS, serum from Chinese HBV-positive (49), LC (52) and HCC patients (39), together with healthy controls (61) was analyzed. All four groups clustered and separated in the OPLS-DA scores plot. Of the top 30 discriminating metabolites, serine, succinate, malate, 5-oxoproline, glutamate, phenylalanine, ornithine, citrate, and tyrosine were all elevated in LC relative to controls. Palmitate was proposed as a biomarker for cirrhosis development in HBV hepatitis, with high sensitivity and specificity in ROC analysis. The purpose of this study however was to examine the progression of hepatitis B to HCC via cirrhosis [142]. Interestingly, a review of metabolomic studies of hepatitis B, HBV-related LC and HBV-related HCC clearly shows the overlap in these three groups in upregulated metabolites [143]. Oxylipins are another group of lipids that have been investigated in HBV-related LC and HCC. UPLC-ESI-TQMS was utilized to quantitate 18 omega-6 fatty acid-derived oxylipins in serum from patients with chronic hepatitis B (34), HBV-related LC (46), HBV-related HCC (38), and healthy controls (50). Compared with healthy controls, LC had statistically significantly elevated 13-HODE, but lower levels of TXB2 [144]. The 13(S)-HODE and 13(R)-HODE enantiomers are produced from linoleic acid by 15-lipoxygenase and are credited with differential effects on cell growth and apoptosis [145]. Unfortunately, it was not determined which enantiomer was elevated in plasma of LC patients [144]. Apparently, patients with HBV-related LC can be classified under the theory of TCM as having one of two typical patterns, Gan Dan Shi Re (GDSR) or Gan Shen Yin

Xu (GSYX). Serum of cases with GDSR (40), GSYX (41), and those with no obvious pattern (called "Latent Pattern" (LP); 30) were investigated using GC-TOFMS metabolomics. Eight metabolites were specific to the GDSR type of HBV cirrhosis, a separate eight were specific to the GSYX type, and a further 10 metabolites were common to both types. The GDSR metabolites were said to be related to abnormalities in linoleic acid metabolism, while the GSYX metabolites were said to arise from abnormalities in glycine, serine, and threonine metabolism. All these 26 metabolites were potential biomarkers for HBV-related cirrhosis [146].

As mentioned earlier, BLA is a neonatal cholestatic condition and is the most life-threatening cholestatic disorder in children. In a Chinese study, liver samples from BLA (52) and IHS (16) were profiled for amino acids and biogenic amines using UPLC-ESI-TQMS. Several amino acids had higher hepatic concentrations in IHS than in BLA. However, histamine was twice as abundant in BLA as in IHS liver. In addition, the degree of fibrosis from F1/F2 to F4 correlated with histamine concentration. Histamine therefore presents a potential target for preventing fibrosis in BLA [147].

Several investigators have used ^{1}H NMR in the search of biomarkers for liver fibrosis and cirrhosis. For example, a Spanish study of LC with minimal hepatic encephalopathy was conducted by ^{1}H NMR, resulting in elevated glucose, lactate, methionine, trimethylamine N-oxide (TMAO), and glycerol [148], none of which is specific to LC or even liver disease. A further Spanish NMR study compared liver biopsies from cirrhosis and chronic hepatitis due to HCV, HBV, alcohol, and autoimmunity. Elevated in cirrhosis were glutamate and phosphoethanolamine [149]. A UK study used ^{1}H NMR metabolite profiling to compare livers removed from patients with either LC associated with ALD (5) or with NASH (14) with healthy donor transplant livers (16). Cirrhotic livers had significantly increased levels of isoleucine, valine, succinate, lactate, and betaine [150]. Another NMR study was conducted on Chinese patients that included those with HCC. The elevated serum metabolites in LC occurred also when the patients had HCC, with the exception of taurine, namely, acetate, pyruvate, glutamine, α-ketoglutarate, glycerol, tyrosine, 1-methylhistidine, and phenylalanine [151]. A French study using ^{1}H NMR examined metabolic differences between alcoholic cirrhotic patients with severe and mild chronic liver failure (CLF) that had been stratified by MELD score. Lactate, pyruvate, glucose, amino acids, and creatinine were significantly higher in patients with severe CLF than mild CLF [152]. These findings cannot be considered as biomarkers of severe CLF, as they are not specific. A Chinese study in compensated cirrhosis (30), decompensated cirrhosis (30), and healthy controls (30) using ^{1}H NMR on serum samples reported that succinate, pyruvate, and phenylalanine increased with cirrhosis progression [153]. Yet, again, these cannot be considered as biomarkers due to their lack of specificity. An earlier Canadian study had been the first to profile metabolites in compensated and decompensated cirrhosis patients with HCV, together with healthy volunteers, but used ^{31}P magnetic resonance spectroscopy performed on the abdomen over the liver. The acquired spectra showed phosphomonoesters (PME), phosphodiesters (PDE), and β-ATP resonances, the last of which was significantly lower in decompensated cirrhosis vs. the other two groups combined, and the PME/PDE ratio was significantly higher in decompensated cirrhosis than controls. This ratio was interpreted based upon published findings as an indicator of a disturbed endoplasmic reticulum membrane in decompensated cirrhosis [154]. Austrian investigators used high-field ^{1}H-MRS and ultrahigh-field ^{31}P-MRS to examine in vivo the livers of NAFLD patients with little or no fibrosis and NASH patients with advanced fibrosis. The ^{1}H-MRS lipid signal was massively increased in NASH livers over NAFLD livers and cross-correlated with histology from liver biopsies. The lipid saturation, polyunsaturation, and monounsaturation indices did not differ between NAFLD and NASH livers. Moreover, ^{31}P-MRS measures of the PME (including phosphoethanolamine) and PDE (including glycerophosphocholine) resonances reflected the severity of fibrosis. Changes in energy metabolism, as reflected by ATP flux, were decreased in advanced fibrosis. This noninvasive real-time profiling technique appeared to be of significant value for investigation of hepatic structure and function [155]. An Italian study combined NMR metabolomics of stool samples with 16S rRNA sequencing of gut microbiota in LC patients (46) and healthy age-matched controls (14). Peripheral blood and liver biopsies were also analyzed together with portal blood from seven cirrhotics and caecal biopsies taken during colonoscopy in 17 LC patients and 6 controls. The metagenomics data demonstrated a marked dysbiosis in LC patients. The principally elevated metabolites in LC feces relative to controls were phenylalanine, threonine, butanoate, methanol, cadaverine, and α-glucose. Using the metagenomics data, eight pathways were underrepresented and two overrepresented in LC. The authors concluded that intervention with prebiotics/probiotics/synbiotics, diet, or fecal microbiota transplant could support development of new customized treatments for LC patients [156]. Interestingly, partial reversal of dysbiosis and metabolomic profile was reported after splenectomy in LC patients (12) [157]. A combined metagenomics and metabolomic investigation of LC was conducted in China with HV (47), compensated LC (49) and decompensated LC (46). Urine was analyzed by UPLC-ESI-QTOFMS and PCA scores plots for total metabolites and a subset of 75 differential metabolites both separated HV from LC urines, with compensated and decompensated LC clustering together. Six metabolites were reported to be lower in LC urine than in HV urine, but none greater [158]. Another combined metagenomics and metabolomics investigation was conducted to compare Turkish patients on a Mediterranean diet (HV, 46; compensated LC, 50; decompensated LC, 43) with American patients on a Western diet (HV, 48; compensated LC, 59; decompensated LC, 50). In this study, ^{1}H NMR was used for plasma metabolomics, which showed higher lactate concentrations in Turkey vs. USA. There were similar trends between decompensated LC and HV in both Turkey and USA, with reduced lipids and phosphocholines. Correlation networks in cirrhotics showed differences between the beneficial taxa *Blautia* and *Oscillispira* in Turkish compared with American patients [159]. The metabolomic differences described in this unique study were disappointing and would have greatly benefitted from analysis using MS-based methodology.

Acute-on-chronic liver failure (ACLF) refers to patients with acute deterioration of liver function in compensated or decompensated but stable cirrhosis. Serum from a group of French compensated and decompensated cirrhosis patients (93) was compared with that from ACLF patients (30) using ^{1}H NMR metabolomics. The latter group showed higher serum lactate, pyruvate, ketone bodies, glutamine, phenylalanine, tyrosine, and creatinine [160], none of which is a specific biomarker. A UK study examined plasma by ^{1}H NMR for stable cirrhotic patients (18), patients with stable cirrhosis during an episode of encephalopathy (18), together with matched controls (17). With the exception of pyruvate, which was significantly higher, glycolysis end-products and gluconeogenesis precursors (pyruvate, alanine, threonine, glycine and aspartate) were significantly lower in cirrhotics with encephalopathy than without and both higher than controls. There was no discernable effect of encephalopathy on branched-chain and aromatic amino acids or on urea cycle intermediates [161]. Yet, again, such NMR-derived metabolites do not show sufficient specificity to be considered as biomarkers. In contrast, a French group compared hepatic encephalopathy (HE) patients (14) with control patients without neurological disease (27) using UPLC-MS analysis of cerebrospinal fluid (CSF) and plasma. A total of 73 metabolites were identified in CSF including amino acids, acylcarnitines, bile acids, and nucleosides. It was further reported that acetylated amino sugars, acetylated amino acids, and metabolites involved in ammonia, amino acid, and energy metabolism were specifically and significantly increased in CSF of HE patients [162]. These findings underscore the superiority of MS-based over NMR-based metabolomics protocols in terms of metabolite identification. Serum analysis by ^{1}H NMR was conducted on a Spanish two groups of HCV patients, one without fibrosis (F0; 30) and the other with cirrhosis (F4; 27). Glucose, citrate, and VLDL1 were significantly elevated, and choline, glutamine, acetoacetate, glycoprotein N-acetyl groups, cysteine, histidine, and LDL1 were significantly depressed in the serum of cirrhotic HCV patients. The authors believed that these results provided new biomarkers to distinguish no fibrosis from severe fibrosis (cirrhosis) in HCV infection [163]. An investigation of Italian patients with chronic HCV attempted to diagnose the degree of fibrosis using ^{1}H NMR on plasma, serum, and urine samples. Remarkably, these investigators did not identify metabolites, but rather, used statistical analysis of their spectra in an attempt to classify and distinguish chronic hepatitis C (little or no fibrosis) from cirrhosis (severe fibrosis) [164]. This study has been severely criticized not only on the basis of the lack of metabolite identification, but also for the statistical methods employed for data analysis [122].

Animal models have also been employed. TAA has been administered i.p. to rats to generate experimental fibrosis and cirrhosis. One such study tracked serum and urine by ^{1}H NMR metabolomics over 7 weeks of TAA administration. Liver injury included fibrosis and cirrhosis. TAA was found to increase 2-oxoglutarate and decrease succinate in both serum and urine, while urinary excretion of fumarate, oxaloacetate, and citrate was increased, leading investigators to conclude that TAA impaired the TCA cycle [165]. These and other reported amino acid changes are not specific to fibrosis or cirrhosis. The i.p. administration of dimethylnitrosamine (DMN) to rats produces histologically confirmed fibrosis. UPLC-ESI-QTOFMS metabolomics on serum from control and DMN-treated rats, together with serum from rats treated with DMN together with Yin-Chen-Hao-Tang decoction (YCHT), a TCM long used in the treatment of liver diseases including fibrosis. Biochemical parameters including serum liver enzymes and total bilirubin, together with liver histology, in the YCHT treated rats were intermediate between the controls and the DMN-treated animals. Moreover, several serum lipids, including LPC(18:1), LPC(18:2), oleic acid (18:1), linoleic acid (18:2), arachidonic acid (20:4), and docosahexaenoic acid (22:6; DHA) that were altered by DMN treatment (LPCs ↑, fatty acids ↓), remained relatively stable with co-administration of YCHT [166]. Despite these lipidomic findings, the antifibrotic mechanism of YCHT remains unclear. Another TCM that has been evaluated in the DMN rat liver fibrosis model is Huangqi Decoction (HQD). In these experiments, 16 individual bile acids were profiled by LC-MS and demonstrated that bile acids were elevated by DMN treatment and that HQD restored these to normal levels. Additionally, gene expression related to bile acid synthesis and transport was examined, and also altered by DMN treatment, but restored by HQD [167].

Carbon tetrachloride (CCl4) is another hepatotoxin that can produce liver fibrosis in rats. Its effects upon the serum metabolome of rats has been reported using UPLC-ESI-QTOFMS. The protocol involved 12 weeks twice weekly s.c. injections of 50% CCl4 in olive oil at a dose of 5 mL/kg. Blood biochemistry and liver histology were consistent with liver fibrosis. Of the many prominent metabolites detected, two, i.e., cervonoyl ethanolamide (8,11,14-eicosatrienoyl ethanolamide) and β-muricholic acid, were defined as biomarker candidates. Pathway analysis proposed that CCl4 induction of liver fibrosis altered glycerophospholipid metabolism, linoleic acid metabolism, α-linoleic acid metabolism, glycine, serine and threonine metabolism, arachidonic acid metabolism, tryptophan metabolism, and aminoacyl-tRNA biosynthesis [168]. This provided a paradigm for chemically-induced liver fibrosis against which other studies could be compared. CCl4 has also been employed to induce decompensated cirrhosis with ascites in rats, using a similar protocol that that described above. In this study, serum and urine were analyzed by Orbitrap UPLC-MS. Aromatic amino acids, alanine, and bile acids were elevated in the CCl4-treated rats, while LPCs, eicosapentaenoic acid, creatine, carnitine, branched-chain amino acids (BCAAs), and arginine were significantly lowered [169].

The TCM used to treat liver fibrosis, Jiaqi Ganxian Granule (JGG), was tested against CCl4-induced hepatic fibrosis in rats. As the mechanism was unknown, detailed UPLC-ESI-QTOFMS metabolomics was conducted on rat serum. Fibrosis markers in serum, namely collagen type IV, procollagen III, hyaluronic acid, and laminin were all significantly increased by CCl4, but normalized by JGG intervention, as was liver histology. Lipid markers that were downregulated by CCl4, but normalized by JGG included sphinganine, dihydroceramide, and monostearoylglycerol. Metabolites that were upregulated by CCl4 but normalized by JGG were the bile acid 3,7-dihydroxy-12-oxocholanoic acid, the phosphatidylinositol PI(18:0/16:0), the ethanolamide metabolite of DHA, LPC(22:6), and PC(20:4/18:2). JGG, therefore, affected sphingolipid and glycerophospholipid metabolism among other pathways [170]. These represent further examples of where metabolomics has informed about the mechanism of action of a TCM on liver disease. A similar study reported in Chinese that *Scutellariae* Radix decoction, prepared from the root of a flowering plant of the mint family, and baicalin, a flavone glycoside purified from *Scutellaria baicalensis*, were effective against liver fibrosis in this rat model. UPLC-ESI-QTOFMS analysis showed that several elevated metabolites in fibrotic rat urine were ameliorated by the decoction treatment, including, L-tryptophan, 3-methyldioxyindole, 5-hydroxyindoleacetylglycine, kynurenic acid, 4-(2-amino-3-hydroxyphenyl)-2,4-dioxobutanoic acid, methylmalonic acid, and L-leucine. Baicalin treatment also reversed these urinary metabolites with the exception of L-leucine [171]. Another rat model of fibrosis uses dimethylnitrosamine (DMN) i.p. administration over a period of 8 weeks. Cultured bear bile powder (CBBP) has been used as a TCM to treat liver diseases for thousands of years. Using Orbitrap UPLC-MS, it was reported that CBBP co-administration (65, 130 and 260 mg/kg) restored the lowered serum concentrations of eicosapentaenoic and docosahexaenoic acids that occurred when DMN provoked fibrosis. CBBP had the additional effect of inducing the expression of the nuclear receptors PPARα and PPARγ. Moreover, expression of four PPARα-regulated genes involved in fatty acid β-oxidation (*Cpt1b*, *Cpt2*, *Mcad*, and *Hadha*) was decreased by DMN treatment but restored by CBBP, suggesting that CBBP may improve fatty acid β-oxidation. By inducing PPARγ, CBBP decreased the downstream expression of the inflammatory cytokine IL-6, while also inhibiting activation of hepatic stellate cells, thereby ameliorating fibrogenesis [172]. Further details of the aforementioned studies appear in Table 3.

Table 3. Metabolomic and lipidomic biomarkers of liver fibrosis and cirrhosis.

Species	Manipulation/Condition	Pathology	Analytical Methodology	Metabolites Reported	Ref.
Human	NAFLD	Fibrosis progression	CE-TOFMS LC-TOFMS	F0/F1→F4 Etiocholanolone sulfate↓ Dehydroepiandrosterone sulfate↓ 16α-hydroxy-dehydroepiandrosterone sulfate↑ (all in serum)	[119]
Human	Fibrosis or Cirrhosis	Significant fibrosis, advanced fibrosis, cirrhosis	^{1}H NMR	No metabolites reported, only multivariate model used to distinguish pathologies.	[121]
Human	Chronic hepatitis B	Cirrhosis	UPLC-QTOFMS	Glycocholic acid↑ Glycochenodeoxycholic acid↑ Taurocholic acid↑ Taurochenodeoxycholic acid↑ (all in serum)	[127]
Human	Chronic hepatitis B	Cirrhosis	GC-MS	Acetate↑ Hexanoate↑ Butanoate↑ Glucose↓ Sorbitol↓ (all in serum)	[128]
Human	Causes not stated	Cirrhosis	2D-GC-TOFMS	D-Alanine↑ D-Proline↑ D-Valine↑ D-Leucine↑ D-Threonine↑ (all in serum)	[129]
Human	HBV, HCV, alcohol	Cirrhosis	UPLC-QTOFMS	Chenodeoxycholic acid↓ 7-Ketolithocholic acid↓ Urobilin↓ Urobilinogen↓ LPC(16:0)↑ LPC(18:0)↑ LPC(18:1)↑ LPC(18:2)↑ (all in feces)	[131]
Human	HBV, alcohol, PBC, cryptogenic cirrhosis	Cirrhosis	UPLC-TQMS	Taurocholic acid↑ Taurochenodeoxycholic acid↑ Tauroursodeoxycholic acid↑ Glycocholic acid↑ Ursodeoxycholic acid↑ Chenodeoxycholic acid↑ Cholic acid↑ Taurolithocholic acid↑ Taurodeoxycholic acid↑ Hyodeoxycholic acid↑ Lithocholic acid↑ Deoxycholic acid↑ (all in serum)	[132]

Table 3. *Cont.*

Species	Manipulation/Condition	Pathology	Analytical Methodology	Metabolites Reported	Ref.
Human	Chronic hepatitis C	Cirrhosis	GC-MS	Proline↑ Serine↑ Glycine↑ Threonine↑ Citrate↑ Xylitol↓ Arabinose↓ Urea↓ **(all in urine)**	[134]
Human	Chronic hepatitis B	Cirrhosis	UPLC-QTOFMS	Phenylalanine↑ Glycochenodeoxycholic acid↑ Oleamide↑ LPC(16:0)↓ PC(16:0/18:2)↓ PC(16:0/22:6)↓ PC(16:0/20:4)↓ PC(18:0/18:2)↓ Canavaninosuccinate↓ **(all in serum)**	[135]
Human	Hepatorenal syndrome	Cirrhosis	UPLC-TQMS	4-Acetamidobutanoate↑ **(in plasma)**	[138]
Human	Chronic hepatitis B	Cirrhosis	^{1}H NMR UPLC-QTOFMS	Tyrosine↑ Oxaloacetate↑ Phenylalanine↑ C16-Sphinganine↑ Phytosphingosine↑ Isobutyrate↑ LPC(18:1) ↑ Linoelaidic acid↑ Bilirubin↑ PC(18:4/20:1)↓ PC(14:1/14:1)↓ LPC(16:0)↓ Formate↓ Ascorbate↓ Carnitine↓ α-CEHC↓ **(all in serum)**	[139]
Human	Causes not stated	Decompensated cirrhosis (90-day mortality vs. survivors)	^{1}H NMR UPLC-QTOFMS	Isoleucine↑ Leucine↑ Lactate↑ Creatinine↑ Urea↑ Tyrosine↑ Histidine↑ Phenylalanine↑ Formate↑ LPC(16:0) ↑ Pyruvate↓ Choline↓ Phosphocholine↓ Glycine↓ Glucose↓ PC(34:2)↓ PC(18:2/18:2)↓ PC(16:0/18:2)↓ PC(18:0/18:2)↓ LPC(18:2)↓ PC(18:2/18:5)↓ PC(22:5/20:4)↓ PI(37:2)↓ PS(41:4)↓ **(all in plasma)**	[140]
Human	Causes not stated	Cirrhosis	UPLC-Orbitrap MS	16α-Hydroxyestrone↑ 4-Androstenedione↓ 17α-Hydroxyprogesterone↓ 18-Hydroxycorticosterone↓ Cortisol↓ Cortexolone↓ Allotetrahydrocortisol↓ Deoxycorticosterone↓ Epitestosterone↓ Testosterone↓ Dehydroepiandrosterone↓ Etiocholanolone↓ Tetrahydrodeoxycortisol↓ Androsterone↓ 17α-Hydroxypregnenolone↓ Epiandrosterone↓ 11-Oxoetiocholanolone↓ 7β-Hydroxy-dehydroepiandrosterone↓ Androstenetriol↓ Androstenediol↓ Pregnanediol↓ **(all in urine)**	[141]
Human	Chronic hepatitis B	Cirrhosis (vs. HBV)	GC-TOFMS	Serine↑ 5-Oxoproline↑ Phenylalanine↑ Tyrosine↑ Ornithine↑ Citrate↑ Palmitic acid↑ Fructose↓ Glutamate↓ Indole-3-acetic acid↓ arachidonic acid↓ 2-Deoxy-D-glucose↓ **(all in serum)**	[142]
Human	Chronic hepatitis B	Cirrhosis (vs. HBV/HV)	UPLC-TQMS	9,10-DiHOME↑ 13-HODE↑ TXB2↓ **(all in serum)**	[144]

Table 3. *Cont.*

Species	Manipulation/Condition	Pathology	Analytical Methodology	Metabolites Reported	Ref.
Human	Chronic hepatitis B	Cirrhosis (GDSR and GSYX patterns, vs. latent pattern (LP))	GC-TOFMS	GDSR vs. LP: Nonanoate↑ Urea↓ Serine↓ 2-Hydroxybutyrate↓ 2-Hydroxyglutarate↓ Phenylalanine↓ Asparagine↓ Citrulline↓ Tyrosine↓ Arabinose↓ Sorbose↓ Fructose↓ Myristate↓ Palmitolate↓ Palmitate↓ Linolate↓ Tryptamine↓ Glycolate↓ Quinate↓ Petroselinate↓ GSYX vs. LP: 1,5-Anhydrosorbitol↑ Fructose↑ 2-Hydroxybutyrate↓ Serine↓ Threonine↓ 5-Oxoglutarate↓ 2-Hydroxyglutarate↓ Phenylalanine↓ Asparagine↓ Tyrosine↓ Arabinose↓ Arabitol↓ Nonanoate↓ Glycerate↓ Pipecolate↓ Glutarate↓ Quinate↓ α-Tocopherol↓ **(all in serum)**	[146]
Human	Biliary atresia (BA) and neonatal hepatitis syndrome (NHS)	Fibrosis F1 to F4	UPLC-TQMS	BA/NHS: Histamine↑ Methionine↓ Phenylalanine↓ Serine↓ Threonine↓ Valine↓ Glutamine↓ Sarcosine↓ Lysine↓ F4>F3>F1/F2 in BA: Histamine↑ **(all in liver homogenates)**	[147]
Human	Alcohol	Cirrhosis ± minimal hepatic encephalopathy (MHE)	¹H NMR	MHE+/MHE-: Lactate↑ Glucose↑ TMAO↑ Glycerol↑ LDL↓ VLDL↓ Isoleucine↓ Leucine↓ Valine↓ Alanine↓ Acetoacetate↓ Choline↓ Glycine↓ **(all in serum)**	[148]
Human	Chronic hepatitis C, Chronic hepatitis B, Alcohol, Autoimmunity	Cirrhosis	MAS ¹H NMR	Phosphoethanolamine↑ Phosphocholine↑ Glutamate↑ Aspartate↓ α-Glucose↓ β-Glucose↓ **(all in liver)**	[149]
Human	ALD, NASH	Cirrhosis	¹H NMR	ALD Cirrhosis: Isoleucine↑ Valine↑ 1,2-Propanediol↑ Succinate↑ Aspartate↑ Betaine↑ Lactate↑ Glucose↑ Uracil↑ Phenylalanine↑ NASH Cirrhosis: Leucine↑ Isoleucine↑ Valine↑ 1,2-Propanediol↑ Succinate↑ Aspartate↑ Betaine↑ Lactate↑ Phenylalanine↑ Uracil↑ Uridine↓ Inosine↓ **(all in liver)**	[150]
Human	Causes not stated	Cirrhosis	¹H NMR	Acetate↑ Pyruvate↑ Glutamine↑ α-Ketoglutarate↑ Taurine↑ Glycerol↑ Tyrosine↑ 1-Methylhistidine↑ Phenylalanine↑ N-Acetylglycoproteins↑ LDL↓ VLDL↓ Isoleucine↓ Leucine↓ Valine↓ Acetoacetate↓ Choline↓ **(all in serum)**	[151]

Table 3. *Cont.*

Species	Manipulation/Condition	Pathology	Analytical Methodology	Metabolites Reported	Ref.
Human	Alcohol	Cirrhosis (mild vs. severe liver failure)	^{1}H NMR	Correlated with severity of liver failure: 3-Hydroxybutyrate↑ Alanine↑ Acetate↑ Choline/Phosphocholine↑ (**all in serum**)	[152]
Human	Chronic hepatitis B	Cirrhosis (compensated vs. decompensated)	^{1}H NMR	Distinguishing between compensated and decompensated cirrhosis: Succinate, Pyruvate, Phenylalanine, Histidine, Lysine, Glutamine, Acetone, Glutamate, Creatine, Alanine (**all in serum**)	[153]
Human	Causes not stated	Cirrhosis	^{1}H NMR	Positively correlated with portal blood proinflammatory cytokines IL6, TNFα and IL1β: Trimethylamine. Negatively correlated with portal blood proinflammatory cytokines IL6, TNFα and IL1β: Acetate, n-Heptanoate. Positively correlated with WBC and platelet counts: Threonine, α-Galactose, β-Glucose (**all in feces**)	[156]
Human	Various liver injuries	Cirrhosis (compensated vs. decompensated)	UPLC-QTOFMS	Lower in LC: N^6-Methyladenosine, 1-Methyluric acid, Cinnamic acid, Decenoylcarnitine, Phenacetylglutamine (**all in urine**)	[158]
Human	Various etiologies, incl. HBV, HCV, alcohol, NASH	Cirrhosis US vs. Turkish (TR) population (dietary)	^{1}H NMR	Lactate (Controls and Decompensated; TR>US), Glucose (Controls and Decompensated; US>TR) (**all in plasma**)	[159]
Human	Alcohol	Acute-on-chronic liver failure (ACLF) vs. stable compensated or decompensated cirrhosis (CLF)	^{1}H NMR	ACLF > CLF: 3-Hydroxybutyrate, Lactate, Acetoacetate, Pyruvate, Glutamine, Glutamate, Creatinine, Tyrosine, Phenylalanine (**all in serum**)	[160]
Human	Causes not stated	Stable cirrhosis (C) ± encephalopathy (E) (C±E) and HV	^{1}H NMR	C±E > HV: Lactate, Pyruvate, Alanine, Threonine, Glycine, Aspartate, Acetoacetate, 3-Hydroxybutyrate, Phenylalanine, Tyrosine, Methionine, Glutamate, Methylamine, Dimethylamine, TMAO, Glycerol. C±E < HV: Valine, Glutamine, Histidine, Arginine. E > HV: Leucine, Isoleucine. C > HV: Myoinositol (**all in plasma**)	[161]

Table 3. *Cont.*

Species	Manipulation/Condition	Pathology	Analytical Methodology	Metabolites Reported	Ref.
Human	Alcohol, HBV or HCV, NASH	Hepatic encephalopathy (HE), cirrhosis (C), neurological patients without liver disease (NP), HV	UPLC-Orbitrap MS	HE > NP: 13x *N*-Acetyl metabolites, 5x Glutamate/Glutamine metabolites, 4x Methionine metabolites, 4x Phenylalanine metabolites, 6x Tryptophan metabolites, 6x Fatty acid metabolites, Pyruvate, 5x Amino acid derivatives, 2x Dipeptides, 3x Bile acids, 3x Nucleoside derivatives, Dihydrothymine, 4x Alcohols and polyols, Ribitol/Arabitol, Cortisol, Pyridoxic acid, Phenyl sulfate HE < NP: Alanine, Taurine, Anhydro sorbitol, Levulinic acid **(both in CSF and plasma)** HE > C: 9x *N*-Acetyl metabolites, Phenacetylglutamine, 2x Methionine metabolites, 2x Phenylalanine metabolites, 3x Tryptophan metabolites, 4x Fatty acid metabolites, Citrulline, 2x Dipeptides, Taurocholic acid, 3x Nucleosides and derivatives, Anhydro sorbitol, 2x Alcohols, Ribitol/Arabitol, Cortisol, Phenyl sulfate HE < C: Methionine sulfoxide, Levulinic acid **(all in plasma)**	[162]
Human	Chronic hepatitis C	Fibrosis (F4 vs. F0)	^{1}H NMR	F4 vs. F0: VLDL↑ Citrate↑ Glucose↑ Phenylalanine↑ LDL↓ HDL↓ Choline↓ Acetoacetate↓ Isoleucine/Leucine↓ Creatinine/Creatine↓ Glutamate↓ Glutamine↓ Asparagine↓ Valine↓ Lysine↓ Cysteine↓ Glycerol↓ Arginine↓ Histidine↓ 3-Hydroxybutyrate↓ **(all in serum)**	[163]
Rat	TAA	Fibrosis/Cirrhosis vs. controls	^{1}H NMR	3-Hydroxybutyrate↑ Acetoacetate↑ Butyrate↑ Choline↑ Glycine↑ Alanine↑ Leucine↑ Lysine↑ Succinate↑ Valine↑ 2-Oxoglutarate↓ Acetate↓ Adipate↓ Dimethylglycine↓ Lactate↓ Pyruvate↓ TMAO↓ Tyrosine↓ **(all in serum)** 1-Methylhistidine↑ 3-Hydroxybutyrate↑ Acetate↑ Alanine↑ Butyrate↑ Choline↑ Creatinine↑ Hippurate↑ Isoleucine↑ Pyruvate↑ Succinate↑ Taurine↑ TMAO↑ Tryptophan↑ Valine↑ 2-Hydroxybutyrate↓ 2-Oxoglutarate↓ Acetoacetate↓ Acetone↓ Adipate↓ Citrate↓ Dimethylamine↓ Dimethylglycine↓ Fumarate↓ Methylamine↓ Oxaloacetate↓ Sarcosine↓ Trimethylamine↓ **(all in urine)**	[165]

Table 3. *Cont.*

Species	Manipulation/Condition	Pathology	Analytical Methodology	Metabolites Reported	Ref.
Rat	Dimethylnitrosamine	Fibrosis	UPLC-QTOFMS	LPC(18:1) ↑ LPC(18:2) ↑ LPC(20:4)↓ FA(22:6)↓ FA(20:4)↓ FA(18:1)↓ FA(18:2)↓ **(all in serum)**	[166]
Rat	Dimethylnitrosamine	Fibrosis	UPLC-QTOFMS	Cholic acid↑ Deoxycholic acid↑ Ursodeoxycholic acid↑ Chenodeoxycholic acid↑ Hyodeoxycholic acid↑ Lithocholic acid↑ Taurocholic acid↑ Taurodeoxycholic acid↑ Tauroursodeoxycholic acid↑ Taurochenodeoxycholic acid↑ Taurohyodeoxycholic acid↑ Taurolithocholic acid↑ Glycocholic acid↑ Glycodeoxycholic acid↑ Glycoursodeoxycholic acid↑ Glycochenodeoxycholic acid↑ **(all in serum)**	[167]
Rat	CCl_4	Fibrosis	UPLC-QTOFMS	Cervonoyl ethanolamide↑ β-Muricholic acid↑ **(all in serum)**	[168]
Rat	CCl_4	Decompensated cirrhosis/ascites	UPLC-Orbitrap MS	Alanine↑ Phenylalanine↑ Tryptophan↑ Tyrosine↑ Nutriacholic acid↑ LPC(16:0)↓ LPC(18:0)↓ LPC(18:2)↓ FA(20:5)↓ Carnitine↓ Creatine↓ Valine↓ Isoleucine↓ Arginine↓ **(all in serum)** Glutamyltaurine↑ 4,6-Dihydroxyquinoline↑ Phenylalanine↑ TMAO↑ 3-Methyldioxyindole↑ 1,2,3-Trihydroxybenzene↑ Tryptophan↑ Histamine↑ Tyrosine↑ Pantothenic acid↑ 2-Phenylglycine↑ Proline↑ N^6,N^6,N^6-Trimethyllysine↑ Dopamine↑ Phenacetylglycine↓ Creatinine↓ Creatine↓ 4-Acetamidobutanoate↓ Indole↓ Carnitine↓ **(all in urine)**	[169]
Rat	CCl_4	Fibrosis	UPLC-QTOFMS	12-Ketochenodeoxycholic acid↑ PI(18:0/16:0) ↑ Cervonoyl ethanolamide↑ LPC(18:2)↑ LPC(22:6)↑ PC(18:1/16:0)↑ PC(18:2/16:0)↑ PC(20:4/18:2)↑ PC(22:6/18:1)↑ Creatine↓ Sphinganine↓ Dihydroceramide↓ 8-HETE↓ LPC(18:0)↓ LPC(20:1)↓ LPC(22:0)↓ **(all in serum)**	[170]
Rat	Dimethylnitrosamine	Fibrosis	UPLC-Orbitrap MS	Leucine↓ LPC(16:0)↓ LPC(16:0)↓ LPC(18:0)↓ LPC(20:1)↓ LPC(20:4)↓ LPC(22:6)↓ FA(16:0)↓ FA(18:0)↓ FA(20:4)↓ FA(20:5)↓ FA(22:6)↓ All-*trans*-retinoic acid↓ Bilirubin↓ **(all in serum)**	[172]
Rat	CCl_4	Fibrosis	^{1}H NMR	2-Oxoglutarate↓ Citrate↓ Dimethylamine↓ Creatinine↓ Phenacetylglycine↓ Hippurate↓ Taurine↑ **(all in urine)**	[123]
Rat	CCl_4	Fibrosis	^{1}H NMR	Glucose↓ Lactate↑ Fumarate↓ NADPH↓ Succinate↑ Acetate↑ 3-Hydroxybutyrate↓ UDP-glucose↑ UDP-galactose↑ **(in serum and liver)**	[125]

5.4. NAFL and NASH

Nonalcoholic fatty liver disease (NAFLD) is the most common liver disorder in Western countries, affecting 17–46% of adults. NAFLD includes two pathologically-distinct conditions with different prognoses: nonalcoholic fatty liver (NAFL) and nonalcoholic steatohepatitis (NASH). "NAFLD is characterized by excessive hepatic fat accumulation, associated with insulin resistance (IR), and defined by the presence of steatosis in >5% of hepatocytes according to histological analysis" [173]. The diagnosis of NAFLD requires the exclusion of chronic alcohol consumption as a cause. NASH is characterized by the presence of steatosis, inflammation, and ballooning degeneration of hepatocytes, with or without fibrosis [174]. NASH can progress to cirrhosis in up to 20% of cases [173,174]. The definitive diagnosis of NASH requires a liver biopsy [173]. A number of biomarkers of NAFLD have been evaluated, including fatty liver index (FLI), NAFLD liver fat score (NAFLD-LFS), hepatic steatosis index (HSI), visceral adiposity index (VAI), and triglyceride x glucose (TyG) index. When steatosis was histologically graded as none (<5%), mild (5–33%), moderate (33-66%), and severe (>66%), with the exception of VAI, all biomarkers showed a linear trend across the steatosis grades. The authors concluded, "More research is needed to identify truly independent and quantitative markers of steatosis" [175]. Metabolomics, therefore, has a role to play in delivering biomarkers for steatosis and its progression. Recently, it has been argued that NAFLD patients should be classified into different subtypes dependent upon perturbation of the principal pathways regulating fatty acid homeostasis. Specific serum lipid signatures can be associated with individual mechanisms of progression from steatosis to NASH, and possibly lead to novel and specific NASH therapies [176]. Such metabolomic approaches that help refine definition of the disease phenotype have now been integrated into orthogonal technologies, such as genomics, proteomics, structural biology, imaging [177], and metagenomics.

Investigation of both NAFL and NASH in a metabolomic context is a relatively recent endeavor. Because of the nature of the disease, many investigators have focused on the lipidome. Until a decade ago, the plasma lipidome of NAFLD and whether or not NASH expressed a distinct lipidomic signature were unknown. An early US study examined plasma lipid profiles in both NAFL and NASH compared to healthy controls (HV), and reported significantly increased monounsaturated fatty acids (MUFAs) with an altered pattern of polyunsaturated fatty acids (PUFAs) in both NAFL and NASH. Moreover, the progression of NAFL to NASH was characterized by an increase in the lipoxygenase metabolites 5-HETE, 8-HETE, and 15-HETE. Interestingly, the nonenzymic oxidation product of arachidonic acid, 11-HETE, was significantly increased only in NASH [178]. A Spanish group reported an altered pattern of serum phosphocholines and potentially antioxidant lyso plasmalogens [PC(P-24:0/0:0) and PC(P-22:0/0:0)] in NASH compared to stage 3 hepatic steatosis. Several sphingolipids were also altered in NAFLD compared with healthy subjects. Furthermore, arachidonic acid and glutamate were both decreased in NASH. Metabolic profiling by these authors of an animal model for NAFLD (glycine N-methyltransferase *Gnmt*-null mice) produced finding consistent with the patient observations [179]. Serum lyso plasmalogens are therefore potential biomarkers for NASH. Another US study of NAFL, NASH and HV found that NAFLD patients had perturbed glutathione metabolism compared to HV, with markedly higher conjugated primary bile acids in plasma. NASH patients displayed lower long-chain fatty acids, higher carnitine and short-chain acyl carnitines, together with several other metabolites. While the metabolomic fingerprints could distinguish NAFL or NASH from HV, they could not distinguish between NAFL and NASH [180]. A ^{1}H NMR-based study in China investigated NAFLD patients and HV, together with mice fed a methionine- and choline-deficient (MCD) diet as a model for NAFLD. Based upon both clinical and animal model findings, four potential biomarkers of NAFLD were proposed: serum glucose, lactate, glutamate/glutamine, and taurine [181]. None of these "usual suspects" provides a basis for evaluating the progression of NAFLD due to lack of specificity. A dietary intervention study in US patients with NAFL examined the effect of insulin sensitivity on the plasma metabolome in NAFL. The pattern of LPCs, in particular LPC(16:0), which was significantly lower in insulin resistant NAFL patients (see Table 4), was put forward to potentially provide biomarkers for NAFL-associated insulin resistance [182]. Serum BA concentrations have also been investigated in

NASH and reported to be elevated both fasting and after a fatty breakfast designed to contract the gall bladder. Elevated fasting BAs included secondary BAs, which are formed by dihydroxylation of primary BAs by gut microbiota species belonging to the orders *Bacteroides, Clostridium,* and *Escherichia,* which may be increased in the dysbiosis associated with NAFLD. Altered patterns of circulating BAs in NASH may contribute to hepatic damage [183]. The pattern of BCAAs and acyl carnitines has been investigated in liver samples from healthy subjects, NAFL, fatty NASH, and nonfatty NASH. Hepatic valine was decreased in NAFL, and all BCAAs and phenylalanine were elevated in NASH, with and without steatosis. Certain carnitine esters were elevated in NAFLD (see Table 4). The findings were interpreted as due to oxidative stress and inflammation in the liver [184]. None of these findings yielded a suitably specific biomarker of NASH or its progression. A US group examined whether or not arachidonic acid-derived eicosanoids could distinguish between NAFL and NASH, since lipotoxicity is a key component of the progression of NAFL to NASH. Several such lipids were altered between NAFL and NASH, including elevated PGE2, 13,14-dihydro-15-keto-PGD2, 11,12-diHETrE, 14,15-diHETrE and attenuated 15-HETE (Table 4). It was reported that 11,12-diHETrE, 13,14-dihydro-15-keto-PGD2 and eicosatetraenedioic acid (20-COOH AA) were the top candidate biomarkers to distinguish NASH from NAFL with an area under the receiver operating characteristic curve (AUROC) of 1 for 11,12-diHETrE and 1 for the combination of 13,14-dihydro-15-keto-PGD2 and 20-COOH AA [185]. If confirmed in other studies, these findings would have great potential as biomarkers for NASH in NAFLD. Another potential distinction between NAFL and NASH are ketone bodies, such as acetoacetate and 3-hydroxybutyrate, which are produced in the liver from fatty acids. NASH patients were found to have lower serum ketone bodies than NAFL patients, with a lower serum total free fatty acid level (Table 4) [186]. Although these findings contribute to an understanding of NASH pathogenesis, they are not useful for the generation of biomarkers of NASH. Examination of increasing severity of NAFL in obese patients revealed α-ketoglutarate as the principal marker of NAFL (Table 4) [187]. With a specificity of only 62.5%, α-ketoglutarate is unlikely to be a biomarker for NAFL. Patients undergoing bariatric surgery that have a wedge liver biopsy taken routinely during surgery have been investigated with lipidomics and metabolomics. Patients were classified histologically as non-NASH, non-NAFLD, NAFL, and NASH. *PNPLA3* I148M (isoleucine→methionine) variant was also determined that is more common in NASH. Discovery and validation cohorts were also used. A strong negative correlation was reported between the number of TG double bonds and the TG concentrations in NASH relative to non-NASH livers, for both discovery and validation cohorts. A "NASH ClinLipMet score" was developed based upon (i) clinical variables, (ii) *PNPLA3* genotype, (iii) lipidomic data and (iv) metabolomic data. This was highest performing combination biomarker with sensitivity of 85.5% and specificity of 72.1% for NASH (Table 4) [188]. In terms of biomarker discovery, the large amount of data were derived only from liver biopsies, and so there are no indications how parts (iii) and (iv) of the aforementioned NASH ClinLipMet score relate to, and can be determined from, serum or plasma. A small clinical study was conducted in liver samples from control, NAFL, and NASH patients in which lipidomic analyses were conducted in liver biopsies. These authors identified a signature comprising 32 lipids that distinguished NASH with 100% specificity and sensitivity. This signature comprised various phospholipids, sphingolipids, fatty acids, triglycerides, and cholesteryl esters, measured by LC-MS, which we do not believe could represent a viable biomarker for NASH due to its complexity. Furthermore, five fatty acids were identified as accumulating in NASH that were demonstrated to be toxic to HepG2 cells and primary human hepatocytes in culture (see Table 4) [189]. A Chinese urinary metabolomics study compared NAFL patients with normal liver function with NASH patients with abnormal liver function. Many discriminating metabolites were reported (Table 4) [190], although none displayed a large fold-change or was seen as highly specific to NASH. An elegant study was reported containing several large clinical cohorts containing biopsy-proven NASH patients that also had liver fat determined by CT. Serum metabolomics identified the top metabolite associated with liver fat as a mass of 202.1185⁺. Databases contained a large number of hits for this mass and so a GWAS strategy was adopted yielding SNPs for the *AGXT2* gene whose expressed enzyme produces a metabolite, dimethylguanidino valeric acid (DMGV), which matched this mass [191]. In terms of a biomarker for NASH or NAFL, DMGV displayed a wide overlap between control and NASH with approx. 20% higher mean value for NASH. This is not a viable biomarker and perhaps other ions in their "Top-20" [191] should be investigated. Other investigators chose a single biomarker for progression of NAFL to NASH, i.e. pyroglutamate (5-oxoproline), based upon a serum metabolomic study. 5-Oxoproline had a higher AUROC value than adiponectin, TNF-α, or IL-8 [192]. The utility of 5-oxoproline as a biomarker for NASH is doubtful, as it is often found to be elevated in relation to hepatic oxidative stress. We have recently reported a highly statistically significant upregulation of 5-oxoproline in HepG2 cells treated with the experimental anti-HCV drug [193], in the liver of whole-body γ-irradiated mice [194] and in γ-irradiated HepG2 cells [195].

An in vivo MRS technique has been applied to patients with biopsy-proven NAFL or NASH. Both high-field ^{1}H and ultra-high-field ^{31}P MRS were employed. Many MRS alterations correlated with NASH, mostly with advanced fibrosis, e.g. phosphoethanolamine/total phosphorus (TP) ratio. ATP/TP declined in advanced fibrosis and ATP flux was lower in NASH [155]. While these rapid noninvasive techniques are useful in a research setting, it is still premature to evaluate their diagnostic potential for NASH. A lipidomic study of patients with chronic hepatitis B virus infection (CHB) with and without NAFLD has been conducted in China. Monounsaturated triacylglycerols (TGs) were found more commonly in NASH patients than non-NASH patients [196]. However, there was considerable overlap between these groups, and examination of the raw data does not support the specificity of monounsaturated TGs, with both saturated and diunsaturated TGs associated with NASH. Patients with steatosis are known to have dysregulation of branched-chain and aromatic amino acids. A metabolomic, transcriptomic and metagenomic study of morbidly obese women with and without steatosis has been reported. The plasma metabolite phenylacetic acid produced from phenylalanine by gut microbiota was the most strongly correlated metabolite to steatosis. Mechanistic studies in human hepatocytes and in mice confirmed this association [197]. Using biopsy-proven patients with normal liver (NL), NAFL, and NASH, serum lipidomics was used to define the pattern of TGs in all three groups. Triglycerides were elevated in the order NAFL > NL $\geq$ NASH. Of the 28 TGs measured, TG(46:0), (48:0), (53:0), (44:1), (48:1), (49:1), (52:1), (53:1), (50:2), (54:5), and (58:2) were always NAFL > NL and NASH < NAFL. Satisfactory AUROC values were obtained for NAFLD vs. NL. Exclusion of patients with glucose > 136 mg/dL improved the sensitivity and specificity for NASH vs. NAFL [198]. As with all studies of this nature, there was considerable overlap between the three different clinical states in serum metabolite profiles. A lipidomic investigation in Greece reported differences between NASH, NAFL, and healthy subjects for several lipid groups and for certain free fatty acids in serum (Table 4). The authors proposed that their bioinformatic methods could distinguish between NASH, NAFL, and healthy status based upon the determination of 36 lipids, 61 glycans, and 23 fatty acids. Moreover, the authors stated that they could differentiate with very high accuracy (up to 90%) using 10–20 total variables between these three conditions. They also reported that they could robustly discriminate between the presence of fibrosis or not using a model containing 10 lipid species [199]. It is unclear to us at this time how such a complex procedure could be adapted to routine clinical diagnosis.

A large study in Germany measured plasma and urine metabolomic profiles across a wide range of liver fat content (LFC) that had been determined by MRI in 769 selected nondiabetic patients. A wide number of metabolites correlated both positively and negatively with LFC (Table 4). Usual positive associations included BCAAs and aromatic amino acids and their metabolites. A more unusual metabolite correlating with LFC was 7α-hydroxy-3-oxo-4-cholestenoate [200], which is a metabolite in the primary bile acid synthesis pathway. Unfortunately, its utility as a potential biomarker for NAFLD is reduced by its occurrence in sterol 27-hydroxylase deficiency, familial hypercholanemia and Zellweger syndrome. A Mexican study targeted 31 acyl carnitines and 7 amino acids in relation to obesity and NAFLD. No biomarkers of NAFLD per se were reported [201]. A search for plasma biomarkers of visceral adipose tissue and hepatic triglyceride content (HTGC) has been reported. A significant number of plasma phospholipids were associated with HTGC (Table 4). Similar findings have been reported by other groups. The aromatic amino acids tyrosine and tryptophan were also positively associated with HTGC [202]. No useful biomarkers for NAFL emerged from this study.

As stated earlier, redox changes in the liver can contribute to both steatosis (NAFL) and hyperuricemia (HU). It has been observed that HU often progresses together with NAFLD, and this has stimulated a metabolomic investigation of HU, HU that progressed to HU with NAFLD within one year, HU with NAFLD, and healthy controls. The principal serum changes were upregulated phosphatidic acid and CE(18:0) and downregulated inosine (Table 4) during progression from HU to HU plus NAFLD [203]. Unfortunately, the exact nature of the phosphatidic acid was not given by the authors, although the empirical formula cited corresponded to PA(16:0/16:0), the exact mass given did not, otherwise this could have been a potential biomarker for NAFLD.

A dual investigation in human and mouse liver was conducted in which GC-MS analysis of both human discovery and validation sets found two hepatic metabolites negatively correlated with nonalcoholic steatosis score, i.e., nicotinic acid and hydroquinone. When HFD was supplemented with nicotinic acid or hydroquinone, nicotinic acid prevented fat accumulation in mouse liver and reduced serum ALT (Table 4). The authors discussed the use of nicotinic acid as a lipid lowering agent and the potential of future such studies in identifying novel therapeutic targets for NAFLD [204]. Another dual human and mouse liver investigation conducted a metabolomic and lipidomic analysis of *Mat1a*-KO and WT mouse liver and serum. MAT1A synthesizes the methylation cofactor *S*-adenosylmethionine. *Mat1a*-KO mice spontaneously develop steatohepatitis. Based upon the *Mat1a*-KO metabolome that is associated with NASH, serum of biopsy proven NAFLD patients was also analyzed and compared with *Mat1a*-KO mouse findings. The metabolomic signature of these mice, comprising high concentrations of triglycerides, diglycerides, fatty acids, ceramides, and oxidized fatty acids, was present in serum of 49% of NAFLD patients, leading to two subtypes of patient, so-called M-subtype and non-M-subtype. Metabolite patterns also distinguished NAFL from NASH. Potential biomarkers might be used to monitor disease progression and identify novel therapeutic targets [205].

A metabolomic study of Chinese NAFLD patients with and without type-2 diabetes mellitus (T2DM) reported elevated bilirubin, various amino acids, and acyl carnitines, together with oleamide [206]. Many of these metabolic changes were confirmatory of published studies. The elevated acyl carnitines reported are consistent with impaired long-chain fatty acid β-oxidation. Interestingly, we had previously reported a three-fold elevation of plasma oleamide in HCV-positive patients versus HCV-negative subjects [207]. Apparently, these authors did not test their patients for HCV, despite the high prevalence of HCV in liver disease patients in China [208].

The metabolomics of NAFLD has also been investigated in children and adolescents. A noninvasive breath test was employed to examine 21 volatile organic compounds (VOCs). Compared with children with a normal liver, children with NAFLD had significantly greater breath concentrations of acetaldehyde, acetone, isoprene, pentane, and trimethylamine. It is highly likely that the gut microbiota plays a role in the generation of both acetaldehyde and trimethylamine. We agree with the authors that breath testing represents a potential for screening with diagnostic biomarkers of pediatric NAFLD [209]. However, many of these VOCs may not be specific to NAFLD because of the 17 VOCs identified in the caecal contents of mice, eight, including acetaldehyde, were reported for mice fed either the MCD diet or normal chow [210]. An Italian study recruited children with biopsy-proven NAFLD (64) and matched healthy controls (64). HPLC was used to measure oxidative stress markers that arose from excessive consumption of GSH [211]. In obese Hispanic-American adolescents, with and without NAFLD, untargeted high resolution mass spectrometry demonstrated changes in lipid and amino acid biochemistry with a particular effect on tyrosine metabolism (see Table 4) [212]. The effect of NAFLD with and without obesity, together with small intestine bacterial overgrowth, on the urinary metabolome was examined in Italian children. Data were reported on multiple perturbed host and gut microbiota pathways (Table 4), and in particular, on elevated urine glucose concentrations in NAFLD [213]. Again, none of the reported changes met criteria for a diagnostic biomarker, in particular, the biochemical distinctiveness of the findings. A further Italian study investigated obese adolescents with and without NAFLD. Plasma metabolomics established increases in branched-chain and aromatic amino acids, together with certain acyl carnitines in NAFLD subjects (Table 4) [214]. Although one of the elevated metabolites in NAFLD (hydroxydecenoylcarnitine) was an unusual finding, the fold difference between the two groups (±NAFLD) was small with large variances and a borderline statistical significance, reducing the opportunity to develop this as a biomarker. Obese adolescents with and without NAFL and with and without metabolic syndrome (MetS) have been studied for their salivary metabolomic changes. Several fatty acids and sugars were reported to differ between these groups (Table 4) [215]. How NAFLD was diagnosed in adolescents, whether by ultrasound or liver enzyme elevations, made a significant difference to the metabolomic findings, especially with lipid profiles, and amino acid and ketone body plasma concentrations [216]. Another NAFLD study in children and adolescents reported changes in certain plasma amino acids and phospholipids (Table 4). These authors generated a model using random forests machine learning with a sensitivity of 73% and specificity of 97% for detecting NAFLD. Random forests was applied to a combination of metabolite and clinical data, such as waist circumference, whole-body insulin sensitivity index (based on an oral glucose tolerance test) and blood triglyceride level [217].

Investigations in animal models have been used frequently to understand the mechanisms of NAFLD and to find biomarkers for disease progression. A mechanistic investigation in MCD diet fed mice with NASH, using UPLC-QTOFMS, reported significant decreases in several serum LPCs with marked increases in tauro-β-muricholate, taurocholate and 12-HETE compared with control mice. These results could be explained by the observed up- and down-regulation of several enzyme and transporter genes. The authors concluded that phospholipid and bile acid metabolism is disrupted in NASH, probably due to enhanced inflammatory signaling in the liver [218]. This group conducted a second study with mice fed MCD, in which they reported an increase in serum oleic and linoleic acids and of nonesterified fatty acids that they attributed to enhanced fatty acid release from white adipose tissue in NASH. They demonstrated that this was due to methionine deficiency and not choline deficiency [219]. Another group fed mice a different NASH-inducing diet based upon lard, cholesterol, and cholic acid. Although this was essentially a proteomic investigation, various key metabolites were measured in liver extracts and found to be altered, including predictable lipid changes, but also perturbations in methionine cycle intermediates (Table 4) [220]. Another strategy for the investigation dietary-induced NASH was reported, whereby livers from mice with a disrupted LDL receptor gene (*Ldlr*-null) that had been fed a western diet (WD; 17% energy as protein, 43% as carbohydrate, 41% as fat, and 0.2% as cholesterol; supplemented with olive oil) were examined. *Ldlr*-null mice fed regular chow served as controls. WD livers displayed a histology and gene expression profile consistent with NASH. Experiments were conducted by replacing the olive oil supplementation with DHA (22:6n-3). As Table 4 shows, multiple lipid classes were either up- or downregulated by WD + olive oil in this genetic/dietary mouse model of NASH. DHA dietary supplementation was effective at protecting against the effects of WD in this mouse line [221]. The effect of NAFLD progression on hepatic BA pools and 70 genes involved in BA homeostasis have been examined in human liver samples. Expression of *CYP7B1* mRNA and protein were highly upregulated in NASH, together with clear changes in glycine- and taurine-conjugated BAs away from the classical BA synthesis pathway towards the alternative BA synthetic pathway (Table 4). These findings were interpreted as an attempt by the liver in NASH to minimize hepatotoxicity [222]. Other investigators have used a 16-week high-fat diet (HFD with 60% calories from fat) in WT mice compared with controls on normal chow (12.7% calories from fat). This HFD regimen produced NAFLD, which was then investigated by ^{1}H NMR metabolomics in serum, liver and urine. Elevations in serum and liver glucose and lipids were reported, together with a decreased urinary excretion of amino acids (BCAAs, aromatic amino acids), energy metabolites and gut microbiota metabolites [223]. A similar study has been reported in which the mouse sera were analyzed by UPLC-QTOFMS and GC-MS. Glucose was elevated and GSH attenuated after HFD-induced NAFL. Several serum metabolites were altered and related to oxidative stress, inflammation, and mitochondrial dysfunction (Table 4) [224]. Although this was a detailed account of the effects of HFD-NAFLD on the metabolome, the findings do not lend themselves readily as biomarkers of NAFLD for reasons of specificity. A different diet feeding regimen has been used to generate NAFLD in the mouse without obesity. This procedure used a high-fat, high-cholesterol, cholate diet (HFDCC) and both liver and plasma were analyzed by GC-TOFMS and UPLC-QTOFMS. Total cholesterol and CE(16:1), (18:1), (18:2), (18:3), (20:1), (20:3), (20:4), (22:5), (22:6) were elevated in liver, together with cholic acid, DGs, TGs, CERs, SMs, LPCs, the PC/PE ratio, while PEs were downregulated. The nonlipid metabolites xylitol, xanthosine, squalene, and phenylethylamine were elevated in liver tissue of HFDCC-fed mice. Citrate, G-1-P, and saccharic acid were all downregulated in these livers. Subtle differences were reported for plasma of HFDCC-fed mice, including elevated total cholesterol, CE(16:1), (18:1), (18:2), (18:3), (20:1), (20:3), (20:4), (22:5), cholic acid, deoxycholic acid, CERs, SMs, and PEs, while FFAs, glycerol, TGs, and LPEs were all diminished in pathological livers [225]. Xanthosine, the ribonucleoside of xanthine, could be a potential biomarker when evaluated in patients. However, it was elevated in liver and its levels in plasma were not reported. Moreover, xanthosine has been reported to be a urinary biomarker for nephropathy in T2DM patients [226] thereby reducing its specificity.

A further means of producing features of NASH in the mouse is with 5-diethoxycarbonyl-1,4-dihydrocollidine (DDC). The three mouse strains A/J, C57BL/6J and PWD/PhJ were placed on a diet supplemented with 0.1% DDC or a control diet for 8 weeks. Livers were analyzed for 44 metabolites by targeted MS methods and also subjected to proteomic and RNA-Seq analyses, which showed that many pathways were altered by DDC treatment, in particular, arachidonic acid and S-adenosylmethionine metabolism. However, after Bonferroni correction of their findings for multiple comparisons, the following hepatic metabolites were elevated by DDC: putrescine, arginine, citrulline, cAMP, 2-oxoglutarate, asparagine, and glutamate (Table 4). In silico modelling was conducted to understand the effect of DDC on eicosanoid metabolism [227]. Livers from mice fed a HFD were compared with controls in a wide-ranging lipidomics study that analyzed diacylglycerols (DAG), cholesterol esters (CE), phospholipids, plasmalogens, sphingolipids, and eicosanoids. A large number of differences between HFD and controls were observed (Table 4) [228]. Another NASH-generating diet has been employed in mice, that of a high-trans-fat, high-fructose diet (TFD) for 8 weeks (steatosis) and 24 weeks (NASH). These experiments sought to examine flux through the hepatic TCA cycle using ^{13}C NMR-based mass isotopomer analysis, which remained normal during steatosis but was two-fold induced in NASH. In parallel to TCA cycle flux induction, ketogenesis was impaired and hepatic diacylglycerols (DGs), ceramides (CERs) and long-chain acyl carnitines accumulated in the liver (Table 4), suggesting inefficient disposal of free fatty acids. The authors concluded that accumulation of "lipotoxic" metabolites could promote inflammation and the metabolic transition to NASH [229]. As serum or plasma was not analyzed, it is not known whether or not any of the accumulated lipids associated with NASH were also present in the circulation and could be evaluated in patients as potential biomarkers for NAFLD progression.

Correlations between specific gut microbiome species and plasma lipids in mice fed HFD that developed NAFL or NASH. *Bacteroides uniformis* species decreased while *Mucispirillum schaedleri* species increased in mice with NASH. Interestingly, *Bacteroides uniformis* correlated positively with TGs and negatively with FFAs. *Mucispirillum schaedleri* correlated positively with FFAs, LPC(20:3), LPC(20:4), and DG(16:1/18:2). Mechanistically, it was claimed that *Bacteroides uniformis* increased specific TGs and decreased hepatic injury and inflammation in diet-induced mice [230]. Clearly, these observations need to be independently evaluated and then investigated in NAFLD patients before potential biomarkers can be proposed.

The db/db mouse model of leptin receptor deficiency is currently the most widely-used mouse model of type-2 diabetes mellitus (T2DB). Another means of examining the metabolic pathways associated with NAFL is to reverse the steatosis. Caloric restriction (CR) was applied to obese diabetic db/db mice with insulin resistance and steatosis, which were also compared pre- and post-CR to nondiabetic heterozygous db/m mice without insulin resistance and steatosis. Compared to db/m mice, db/db mice had elevated hepatic ketone bodies, lactate, acetate, glutathione, and various glycerolipids, in particular, diglycerides and triglycerides, many of which were reversed by CR (Table 4). The transcriptomic findings were consistent with these observations [231]. In addition to the db/db mouse, a leptin-deficient obese mouse (ob/ob) has also been developed, which is a model for NAFLD. Homozygous ob/ob mice have been compared with nonsteatotic heterozygous ob/+ mice using high resolution magic-angle spinning (HR MAS) ^{1}H NMR. ^{1}H signals from lipids were highly statistically significantly elevated in ob/ob livers, as expected. Several other molecules involved in betaine (N,N,N-trimethylglycine) metabolism were altered (Table 4) [232].

Rats have also been fed a HFD to induce NASH and serum analyzed by UPLC-QTOFMS. Elevated glucose, triglycerides and cholesterol were indicative of insulin resistance. Altered lipid metabolites involved sphingomyelin (SM), phosphatidylcholine (PC), 13-hydroperoxy-9,11-octadecadienoic acid (13-HpODE), and fatty acids (FA) 20:3, 22:3, 20:1 and phytomonic acid (11,12-methyleneoctadecanoic acid) (Table 4) [233]. This last fatty acid is an unusual finding and, if confirmed, could be evaluated in human samples as a potential biomarker for NASH. Another rat study designed to evaluate the effect of turmeric extract on experimental NASH compared HFD-fed with control-fed rats. UPLC-QTOFMS analysis or serum revealed relatively few upregulated metabolites and a much greater number of downregulated lipids, in particular several steroids, including androgen and corticosteroid metabolites (Table 4) [234]. The only highly statistically significant upregulated metabolite was the fatty acid FA(28:8), which has been described as a marine ω-3 fatty acid [235] derived from dinoflagellate species [236]. If confirmed and a mechanism for its formation in human liver by fatty acid elongases and desaturases can be described, this would represent a potential NASH biomarker. A study was conducted comparing metabolomic profiles of rat and human liver, and, of particular interest, MCD diet-fed rat liver (model for NASH) and liver from NASH patients. Despite the large number of metabolic differences reported between treated and control rat liver and NASH liver and healthy patient liver, very few metabolites corresponded between MCD rat liver and human NASH liver. In fact, in the scores plot presented, healthy rat liver was closer to diseased rat liver than to healthy human liver, which was itself closer to diseased human liver. Asparagine, citrulline, and lysine, together with stearoyl carnitine, were the only metabolites upregulated in both rat MCD liver and human NASH liver (Table 4) [237]. Interestingly, stearoyl carnitine together with (9E)-octadecenoyl carnitine, docosapentaenoic acid and vitamin D2 were elevated in serum of rats fed either HFD (NAFL), MCD diet (NASH), or HFD plus streptozocin (NASH plus T2DM) [238]. These rat observations reduce the potential value of long-chain fatty acyl carnitines, like stearoyl carnitine, as potential biomarkers for clinical NASH or NAFLD progression. Another investigation was conducted in rats focusing on fatty acid profiles in blood cells and the liver of rats fed either a control diet or a HFD/cholesterol diet. Correlations between certain MUFAs and PUFAs were reported for both diets [239]. None of these fatty acids changes were specific enough to be evaluated as biomarkers of NAFLD in patients. Finally, an investigation of the pattern of BAs in serum, liver, and caecal contents was undertaken in rats fed HFD and control diet. Metagenomic analyses established that hyodeoxycholate, which was decreased in both serum and caecal contents of rats fed HFD, was related to the level of the *Bacteroidetes* phylum. The concentration of cholate that was increased in the caecal contents of rats fed HFD, was correlated with levels of *Firmicutes* and *Verrucomicrobia* phyla, but correlated inversely with *Bacteroidetes* [240]. As the BA pattern appeared to be dependent upon the status of the gut microbiota, the data obtained were not useful for evaluation as biomarkers of NAFLD.

Table 4. Metabolomic and lipidomic biomarkers of NAFL and NASH.

Species	Manipulation/Condition	Pathology	Analytical Methodology	Metabolites Reported	Ref.
Human	Obesity/metabolic syndrome	NAFL and NASH NAFL→NASH	HPLC-TQMS	FA(14:0)↑ FA(16:0)↑ FA(14:1n5)↑ FA(16:1n7)↑ FA(18:2n6)↓ FA(18:3n6)↑ FA(20:3n6)↑ FA(22:6n3)/FA(22:5n3) in PC and PE pools↓ 5-HETE↑ 8-HETE↑ 15-HETE↑ **(all in plasma)**	[178]
Human	Nondiabetic. NAFLD confirmed by liver biopsy	NAFLD vs. HV	UPLC-TQMS GC-MS	Glycocholate↑ Taurocholate↑ Glycochenodeoxycholate↑ Homocysteine↑ Cysteine↑ GSH↓ Glutamylvaline↑ γ-Glutamylleucine↑ γ-Glutamylphenylalanine↑ γ-Glutamyltyrosine↑ Cysteine-glutathione-disulfide↓ Carnitine↑ Propionylcarnitine↑ 2-Methylbutanoylcarnitine↑ Butanoylcarnitine↑ Tyrosine↑ Glutamate↑ Isoleucine↑ Leucine↑ Valine↑ Taurocholate↑ **(all in plasma)**	[180]
Human	Liver samples from normal (17), steatosis (4), NASH (fatty) (14) and NASH (not fatty) (23)	NAFL→NASH	UPLC Orbitrap-MS	Taurocholate↑ Taurodeoxycholate↑ Glycochenodeoxycholate↑ Taurine↑ Cholic acid↓ Glycodeoxycholate↓ **(all in liver)** Gene expression data consistent with the above (CYP7B1↑)	[222]
Human	Dietary intervention study, unrelated healthy surgical liver samples	NAFL (20 insulin-resistant/20 insulin sensitive) vs. control	UPLC-TQMS GC-MS	Insulin-resistant NAFL vs. insulin-sensitive NAFL: Total LPCs↓ LPC(16:0)↓ **(all in plasma)**	[182]
Human	NASH and healthy subjects given high-fat meal to stimulate gall bladder contraction	Fasting and postprandial serum from NASH and healthy subjects	UPLC-TQMS	NASH vs. control (preprandial): Total BAs↑ Glyco-BAs↑ Tauro-BAs↑ NASH vs. control (postprandial): Mainly Total BAs↑ Glyco-BAs↑ **(all in serum)**	[183]
Human	Normal, Steatosis, NASH with steatosis, NASH without steatosis livers	Normal, NAFL, fatty NASH, nonfatty-NASH	UPLC Orbitrap-MS	Control→NAFL: Acetyl carnitine↑ Lauroyl carnitine↑ Butanoyl carnitine↑ Palmitoyl carnitine↑ Hexanoyl carnitine↓ Valine↓ NAFL→NASH: Leucine↑ Isoleucine ↑ Tyrosine↑ Valine↑ Phenylalanine↑ **(all in liver)**	[184]

Table 4. *Cont.*

Species	Manipulation/Condition	Pathology	Analytical Methodology	Metabolites Reported	Ref.
Human	Biopsy-proven NAFL, biopsy-proven NASH and normal controls with MRI fat fraction <5%	Normal, NAFL and NASH	UPLC-QTRAP MS/MS	NAFL→NASH: PGE2↑ 13,14-dihydro-15-keto-PGD2↑ 11,12-diHETrE↑ 14,15-diHETrE↑ 15-HETE↓ [all AA-derived] **(all in plasma)**	[185]
Human	Obese normal liver, obese NAFL and obese NASH	Normal, NAFL and NASH	^{1}H NMR	LDL-cholesterol↑ Alanine↑ Histidine↑ Phenylalanine↑ Tyrosine↑ Leucine↑ Free fatty acids↓ Citrate↓ 3-Hydroxybutyrate↓ Acetoacetate↓ **(all in serum)**	[186]
Human	Morbid obesity with and without NAFL	Obesity without NAFL, mild NAFL, moderate NAFL, severe NAFL	UPLC-LITMS GC-TOFMS Metabolon, Inc.	α-Ketoglutarate principal plasma marker with AUROC of 0.743, sensitivity of 80%, specificity of 62.5%. **(all in plasma)**	[187]
Human Mouse	Liver biopsies from patients with normal liver and NAFLD HFD, HFD + nicotinic acid, HFD + hydroquinone, HFD + *tert*-butylhydroquinone	NASH vs. NAFL vs. control	GC-MS	Nicotinic acid and hydroquinone negatively correlated with steatosis (NAS) score. Nicotinic acid supplementation of HFD prevented fat accumulation and improved serum ALT. **(all in liver)**	[204]
Human	NAFLD, NAFLD + T2DM, control, evaluated by ultrasound	NAFLD, NAFLD + T2DM, control	UPLC-QTOFMS	NAFLD vs. control: Proline↑ Phenylalanine↑ Oleamide↑ Bilirubin↑ Palmitoyl carnitine↑ LPC(20:5)↑ Lyso-PAF C-18↓ NAFLD + T2DM vs. control: Leucine↑ Oleamide↑ LPC(14:0)↑ Bilirubin↑ Tetradecenoyl carnitine↑ Linoleoyl carnitine↑ Tetradecadienoyl carnitine↑ (all in serum)	[206]
Human	Hyperuricemia (HU), HU+NAFLD, HU progressed to HU+NAFLD, healthy controls	HU, initial HU+NAFLD, initial HU→outcome HU+NAFLD, healthy controls	UPLC-QTOFMS	HU vs. control: Phosphatidic acid↑ 3,4-Dihydroxyphenylglycol↑ Valine↑ CE(18:0)↑ Uric acid↑ Acetyl carnitine↑ Inosine↓ 5-Hydroxyindoleacetic acid↓ 5-Aminoimidazole ribotide↓ Pyrrolidonecarboxylic acid↓ Glycerophosphocholine↓ HU vs. outcome HU+NAFLD: Phosphatidic acid↑ Inosinic acid↑ Tryptophan↑ Valine↑ Alanine↑ Lactate↑ CE(18:0)↑ Uric acid↑ Trimethylamine↑ Acetyl carnitine↑ 5-Methoxyindoleacetic acid↑ Acetoin↑ Inosine↓ Kynurenine↓ 5-Hydroxyindoleacetic acid↓ Pyrrolidonecarboxylic acid↓ 4-Fumarylacetoacetate↓ Pregnenolone sulfate↓ **(all in serum)**	[203]

Table 4. *Cont.*

Species	Manipulation/Condition	Pathology	Analytical Methodology	Metabolites Reported	Ref.
Human	Bariatric surgery patients with wedge liver biopsy during surgery classified histologically as non-NASH, non-NAFLD, NAFL and NASH. *PNPLA3* I148M variant also determined (more common in NASH). Discovery and validation cohorts used.	non-NASH vs. non-NAFLD vs. NAFL vs. NASH	UPLC-QTOFMS 2D-GC-TOFMS	Strong negative correlation between number of TG double bonds to TG concentrations in NASH relative to non-NASH for both discovery and validation cohorts. A "NASH ClinLipMet score" was developed based upon (i) clinical variables, (ii) *PNPLA3* genotype, (iii) lipidomic data and (iv) metabolomic data. This was highest performing combination biomarker with sensitivity of 85.5% and specificity of 72.1% for NASH. **(all in liver)**	[188]
Human	Normal liver, NAFL liver, NASH liver	NASH vs. NAFLD vs. control lipidomics	UPLC-TQMS GC-MS	Thirty-two lipids discriminated NASH with 100% sensitivity and specificity. Accumulated hepatotoxic lipids in NASH included FA(14:0), FA(16:0), FA(16:1n-7), FA(18:1n-7) and FA(18:1n-9). Reduced in NASH: FA(20:4n-6), FA(20:5n-3), FA(22:6n-3), total CER, total SM, total PI, total PS, total PE, total PC. **(all in liver)**	[189]
Human	Nondiabetic NAFL patients with normal liver function, NASH with abnormal liver function, healthy controls.	NASH vs. NAFL vs. control urines.	LC-TQMS	NASH vs. control: Lysine↑ Valine↑ Citrulline↑ Arginine↑ Threonine↑ Tyrosine↑ Leucine↑ Hippurate↑ 3-Indoleacetate↑ 5-Hydroxyindoleacetate↓ 3-Indoleformate↓ Cortisol↓ NASH vs. NAFL: Methyl xanthine↑ Tryptophan↑ 3-Indoleacetate↑ Gluconate↑ Proline↓ **(all in urine)**	[190]
Human	Several large clinical cohorts with CT-defined liver fat plus NASH patients.	NASH vs. controls	UPLC-Q-Orbitrap-MS	Top metabolite correlated with liver fat was 202.1185$^+$, which produced 24 hits in HMDB. Dimethylguanidino valeric acid (DMGV) chosen on basis of GWAS, which found SNPs for AGXT2 that produces DMGV. **(all in plasma)**	[191]
Human	NAFLD criteria met/not met at baseline, after dietary manipulation.	Non-NAFLD, Non-NAFLD→ NAFLD, NAFLD→ Non-NAFLD	UPLC-QTOFMS	Phospholipid and sphingolipid changes not of great statistical significance. Also lipid groups, not individual lipids, given only. **(all in serum)**	[241]

Table 4. *Cont.*

Species	Manipulation/Condition	Pathology	Analytical Methodology	Metabolites Reported	Ref.
Human	NAFL and NASH based upon liver biopsy, healthy controls.	NASH vs. NAFL vs. controls	HPLC-Orbitrap-MS	Five metabolites increased control→NAFL→NASH – Uracil, α-Linolenic acid (all-*cis*-9,12,15-octadecatrienoic acid), Glutamate, Glutamine and 5-Oxoproline, which was chosen as a biomarker with a better AUROC for NASH vs. NAFL, than adiponectin, TNF-α, or IL-8. **(all in serum)**	[192]
Human	NAFL and NASH confirmed by liver biopsy	NASH vs. NAFL	High-field ^{1}H MRS and ultra-high-field ^{31}P MRS (*in vivo*)	Many MRS alterations correlated with NAFL→NASH, mostly with advanced fibrosis, e.g. phosphoethanolamine/total phosphorus (TP) ratio. ATP/TP↓ in advanced fibrosis and ATP flux↓ in NASH	[155]
Human	Chronic hepatitis B (CHB) with biopsy-proven NAFLD and without NAFLD, healthy controls	CHB +NAFLD vs. CHB-NAFLD vs. controls	UPLC-QTOFMS	Most neutral lipids and ceramides were elevated in CHB+NAFLD but decreased in CHB-NAFLD vs. healthy controls. Monounsaturated TGs were a good predictor of NASH, superior to cytokeratin-18 or ALT.	[196]
Human	Hepatic steatosis in morbidly obese women	Metagenomic signature of hepatic steatosis	^{1}H NMR (urine and plasma) UPLC-TQMS (plasma)	Microbiota metabolite produced from phenylalanine, phenylacetic acid (PAA) associated with steatosis.	[197]
Human	Biopsy-proven subjects with normal liver (NL), NAFL and NASH	NASH vs. NAFL vs. NL discovery and validation cohorts	UPLC-QTOFMS	Triglycerides are elevated NAFL > NL ≥ NASH. Of the 28 TGs measured, TG(46:0), (48:0), (53:0), (44:1), (48:1), (49:1), (52:1), (53:1), (50:2), (54:5) and (58:2) were always NAFL > NL and NASH < NAFL. **(all in serum)**	[198]
Human	Large study of 769 nondiabetic patients with liver fat content measured by MRI and correlated with metabolite profiles of urine and fasting plasma	613 plasma and 587 urine samples across a range of liver pathologies (34.7% with steatosis)	UPLC-LITMS ^{1}H NMR	Associations in plasma with LFC: BCAAs↑ Aromatic amino acids↑ Dipeptides↑ Proline↑ Tryptophan↑ Indoleacetate↑ Urate↑ Piperine↑ 7α-Hydroxy-3-oxo-cholestenoate↑ Ether-PCs↓ 3-Phenylpropionate↓ Proline betaine↓ Associations in urine with LFC: BCAA derivatives↑ Lactate↑ Isovalerylglycine↓ Isobutyrylglycine↓ γ-Glutamylthreonine↓ 4-Vinylphenol sulfate↓ Hippurate↓ Cinnamoylglycine↓	[200]

Table 4. *Cont.*

Species	Manipulation/Condition	Pathology	Analytical Methodology	Metabolites Reported	Ref.
Human	NAFLD determined by hepatic ultrasound	BMI < 25 vs. BMI > 30 vs. BMI > 30 with NAFLD	TQMS for 31 acyl carnitines and 7 amino acids	Family history predicted obesity correlating with amino acids that contributed to an increase in specific acyl carnitines. Excess FFAs related to obesity were associated with NAFLD.	[201]
Human	Patients with normal fasting glucose. Visceral adipose tissue (VAT) assessed by MRI. Hepatic TG content (HTGC) determined by proton-MR spectroscopy.	Range of VAT and HTGC	ESI-FIA-MS/MS	Associated with HTGC: LPC(14:0), PC(28:1), PC(30:0), PC(32:1), PC(32:2), PC(34:1), PC(34:3), PC(34:4), PC(36:1), PC(36:2), PC(36:3), PC(36:6), PC(38:3), PC(38:5), PC(40:4), PC(40:5), SM(22:3), Tryptophan, Tyrosine **(all in plasma)**	[202]
Human	NAFL and NASH determined by liver biopsy and healthy controls by ultrasound and liver enzymes	NASH vs. NAFL vs. controls	UPLC-Orbitrap-MS GC	Lipid group trends: DG: NASH > NAFL > healthy PG: NASH ≈ NAFL > healthy PA: NASH ≈ NAFL > healthy AcCa: NASH < NAFL ≈ healthy CE: NASH < NAFL < healthy LPC: NASH < NAFL ≈ healthy SM: NASH < NAFL ≈ healthy FA(16:0): NASH > NAFL > healthy FA(16:1n-7*cis*): NASH > NAFL > healthy FA(18:1n-9*cis*): NASH > NAFL > healthy FA(18:2n-6): NASH < NAFL < healthy FA(20:4n-6): NASH < NAFL < healthy	[199]
Human	Children, overweight or obese, with or without clinical/radiological signs of NAFLD	NAFLD vs. control	Selective ion flow tube mass spectrometry (SIFT-MS)	Acetaldehyde↑ Acetone↑ Isoprene↑ Pentane↑ Trimethylamine↑ **(all in breath)**	[209]
Human	Children with biopsy-proven NAFLD and matched healthy controls	NAFLD vs. control	HPLC	Homocysteine↑ Cysteine↑ CysGly↑ GSH↓ **(all in plasma)**	[211]
Human	Children with obesity and NAFL confirmed by MRS and matched obese controls	NAFL vs. control	UPLC-Q-Orbitrap-MS	Tyrosine↑ Glutamate↑ Octanoic acid↑ Linoleic acid↓ **(all in plasma)**	[212]
Human	Children with obesity, NAFL, NASH and healthy controls	NASH vs. NAFL vs. control	GC-MS	1-Butanol↑ (in NAFL) 1-Pentanol↑ (in NAFL) ↓ (in NASH) Phenol↑ (in NAFL) 2-Butanone↑ (in NAFL and NASH) 4-Methyl-2-pentanone↓ (in NAFL)↑ (in NASH) **(all in feces)** Metagenomics also conducted. Correlations with NAFLD and certain VOCs reported	[242]

Table 4. *Cont.*

Species	Manipulation/Condition	Pathology	Analytical Methodology	Metabolites Reported	Ref.
Human	Children with NAFLD, with or without obesity	Obese − NAFL, obese + NAFL, normal weight healthy controls	GC-MS	NAFL vs. control: Glucose↑ 1-Methylhistidine↑ Pseudouridine↑ Glycolic acid↑ Mannose↓ *p*-Cresol sulfate↓ Kynurenine↓ Hydroquinone↓ Adipate↓ Phenylacetic acid↓ Small intestine bacterial overgrowth (SIBO): Glycolic acid↑ Mannose↑ Valine↓ *p*-Cresol sulfate↓ Butanoate↓ Adipate↓ (all in urine)	[213]
Human	Children with obesity, with and without NAFLD assessed by MRI	Obese + NAFLD vs. obese − NAFLD	UPLC-QTRAP-MS	Isoleucine↑ Leucine↑ Valine↑ C4-carnitine↑ C5-carnitine↑ C14:1-OH-carnitine↑ Tryptophan↑ Lysine↑ Glutamate↑ PC(32:1)↑ (all in plasma)	[214]
Human	Children with obesity, with and without NAFL assessed by ultrasound (US), with and without metabolic syndrome (MetS) and nonobese controls	Obese + NAFL vs. obese − NAFL Obese + MetS vs. obese − MetS	GC-MS	Obese − NAFL vs. controls: Palmitate↑ Myristate↑ Urea↑ *N*-Acetylgalactosamine↑ Maltose↑ Gluconate↑ Isoleucine↑ Hydroxybutanoate↓ Malate↓ Obese + NAFL vs. controls: Laurate↑ Maltose↑ (all in saliva)	[215]
Human	Adolescents with NAFLD assessed by US or ALT/AST	US vs. ALT vs. AST diagnostic methods	Biochemical lipid analysis ^{1}H NMR	Many differences in lipid profiles, amino acids (alanine, glutamine, histidine; BCAAs; aromatic amino acids) and ketone bodies (acetate, acetoacetate, β-hydroxybutyrate) (all in plasma)	[216]
Human	Adolescents with obesity and with or without NAFLD confirmed by MRI	NAFLD vs. non-NAFLD	UPLC-Q-Orbitrap-MS	Leucine/Isoleucine↑ Tryptophan↑ Serine↓ Dihydrothymine↓ LPE(20:0)↓ LPC(18:1)↓ (all in plasma)	[217]
Human	Children with or without NAFLD confirmed by ultrasound and liver enzymes	NAFLD vs. non-NAFLD	GC-MS	24-h Urinary steroid profiles: Cortisol (obese controls)↑ Tetrahydrocortisone (NAFLD)↑ Overall data pointed to 5α-reductase↑, 21-hydroxylase↑ and 11β-hydroxysteroid dehydrogenase 1↓	[243]
Human Mouse	Morbidly obese, nondiabetic *Gnmt*-null vs. WT	NAFL→NASH NASH vs. control	UPLC-QTOFMS	PC(14:0/20:4)↑ LPC(18:1)↑ PC(P-24:0/0:0)↓ PC(P-22:0/0:0)↓ PC(O-20:0/0:0)↓ FA(20:4)↓ Glutamate↓ (all in serum) Results consistent with human studies	[179]

Table 4. *Cont.*

Species	Manipulation/Condition	Pathology	Analytical Methodology	Metabolites Reported	Ref.
Mouse Human	Methionine and choline deficient diet (MCD) HBV-negative, NAFLD confirmed by liver biopsy	NASH vs. NAFL vs. control	^{1}H NMR	Glucose↑ Lactate↑ Glutamate↑ Taurine↑ TG↑ Total cholesterol↑ LDL cholesterol↑ Glucose↑ Lactate↑ Glutamate↑ Taurine↑ **(all in serum)**	[181]
Mouse Human	*Mat1a*-KO vs. WT mouse liver and serum metabolome NAFL and NASH discovery and validation cohorts	*Mat1a*-KO vs. WT Clustering analysis into M-subtype and Non-M-subtype based upon mouse metabolomes	UPLC-QTOFMS	M-subtype NASH biomarkers: Amino acids (5), Fatty acyls (8), Triglycerides (3), Glycerophospholipids (37), Sphingomyelins (1) Non-M-subtype NASH biomarkers: Amino acids (1), Fatty acids (1), Bile acids (1), Triglycerides (3) M-subtype patients: 34% NASH Non-M-subtype patients: 39% NASH	[205]
Mouse	MCD	NASH vs. control	UPLC-QTOFMS	Tauro-β-muricholate↑ Taurocholate↑ 12-HETE↑ LPC(16:0)↓ LPC(18:0)↓ LPC(18:1)↓ **(all in serum)**	[218]
Mouse	MCD vs. choline-supplemented MCD (MCS)	Differential effects of methionine and choline deficiency	UPLC-QTOFMS	MCD vs MCS: Oleic acid↑ Linoleic acid↑ Total nonesterified fatty acids↑ **(all in serum)**	[219]
Mouse	NASH-inducing diet (35% lard, 1.25% cholesterol, 0.5% sodium cholate)	NAFLD vs. control	HPLC-TQMS	Glycerol↑ Free cholesterol↑ Esterified cholesterol↑ Putrescine↑ N^8-Acetylspermidine↓ Spermine↓ Adenine↓ Adenosine↓ Homocysteine↓ Methylthioadenosine↓ S-Adenosylhomocysteine↓ S-Adenosylmethionine↓ Proteomic findings were consistent with the above **(all in liver)**	[220]
Mouse	*Ldlr*-null mice fed a Western diet (energy as 17% protein, 43% carbohydrate, 41% fat, 0.2% cholesterol) + olive oil (WD + O)	NAFLD/NASH vs. control	UPLC-LITMS GC-MS Metabolon, Inc.	Saturated fatty acids↑ MUFAs↑ Palmitoyl-sphingomyelin↑ Cholesterol↑ n-6 PUFA↑ 12-HETE↑ C_{20-22} n-3 PUFA↓ 18-HEPE↓ 17,18-diHETE↓ S-Lactoyl-glutathione↓ **(all in liver)** F3-Isoprostanes↓ **(in urine)**	[221]

Table 4. *Cont.*

Species	Manipulation/Condition	Pathology	Analytical Methodology	Metabolites Reported	Ref.
Mouse	HFD (60% calories from fat) and normal chow (12.7% calories from fat)	NAFLD vs. control	^{1}H NMR	Glucose↑ Total cholesterol↑ HDL-cholesterol↑ AST↑ ALT↑ Phosphatidylcholine↑ Pyruvate↓ Acetate↓ Lactate↓ Citrate↓ Arginine↓ Ornithine↓ Acetoacetate↓ 3-Hydroxybutyrate↓ Isoleucine↓ Leucine↓ Valine↓ Glutamate↓ Glutamine↓ Tyrosine↓ Phenylalanine↓ Alanine↓ Lysine↓ Glycine↓ Betaine↓ Isobutanoate↓ 1-Methylhistidine↓ **(all in serum)** Total cholesterol↑ Triglycerides↑ Fatty acids↑ PUFA/MUFA↓ **(all in liver)** Pyruvate↑ Creatinine↑ Taurine↑ Glycine↑ Formate↑ Butanoate↑ Guanidinoacetate↑ Glucose↑ 1-Methylnicotinamide↑ Nicotinamide *N*-oxide↑ Acetoacetate↓ Succinate↓ Citrate↓ 2-Oxoglutarate↓ Trimethylamine↓ *Trans*-aconitate↓ Hippurate↓ Trigonelline↓ Niacinamide↓ Tyrosine↓ 1-Methylhistidine↓ Phenylalanine↓ **(all in urine)**	[223]
Mouse	HFD (60% calories from fat) and normal chow (13.5% calories from fat)	NAFLD vs. control	UPLC-QTOFMS GC-MS	Methylhippurate↑ Glycerol 3-phosphate↑ Mannose↑ Ketoleucine↑ 2-Ketohexanoate↑ Hydroxyphenyllactate↑ Succinate↑ Xylose/Ribose/Arabinose↓ Glucuronate↓ Catechol↓ 4-Coumarate↓ Hippurate↓ Taurocholate↓ Glycochenodeoxycholate↓ Glycocholate↓ Histamine↓ **(all in serum)**	[224]
Mouse	A/J, C57BL/6J and PWD/PhJ strains fed standard diet with 0.1% DDC	DDC-treated vs. control	UPLC-Q-LITMS	Putrescine↑ Arginine↑ Citrulline↑ cAMP↑ 2-Oxoglutarate↑ Asparagine↑ Glutamate↑ **(all in liver)**	[227]
Mouse	HFD-fed mice (42% calories from fat, 43% from carbohydrates, 15% from protein) vs. standard chow (17% from fat, 58% from carbohydrates, 25% from protein)	NAFLD vs. control	UPLC-Q-LITMS	SFA-DAGs↑ MUFA-DAGs↑ PUFA-DAGs↓ SFA-CEs↑ MUFA-CEs↑ PAs↑ PGs↑ SFA-CERs↑ Sphingosine↑ Sphingosine-1-phosphate↑ Dihydrosphingosine↑ Dihydrosphingosine-1-phosphate↑ Galactosylceramide↓ Glucosylceramide↓ Lactosylceramide↑ Globotrioseacylceramide↑ TxB2↑ PGF2α↑ All other eicosanoids↓ Pattern changed from weeks 16-52. **(all in liver)**	[228]

Table 4. *Cont.*

Species	Manipulation/Condition	Pathology	Analytical Methodology	Metabolites Reported	Ref.
Mouse	db/db leptin receptor-deficient mice with insulin resistance and steatosis subjected to caloric restriction (CR), db/m mice without insulin resistance and steatosis	db/db, pre- and post-caloric restriction, db/m	^{1}H NMR UPLC-QTOFMS	db/db vs. db/m: Acetone↑ 3-Hydroxybutyrate↑ Lactate↑ Acetate↑ Glutathione↑ Ascorbate↑ Many glycerolipids↑ db/db + CR vs. db/db: 3-Hydroxybutyrate↓ Ascorbate↓ Many glycerolipids↓ RT-PCR findings consistent with metabolomic data **(all in liver)**	[231]
Mouse	Leptin-deficient obese *ob/ob* mice and nonsteatotic *ob/+* heterozygous mice	Intact liver tissues of two mouse lines compared	HR-MAS ^{1}H NMR	Many lipid ^{1}H signals highly statistically significantly elevated in steatotic *ob/ob* livers compared with nonsteatotic *ob/+* livers, as expected. *ob/ob* livers vs. *ob/+* livers: Betaine↑ Phenylalanine↑ Uridine↑ Creatinine↓ Glutamate↓ Glycine↓ Glycolate↓ Trimethylamine N-oxide↓ N,N-Dimethylglycine↓ ADP↓ AMP↓	[232]
Mouse	High-*trans*-fat high-fructose diet (TFD) for 8 weeks (steatosis) and 24 weeks (NASH)	TFD-fed, normal diet-fed	Fasting hepatic mitochondrial flux by ^{13}C NMR isotopomer analysis. LC-TQMS lipidomics	8-week (steatosis) vs. 24-week (NASH): Endogenous glucose production↑ TCA cycle flux↑ Anaplerosis↑ Pyruvate cycling↑ Control vs. 8-week (steatosis): Total diacylglycerols↑ Total ceramides↑ C8-acyl carnitine↑ C16-acyl carnitine↑ 8-week (steatosis) vs. 24-week (NASH): DG(16:1/16:1)↑ DG(16:0/18:1)↑ DG(34:2)↑ DG(18:1/18:1)↑ DG(18:1/18:2)↑ DG(18:2/18:2)↑ DG(16:0/20:4)↑ DG(18:0/20:4)↑ DG(18:1/20:4)↑ DG(18:2/20:4)↑ DG(18:2/20:2)↑ DG(16:1/22:6)↑ DG(18:1/22:6)↑ C6-acyl carnitine↑ C8-acyl carnitine↑ C14-acyl carnitine↑ C16-acyl carnitine↑ CER(20:0)↓ CER(22:0)↓ **(all in liver)**	[229]

Table 4. *Cont.*

Species	Manipulation/Condition	Pathology	Analytical Methodology	Metabolites Reported	Ref.
Mouse	High-fat, high-cholesterol, cholate (HFDCC)-fed mice with NAFLD without obesity	HFDCC vs. control	GC-TOFMS UPLC-QTOFMS	Total cholesterol↑ CE(16:1), (18:1), (18:2), (18:3), (20:1), (20:3), (20:4), (22:5), (22:6)↑ Cholic acid↑ DGs↑ TGs↑ CERs↑ SMs↑ LPCs↑ PC/PE↑ PEs↓ Xylitol↑ Xanthosine↑ Squalene↑ Phenylethylamine↑ Citrate↓ G-1-P↓ Saccharic acid↓ **(all in liver)** Total cholesterol↑ CE(16:1), (18:1), (18:2), (18:3), (20:1), (20:3), (20:4), (22:5)↑ Cholic acid↑ Deoxycholic acid↑ CERs↑ SMs↑ PEs↑ FFAs↓ Glycerol↓ TGs↓ LPEs↓ **(all in plasma)**	[225]
Rat	HFD-induced NASH	HFD vs. control diet	UPLC-QTOFMS	Glucose↑ Triglycerides↑ LDL-cholesterol↑ SM(36:1)↑ LPC(18:1)↑ LPC(20:2)↑ SM(34:2)↑ PC(34:1)↑ PC(38:4)↑ PC(38:3)↑ LPC(17:1)↑ PC(35:2)↑ FA(20:1)↑ FA(20:3)↑ FA(22:3)↑ Phytomonate↑ LPC(14:0)↑ 13-HpODE↑ PC(37:4)↓ PC(38:4)↓ PC(38:6)↓ SM(34:1)↓ SM(34:2)↓SM(42:3)↓ SM(40:1)↓ PC(40:5)↓ PC(40:6)↓ PC(40:8)↓ Creatine↓ Indoxyl sulfate↓ **(all in serum)**	[233]
Rat	HFD-induced NASH, positive controls (methionine plus choline supplementation), control diet	HFD vs. positive control vs. control diet	UPLC-QTOFMS	HFD vs. control: FA(28:8)↑ CE(12:0)↑ PG(14:0/18:1)↑ Cortisone↓ Antrosta-1,4-diene-3,17-dione↓ All-*trans*-retinoyl-β-glucuronide↓ LPA(18:2)↓ PE(15:0/22:2)↓ Cortol↓ 21-Hydroxypregnenolone↓ Cortolone↓ Urobilin↓ LPA(18:1)↓ PA(P-20:0/14:0)↓ **(all in serum)**	[234]
Rat Human	Rats fed HFD to lead to steatosis, rats fed MCD diet to lead to NASH, rats fed methionine and choline sufficient diet as controls→liver samples NASH (fatty), NASH (not fatty), steatosis, healthy liver samples	NASH vs. NAFL vs. control (rat and human)	UPLC Orbitrap-MS	Bile acid metabolomics: Significant BA profile differences between rat MCD and human NASH. Amino acid metabolomics: Asparagine↑ Citrulline↑ Lysine↑ comparable between rat MCD and human NASH. Fatty acid, carnitine and LPC metabolomics: Stearoyl carnitine↑ only lipid in both rat MCD and human NASH	[237]
Rat	HFD, MCD diet and streptozocin (STZ) in rats. Metabolomics and transcriptomics on serum and liver.	NAFL vs. NASH vs. NAFL + T2DM	UPLC-QTOFMS	Venn diagram for HFD, MCD and HFD+STZ serum: Stearoyl carnitine↑ (9E)-octadecenoyl carnitine↑ docosapentaenoic acid↑ vitamin D2↑	[238]

Table 4. *Cont.*

Species	Manipulation/Condition	Pathology	Analytical Methodology	Metabolites Reported	Ref.
Rat	HFD/cholesterol diet vs. normal diet	Stage of steatosis, inflammation and fibrosis determined histologically	GC	Correlation between liver and blood cell total fatty acids for control diet: FA(16:1), FA(22:6), FA(18:1n-7), FA(22:5) Correlation between liver and blood cell total fatty acids for HFD/cholesterol diet: FA(22:6), FA(18:1n-7)	[239]
Rat	HFD vs. normal diet	NAFLD established by histology and liver enzymes	UPLC-TQMS	BAs in liver: Taurocholate↑ Taurohyodeoxycholate↓ Ursodeoxycholate↓ BAs in caecal contents: Cholate↑ Hyodeoxycholate↓ Muricholate↓ BAs in serum: Taurocholate↑ Hyodeoxycholate↓ Taurohyodeoxycholate↓	[240]

Overall Summary

A summary of metabolic, metabolomic, and lipidomic investigations into ALD is given in Table 1. It is clear that the hepatic metabolic phenotypes and therefore biomarkers of both chronic alcohol consumption and ALD are far from being defined. Despite the considerable number of published investigations, large variations in study design, species investigated, experimental methodologies and metabolic findings render a consensus opinion difficult to formulate. Nevertheless, it is becoming clear that various lipid classes may play a role in both ALD etiology and in shaping the resultant hepatic metabolic phenotype. Moreover, the recent attention to gut microbiota-liver cross talk offers new avenues to solving the mechanisms of ALD and providing effective predictive biomarkers. The effects of alcohol on lipid metabolism has recently been reviewed [52], as has the Lieber-DeCarli diet as a model for experimental liver disease [55].

Regarding cholestasis, it is well known to be associated with elevated hepatic and serum bile acids, and can occur in the diseases PBC and PSC, as well as in pregnancy and in the neonatal period. Metabolomics has revealed that not just the expected primary BAs are elevated in these conditions, but also BA removal is enhanced by sulfation, with various sulfate conjugates found in the urine. More mechanistic investigations were generally conducted in rats, predominantly by administration of the hepatotoxin ANIT. This protocol has found particular utility in the screening of TCMs that have been used for centuries to treat jaundice in China. Attesting to the efficacy of these treatments, the metabolomic signature of ANIT-induced cholestasis was attenuated in all cases. In addition, a number of combination biomarkers have been evaluated for the various manifestations of both clinical and experimental cholestasis, but it remains to be seen if any of these are adopted into routine clinical practice (Table 2).

In the case of fibrosis and cirrhosis, a total of 38 studies are summarized in Table 3, i.e., 22 conducted by MS and 16 by NMR. Nine investigations were conducted in rats and 29 in patients and volunteers. Considering first the NMR-based studies, it should be noted that these investigations in general identify in liver samples, serum, plasma, or urine relatively high concentration metabolites, such as Krebs cycle intermediates, amino acids and simple sugars that have been described as "the usual suspects" [244]. This simple fact renders these targets unsuitable as biomarker candidates for the detection or progression of fibrosis because of their ubiquitous nature. Although ^{1}H NMR-based metabolomic studies are seen as having many advantages, such as simplicity, rapidity, and reproducibility, they suffer from modest resolution and sensitivity. MS-based methodologies, in contrast, are able to resolve, identify and quantitate hundreds of molecules in a sample, rather than tens of metabolites by NMR. They have the distinct advantage in the realm of the relatively low concentration constituents of the metabolome. As Table 3 demonstrates, fibrosis progression in NAFLD could be evaluated in terms of decreasing serum concentrations of etiocholanolone sulfate (E) and dehydroepiandrosterone sulfate (D), with concomitant increasing concentration of 16α-hydroxy-dehydroepiandrosterone sulfate (16). Discovery of these molecules as potential biomarkers was assessed in a validation cohort [119]. The ratios 16/D and 16/E exhibited clear statistically significant trends across F0-1, F2, F3, to F4, with sensitivities/specificities of 81%/80% and 76%/85%, respectively [119]. More commonly, MS-based methods have shown elevations in specific serum bile acids in human liver cirrhosis [128,132,135], together with fluctuations in a broad range of urinary steroids [141]. Another common finding were alterations in serum phospholipids in both human liver cirrhosis [135,139,140] and in animal models [169,170,172]. In both the human and animal model investigations, perturbations in metabolic intermediates, akin to those revealed by NMR, have also been described. We consider that only metabolites that appear unique to fibrosis and/or cirrhosis, such as etiocholanolone sulfate, dehydroepiandrosterone sulfate, and 16α-hydroxy-dehydroepiandrosterone sulfate should be evaluated as biomarkers. The unusual metabolite cervonoyl ethanolamide (8,11,14-eicosatrienoyl ethanolamide) was elevated in the rat CCl4 fibrosis model, but has so far not been evaluated in patients with liver fibrosis. However, this fatty acid amide was also elevated in hyperlipidemic rats [245], reducing its potential as a biomarker for fibrosis.

A total of 30 studies involving adult patients, nine involving adolescents or children, and 21 studies that involve mouse or rat investigations of NAFLD, are included in Table 4. Of these, a total of 49 investigations used mass spectrometry-based methodologies and ten used NMR-based methods. A large quantity of literature has described a wealth of metabolomic and lipidomic investigations into steatosis (NAFL) and NASH, together with experiments in laboratory rodent models. In the most part, this accumulated information largely describes potential mechanisms by which the liver accumulates lipid droplets and the transition to an accompanied inflammation that defines NASH. As Table 4 shows, there is a wealth of information regarding up- and down-regulated molecules in plasma/serum, urine and liver itself. The question is: how useful are these data for the generation of biomarkers of NAFL or NASH, or the progression of NAFL to NASH? The metabolic profiles of liver that have been determined in certain investigations are not immediately useful for biomarker evaluation unless serum/plasma or urine was also investigated. The purpose of a biomarker for liver disease is to avoid liver biopsy. The increase in peripheral fatty acids and acyl carnitines are consistent with the known etiology of fatty liver disease. Elevated concentrations of BAs, BCAAs, and aromatic amino acids are also well-known characteristics of these diseases. The issue is specificity, especially as many of the studies involved obese patients and those with diabetes and insulin resistance, all of which factors could confound the NAFLD findings. In a study of nondiabetic patients with steatosis and NASH, an interesting candidate biomarker emerged, γ-glutamyltyrosine, but unfortunately the change between control subjects and NAFLD patients was small (1.2–1.3-fold, but highly statistically significant) with a number of outliers [180]. Larger fold-changes were observed for acyl carnitines. Lauroyl carnitine was four-fold increased over controls in steatosis and NASH and hexanoyl carnitine was 3.5-fold elevated in NASH but 2.5-fold decreased in steatosis [184]. As no other study reported these acyl carnitine changes in NAFLD, they would need to be independently verified. Nevertheless, acyl carnitine patterns represent potential biomarkers for progression from steatosis to NASH. We have already discussed above 7α-hydroxy-3-oxo-4-cholestenoate [200] as a potential biomarker for steatosis. Providing that the patients under investigation were negative for sterol 27-hydroxylase deficiency, familial hypercholanemia and Zellweger syndrome, with which this BA intermediate is also associated, it could be further evaluated as a potential biomarker for steatosis. Regarding NAFL in children and adolescents, almost all patient groups in Table 4 were also obese. These studies did not appear to yield potential biomarkers of pediatric NAFLD.

NAFLD does not have a natural history in almost all laboratory rodent studies; rather, it is induced with specialized diets or occurs in genetically modified mice, such as leptin-deficient obese mice (ob/ob) or leptin receptor-deficient mice (db/db) (Table 4). Unusual metabolites such as the globotrioseacylceramide Gb3(d18:1/22:1), which was highly statistically significantly elevated in the livers of mice fed a high-fat high-cholesterol diet [228], could not be further evaluated because their serum concentrations were not determined. Another unusual metabolite, phytomonic acid (11,12-methyleneoctadecanoic acid), reported in serum of HFD-induced NASH in rats [233] may also not be useful as human biomarkers of NAFLD, because it may be produced by the gut microbiota, given that its older name is lactobacillic acid. The C8 and C16 acyl carnitines were elevated in liver tissue of mice fed a high-fructose high-trans-fat diet [229] similar to human findings referred to above [184]. However, again there were no serum/plasma data from which to evaluate the potential of acyl carnitines as biomarkers of human NAFLD. Other data from rats with different NAFLD phenotypes pointed to the elevation of stearoyl and elaidoyl [(9E)-octadecenoyl] carnitine in serum, with palmitoyl and stearoyl carnitine upregulated in liver tissue [238]. In summary, an abundance of metabolomic data from human and animal model studies of NAFLD provide a number of leads for evaluation of biomarkers in independent trials.

Author Contributions: Conceptualization, D.B. and J.R.I.; Literature Analysis, D.B. and J.R.I.; Writing—original draft preparation, D.B. and J.R.I.; Writing—review and editing, D.B. and J.R.I. All authors have read and agreed to the published version of the manuscript.

References

1. Massarweh, N.N.; El-Serag, H.B. Epidemiology of Hepatocellular Carcinoma and Intrahepatic Cholangiocarcinoma. *Cancer Control* **2017**, *24*, 1073274817729245. [CrossRef]

2. Severi, T.; van Malenstein, H.; Verslype, C.; van Pelt, J.F. Tumor initiation and progression in hepatocellular carcinoma: Risk factors, classification, and therapeutic targets. *Acta Pharmacol. Sin.* **2010**, *31*, 1409–1420. [CrossRef]

3. Altekruse, S.F.; Devesa, S.S.; Dickie, L.A.; McGlynn, K.A.; Kleiner, D.E. Histological classification of liver and intrahepatic bile duct cancers in SEER registries. *J. Registry Manag.* **2011**, *38*, 201–205.

4. Baecker, A.; Liu, X.; La Vecchia, C.; Zhang, Z.F. Worldwide incidence of hepatocellular carcinoma cases attributable to major risk factors. *Eur. J. Cancer Prev.* **2018**, *27*, 205–212. [CrossRef]

5. Uhlen, M.; Fagerberg, L.; Hallstrom, B.M.; Lindskog, C.; Oksvold, P.; Mardinoglu, A.; Sivertsson, A.; Kampf, C.; Sjostedt, E.; Asplund, A.; et al. Proteomics. Tissue-based map of the human proteome. *Science* **2015**, *347*, 1260419. [CrossRef]

6. Ben-Moshe, S.; Itzkovitz, S. Spatial heterogeneity in the mammalian liver. *Nat. Rev. Gastroenterol. Hepatol.* **2019**, *16*, 395–410. [CrossRef]

7. Zhang, D.Y.; Goossens, N.; Guo, J.; Tsai, M.C.; Chou, H.I.; Altunkaynak, C.; Sangiovanni, A.; Iavarone, M.; Colombo, M.; Kobayashi, M.; et al. A hepatic stellate cell gene expression signature associated with outcomes in hepatitis C cirrhosis and hepatocellular carcinoma after curative resection. *Gut* **2016**, *65*, 1754–1764. [CrossRef]

8. Verhulst, S.; Roskams, T.; Sancho-Bru, P.; van Grunsven, L.A. Meta-Analysis of Human and Mouse Biliary Epithelial Cell Gene Profiles. *Cells* **2019**, *8*, 1117. [CrossRef]

9. Aguilar-Bravo, B.; Sancho-Bru, P. Laser capture microdissection: Techniques and applications in liver diseases. *Hepatol. Int.* **2019**, *13*, 138–147. [CrossRef]

10. Nicholson, J.K.; Lindon, J.C.; Holmes, E. 'Metabonomics': Understanding the metabolic responses of living systems to pathophysiological stimuli via multivariate statistical analysis of biological NMR spectroscopic data. *Xenobiotica* **1999**, *29*, 1181–1189. [CrossRef]

11. Idle, J.R.; Gonzalez, F.J. Metabolomics. *Cell Metab.* **2007**, *6*, 348–351. [CrossRef]

12. Beyoglu, D.; Zhou, Y.; Chen, C.; Idle, J.R. Mass isotopomer-guided decluttering of metabolomic data to visualize endogenous biomarkers of drug toxicity. *Biochem. Pharmacol.* **2018**, *156*, 491–500. [CrossRef]

13. Nicholson, J.K.; Lindon, J.C. Systems biology: Metabonomics. *Nature* **2008**, *455*, 1054–1056. [CrossRef]

14. Gika, H.; Virgiliou, C.; Theodoridis, G.; Plumb, R.S.; Wilson, I.D. Untargeted LC/MS-based metabolic phenotyping (metabonomics/metabolomics): The state of the art. *J. Chromatogr. B Anal. Technol. Biomed. Life Sci.* **2019**, *1117*, 136–147. [CrossRef]

15. Roy, C.; Tremblay, P.Y.; Bienvenu, J.F.; Ayotte, P. Quantitative analysis of amino acids and acylcarnitines combined with untargeted metabolomics using ultra-high performance liquid chromatography and quadrupole time-of-flight mass spectrometry. *J. Chromatogr. B Anal. Technol. Biomed. Life Sci.* **2016**, *1027*, 40–49. [CrossRef]

16. Sinclair, K.; Dudley, E. Metabolomics and Biomarker Discovery. *Adv. Exp. Med. Biol.* **2019**, *1140*, 613–633. [CrossRef]

17. Bartel, J.; Krumsiek, J.; Theis, F.J. Statistical methods for the analysis of high-throughput metabolomics data. *Comput. Struct. Biotechnol. J.* **2013**, *4*, e201301009. [CrossRef]

18. Considine, E.C.; Thomas, G.; Boulesteix, A.L.; Khashan, A.S.; Kenny, L.C. Critical review of reporting of the data analysis step in metabolomics. *Metabolomics* **2017**, *14*, 7. [CrossRef]

19. Rosato, A.; Tenori, L.; Cascante, M.; De Atauri Carulla, P.R.; Martins Dos Santos, V.A.P.; Saccenti, E. From correlation to causation: Analysis of metabolomics data using systems biology approaches. *Metabolomics* **2018**, *14*, 37. [CrossRef]

20. Wishart, D.S.; Lewis, M.J.; Morrissey, J.A.; Flegel, M.D.; Jeroncic, K.; Xiong, Y.; Cheng, D.; Eisner, R.; Gautam, B.; Tzur, D.; et al. The human cerebrospinal fluid metabolome. *J. Chromatogr. B Anal. Technol. Biomed. Life Sci.* **2008**, *871*, 164–173. [CrossRef]

21. Psychogios, N.; Hau, D.D.; Peng, J.; Guo, A.C.; Mandal, R.; Bouatra, S.; Sinelnikov, I.; Krishnamurthy, R.; Eisner, R.; Gautam, B.; et al. The human serum metabolome. *PLoS ONE* **2011**, *6*, e16957. [CrossRef] [PubMed]

22. Bouatra, S.; Aziat, F.; Mandal, R.; Guo, A.C.; Wilson, M.R.; Knox, C.; Bjorndahl, T.C.; Krishnamurthy, R.; Saleem, F.; Liu, P.; et al. The human urine metabolome. *PLoS ONE* **2013**, *8*, e73076. [CrossRef] [PubMed]

23. Karu, N.; Deng, L.; Slae, M.; Guo, A.C.; Sajed, T.; Huynh, H.; Wine, E.; Wishart, D.S. A review on human fecal metabolomics: Methods, applications and the human fecal metabolome database. *Anal. Chim. Acta* **2018**, *1030*, 1–24. [CrossRef]

24. Wishart, D.S.; Feunang, Y.D.; Marcu, A.; Guo, A.C.; Liang, K.; Vazquez-Fresno, R.; Sajed, T.; Johnson, D.; Li, C.; Karu, N.; et al. HMDB 4.0: The human metabolome database for 2018. *Nucleic Acids Res.* **2018**, *46*, D608–D617. [CrossRef]

25. Scalbert, A.; Brennan, L.; Manach, C.; Andres-Lacueva, C.; Dragsted, L.O.; Draper, J.; Rappaport, S.M.; van der Hooft, J.J.; Wishart, D.S. The food metabolome: A window over dietary exposure. *Am. J. Clin. Nutr.* **2014**, *99*, 1286–1308. [CrossRef]

26. Lydic, T.A.; Goo, Y.H. Lipidomics unveils the complexity of the lipidome in metabolic diseases. *Clin. Transl. Med.* **2018**, *7*, 4. [CrossRef]

27. Garcia-Ortega, L.F.; Martinez, O. How Many Genes Are Expressed in a Transcriptome? Estimation and Results for RNA-Seq. *PLoS ONE* **2015**, *10*, e0130262. [CrossRef]

28. Wilhelm, M.; Schlegl, J.; Hahne, H.; Gholami, A.M.; Lieberenz, M.; Savitski, M.M.; Ziegler, E.; Butzmann, L.; Gessulat, S.; Marx, H.; et al. Mass-spectrometry-based draft of the human proteome. *Nature* **2014**, *509*, 582–587. [CrossRef]

29. Zanger, U.M.; Schwab, M. Cytochrome P450 enzymes in drug metabolism: Regulation of gene expression, enzyme activities, and impact of genetic variation. *Pharmacol. Ther.* **2013**, *138*, 103–141. [CrossRef]

30. Aslebagh, R.; Wormwood, K.L.; Channaveerappa, D.; Wetie, A.G.N.; Woods, A.G.; Darie, C.C. Identification of Posttranslational Modifications (PTMs) of Proteins by Mass Spectrometry. *Adv. Exp. Med. Biol.* **2019**, *1140*, 199–224. [CrossRef]

31. Menetski, J.P.; Hoffmann, S.C.; Cush, S.S.; Kamphaus, T.N.; Austin, C.P.; Herrling, P.L.; Wagner, J.A. The Foundation for the National Institutes of Health Biomarkers Consortium: Past Accomplishments and New Strategic Direction. *Clin. Pharmacol. Ther.* **2019**, *105*, 829–843. [CrossRef] [PubMed]

32. Booth, J. A short history of blood pressure measurement. *Proc. R. Soc. Med.* **1977**, *70*, 793–799. [CrossRef] [PubMed]

33. Dobson, M. Nature of the urine in diabetes. *Med. Obs. Inqu.* **1776**, *5*, 298–310.

34. Garrod, A.E. *Inborn Errors of Metabolism*; Henry Frowde and Hodder & Stoughton: London, UK, 1909.

35. Garrod, A.E. The incidence of alkaptonuria: A study in chemical individuality. *Lancet* **1902**, *ii*, 1616–1620. [CrossRef]

36. Piro, A.; Tagarelli, G.; Lagonia, P.; Quattrone, A.; Tagarelli, A. Archibald Edward Garrod and alcaptonuria: "Inborn errors of metabolism" revisited. *Genet. Med.* **2010**, *12*, 475–476. [CrossRef]

37.   Perlman, R.L.; Govindaraju, D.R. Archibald E. Garrod: The father of precision medicine. *Genet. Med.* **2016**, *18*, 1088–1089. [CrossRef]

38.   Phornphutkul, C.; Introne, W.J.; Perry, M.B.; Bernardini, I.; Murphey, M.D.; Fitzpatrick, D.L.; Anderson, P.D.; Huizing, M.; Anikster, Y.; Gerber, L.H.; et al. Natural history of alkaptonuria. *N. Engl. J. Med.* **2002**, *347*, 2111–2121. [CrossRef]

39.   Ranganath, L.R.; Khedr, M.; Milan, A.M.; Davison, A.S.; Hughes, A.T.; Usher, J.L.; Taylor, S.; Loftus, N.; Daroszewska, A.; West, E.; et al. Nitisinone arrests ochronosis and decreases rate of progression of Alkaptonuria: Evaluation of the effect of nitisinone in the United Kingdom National Alkaptonuria Centre. *Mol. Genet. Metab.* **2018**, *125*, 127–134. [CrossRef]

40.   Adinolfi, M. Embryonic antigens. In *Encyclopedia of Immunology*, 2nd ed.; Delves, P.J., Ed.; Academic Press: Cambridge, MA, USA, 1998; pp. 798–802.

41.   Abelev, G.I.; Perova, S.D.; Khramkova, N.I.; Postnikova, Z.A.; Irlin, I.S. Production of embryonal alpha-globulin by transplantable mouse hepatomas. *Transplantation* **1963**, *1*, 174–180. [CrossRef]

42.   Chan, S.L.; Chan, A.W.H.; Yu, S.C.H. Alpha-Fetoprotein as a Biomarker in Hepatocellular Carcinoma: Focus on Its Role in Composition of Tumor Staging Systems and Monitoring of Treatment Response. In *Biomarkers in Disease: Methods, Discoveries and Applications*; Patel, V.B., Preedy, V.R., Eds.; Springer Science+Business Media: Dordrecht, The Netherlands, 2017; pp. 623–635. [CrossRef]

43.   Wu, M.; Liu, H.; Liu, Z.; Liu, C.; Zhang, A.; Li, N. Analysis of serum alpha-fetoprotein (AFP) and AFP-L3 levels by protein microarray. *J. Int. Med. Res.* **2018**, *46*, 4297–4305. [CrossRef]

44.   Derosa, G.; Maffioli, P. Traditional markers in liver disease. In *Biomarkers in Disease: Methods, Discoveries and Applications*; Patel, V.B., Preedy, V.R., Eds.; Springer Science+Business Media: Dordrecht, The Netherlands, 2017. [CrossRef]

45.   Lou, J.; Zhang, L.; Lv, S.; Zhang, C.; Jiang, S. Biomarkers for Hepatocellular Carcinoma. *Biomark. Cancer* **2017**, *9*, 1–9. [CrossRef] [PubMed]

46.   Bruha, R. Osteopontin as a biomarker in liver disease. In *Biomarkers in Liver Disease: Methods, Discoveries and Applications*; Patel, V.B., Preedy, V.R., Eds.; Springer Science+Business Media: Dordrecht, The Netherlands, 2017. [CrossRef]

47.   Crandall, D.I.; Halikis, D.N. Homogentisic acid oxidase. I. Distribution in animal tissue and relation to tyrosine metabolism in rat kidney. *J. Biol. Chem.* **1954**, *208*, 629–638.

48.   Bernardini, G.; Laschi, M.; Geminiani, M.; Braconi, D.; Vannuccini, E.; Lupetti, P.; Manetti, F.; Millucci, L.; Santucci, A. Homogentisate 1,2 dioxygenase is expressed in brain: Implications in alkaptonuria. *J. Inherit. Metab. Dis.* **2015**, *38*, 807–814. [CrossRef] [PubMed]

49.   Hartmann, P.; Seebauer, C.T.; Schnabl, B. Alcoholic liver disease: The gut microbiome and liver cross talk. *Alcohol. Clin. Exp. Res.* **2015**, *39*, 763–775. [CrossRef] [PubMed]

50.   Osna, N.A.; Donohue, T.M., Jr.; Kharbanda, K.K. Alcoholic Liver Disease: Pathogenesis and Current Management. *Alcohol. Res.* **2017**, *38*, 147–161. [PubMed]

51.   Lieber, C.S.; Teschke, R.; Hasumura, Y.; Decarli, L.M. Differences in hepatic and metabolic changes after acute and chronic alcohol consumption. *Fed. Proc.* **1975**, *34*, 2060–2074.

52.   You, M.; Arteel, G.E. Effect of ethanol on lipid metabolism. *J. Hepatol.* **2019**, *70*, 237–248. [CrossRef]

53.   Lieber, C.S.; Jones, D.P.; Decarli, L.M. Effects of Prolonged Ethanol Intake: Production of Fatty Liver Despite Adequate Diets. *J. Clin. Investig.* **1965**, *44*, 1009–1021. [CrossRef]

54.   Lieber, C.S.; DeCarli, L.M. Liquid diet technique of ethanol administration: 1989 Update. *Alcohol Alcohol.* **1989**, *24*, 197–211.

55.   Guo, F.; Zheng, K.; Benede-Ubieto, R.; Cubero, F.J.; Nevzorova, Y.A. The Lieber-DeCarli Diet-A Flagship Model for Experimental Alcoholic Liver Disease. *Alcohol Clin. Exp. Res.* **2018**, *42*, 1828–1840. [CrossRef]

56.   Kim, S.J.; Jung, Y.S.; Kwon, D.Y.; Kim, Y.C. Alleviation of acute ethanol-induced liver injury and impaired metabolomics of S-containing substances by betaine supplementation. *Biochem. Biophys. Res. Commun.* **2008**, *368*, 893–898. [CrossRef] [PubMed]

57.   Zivkovic, A.M.; Bruce German, J.; Esfandiari, F.; Halsted, C.H. Quantitative lipid metabolomic changes in alcoholic micropigs with fatty liver disease. *Alcohol Clin. Exp. Res.* **2009**, *33*, 751–758. [CrossRef]

58. Manna, S.K.; Patterson, A.D.; Yang, Q.; Krausz, K.W.; Li, H.; Idle, J.R.; Fornace, A.J., Jr.; Gonzalez, F.J. Identification of noninvasive biomarkers for alcohol-induced liver disease using urinary metabolomics and the Ppara-null mouse. *J. Proteome Res.* **2010**, *9*, 4176–4188. [CrossRef] [PubMed]

59. Manna, S.K.; Patterson, A.D.; Yang, Q.; Krausz, K.W.; Idle, J.R.; Fornace, A.J.; Gonzalez, F.J. UPLC-MS-based urine metabolomics reveals indole-3-lactic acid and phenyllactic acid as conserved biomarkers for alcohol-induced liver disease in the Ppara-null mouse model. *J. Proteome Res.* **2011**, *10*, 4120–4133. [CrossRef]

60. Fernando, H.; Bhopale, K.K.; Kondraganti, S.; Kaphalia, B.S.; Shakeel Ansari, G.A. Lipidomic changes in rat liver after long-term exposure to ethanol. *Toxicol. Appl. Pharmacol.* **2011**, *255*, 127–137. [CrossRef]

61. Suciu, A.M.; Crisan, D.A.; Procopet, B.D.; Radu, C.I.; Socaciu, C.; Tantau, M.V.; Stefanescu, H.O.; Grigorescu, M. What's in Metabolomics for Alcoholic Liver Disease? *J. Gastrointestin. Liver Dis.* **2018**, *27*, 51–58. [CrossRef]

62. Shi, X.; Yao, D.; Chen, C. Identification of N-acetyltaurine as a novel metabolite of ethanol through metabolomics-guided biochemical analysis. *J. Biol. Chem.* **2012**, *287*, 6336–6349. [CrossRef]

63. Johnson, C.H.; Patterson, A.D.; Krausz, K.W.; Lanz, C.; Kang, D.W.; Luecke, H.; Gonzalez, F.J.; Idle, J.R. Radiation metabolomics. 4. UPLC-ESI-QTOFMS-Based metabolomics for urinary biomarker discovery in gamma-irradiated rats. *Radiat. Res.* **2011**, *175*, 473–484. [CrossRef]

64. Johnson, C.H.; Patterson, A.D.; Krausz, K.W.; Kalinich, J.F.; Tyburski, J.B.; Kang, D.W.; Luecke, H.; Gonzalez, F.J.; Blakely, W.F.; Idle, J.R. Radiation metabolomics. 5. Identification of urinary biomarkers of ionizing radiation exposure in nonhuman primates by mass spectrometry-based metabolomics. *Radiat. Res.* **2012**, *178*, 328–340. [CrossRef]

65. Luginbuhl, M.; Rutjens, S.; Konig, S.; Furrer, J.; Weinmann, W. N-Acetyltaurine as a novel urinary ethanol marker in a drinking study. *Anal. Bioanal. Chem.* **2016**, *408*, 7529–7536. [CrossRef]

66. Luginbuhl, M.; Konig, S.; Schurch, S.; Weinmann, W. Evaluation of N-acetyltaurine as an ethanol marker in human blood. *Alcohol* **2017**, *65*, 11–18. [CrossRef]

67. Xie, G.; Zhong, W.; Li, H.; Li, Q.; Qiu, Y.; Zheng, X.; Chen, H.; Zhao, X.; Zhang, S.; Zhou, Z.; et al. Alteration of bile acid metabolism in the rat induced by chronic ethanol consumption. *FASEB J.* **2013**, *27*, 3583–3593. [CrossRef]

68. Xie, G.; Zhong, W.; Zheng, X.; Li, Q.; Qiu, Y.; Li, H.; Chen, H.; Zhou, Z.; Jia, W. Chronic ethanol consumption alters mammalian gastrointestinal content metabolites. *J. Proteome Res.* **2013**, *12*, 3297–3306. [CrossRef]

69. Chen, P.; Torralba, M.; Tan, J.; Embree, M.; Zengler, K.; Starkel, P.; van Pijkeren, J.P.; DePew, J.; Loomba, R.; Ho, S.B.; et al. Supplementation of saturated long-chain fatty acids maintains intestinal eubiosis and reduces ethanol-induced liver injury in mice. *Gastroenterology* **2015**, *148*, 203–214. [CrossRef]

70. Fang, H.; Zhang, A.H.; Sun, H.; Yu, J.B.; Wang, L.; Wang, X.J. High-throughput metabolomics screen coupled with multivariate statistical analysis identifies therapeutic targets in alcoholic liver disease rats using liquid chromatography-mass spectrometry. *J. Chromatogr. B Anal. Technol. Biomed. Life Sci.* **2019**, *1109*, 112–120. [CrossRef]

71. Zhang, T.; Zhang, A.; Qiu, S.; Sun, H.; Guan, Y.; Wang, X. High-throughput metabolomics approach reveals new mechanistic insights for drug response of phenotypes of geniposide towards alcohol-induced liver injury by using liquid chromatography coupled to high resolution mass spectrometry. *Mol. Biosyst.* **2017**, *13*, 73–82. [CrossRef]

72. Deda, O.; Virgiliou, C.; Orfanidis, A.; Gika, H.G. Study of Fecal and Urinary Metabolite Perturbations Induced by Chronic Ethanol Treatment in Mice by UHPLC-MS/MS Targeted Profiling. *Metabolites* **2019**, *9*, 232. [CrossRef]

73. He, L.; Li, F.; Yin, X.; Bohman, P.; Kim, S.; McClain, C.J.; Feng, W.; Zhang, X. Profiling of Polar Metabolites in Mouse Feces Using Four Analytical Platforms to Study the Effects Of Cathelicidin-Related Antimicrobial Peptide in Alcoholic Liver Disease. *J. Proteome Res.* **2019**, *18*, 2875–2884. [CrossRef]

74. Gao, B.; Lang, S.; Duan, Y.; Wang, Y.; Shawcross, D.L.; Louvet, A.; Mathurin, P.; Ho, S.B.; Starkel, P.; Schnabl, B. Serum and Fecal Oxylipins in Patients with Alcohol-Related Liver Disease. *Dig. Dis. Sci.* **2019**, *64*, 1878–1892. [CrossRef]

75. Michelena, J.; Alonso, C.; Martinez-Arranz, I.; Altamirano, J.; Mayo, R.; Sancho-Bru, P.; Bataller, R.; Gines, P.; Castro, A.; Caballeria, J. Metabolomics Discloses a New Non-invasive Method for the Diagnosis and Prognosis of Patients with Alcoholic Hepatitis. *Ann. Hepatol.* **2019**, *18*, 144–154. [CrossRef]

76. Keitel, V.; Droge, C.; Haussinger, D. Targeting FXR in Cholestasis. *Handb. Exp. Pharmacol.* **2019**, *256*, 299–324. [CrossRef]

77. Ishihara, K.; Katsutani, N.; Asai, N.; Inomata, A.; Uemura, Y.; Suganuma, A.; Sawada, K.; Yokoi, T.; Aoki, T. Identification of urinary biomarkers useful for distinguishing a difference in mechanism of toxicity in rat model of cholestasis. *Basic Clin. Pharmacol. Toxicol.* **2009**, *105*, 156–166. [CrossRef]

78. Cho, J.Y.; Matsubara, T.; Kang, D.W.; Ahn, S.H.; Krausz, K.W.; Idle, J.R.; Luecke, H.; Gonzalez, F.J. Urinary metabolomics in Fxr-null mice reveals activated adaptive metabolic pathways upon bile acid challenge. *J. Lipid Res.* **2010**, *51*, 1063–1074. [CrossRef]

79. Passmore, I.J.; Letertre, M.P.M.; Preston, M.D.; Bianconi, I.; Harrison, M.A.; Nasher, F.; Kaur, H.; Hong, H.A.; Baines, S.D.; Cutting, S.M.; et al. Para-cresol production by Clostridium difficile affects microbial diversity and membrane integrity of Gram-negative bacteria. *PLoS Pathog* **2018**, *14*, e1007191. [CrossRef]

80. Matsubara, T.; Tanaka, N.; Sato, M.; Kang, D.W.; Krausz, K.W.; Flanders, K.C.; Ikeda, K.; Luecke, H.; Wakefield, L.M.; Gonzalez, F.J. TGF-beta-SMAD3 signaling mediates hepatic bile acid and phospholipid metabolism following lithocholic acid-induced liver injury. *J. Lipid Res.* **2012**, *53*, 2698–2707. [CrossRef]

81. Aoki, M.; Konya, Y.; Takagaki, T.; Umemura, K.; Sogame, Y.; Katsumata, T.; Komuro, S. Metabolomic investigation of cholestasis in a rat model using ultra-performance liquid chromatography/tandem mass spectrometry. *Rapid Commun. Mass Spectrom.* **2011**, *25*, 1847–1852. [CrossRef]

82. Yamazaki, M.; Miyake, M.; Sato, H.; Masutomi, N.; Tsutsui, N.; Adam, K.P.; Alexander, D.C.; Lawton, K.A.; Milburn, M.V.; Ryals, J.A.; et al. Perturbation of bile acid homeostasis is an early pathogenesis event of drug induced liver injury in rats. *Toxicol. Appl. Pharmacol.* **2013**, *268*, 79–89. [CrossRef]

83. Chen, Z.; Zhu, Y.; Zhao, Y.; Ma, X.; Niu, M.; Wang, J.; Su, H.; Wang, R.; Li, J.; Liu, L.; et al. Serum Metabolomic Profiling in a Rat Model Reveals Protective Function of Paeoniflorin Against ANIT Induced Cholestasis. *Phytother. Res.* **2016**, *30*, 654–662. [CrossRef]

84. Ma, X.; Chi, Y.H.; Niu, M.; Zhu, Y.; Zhao, Y.L.; Chen, Z.; Wang, J.B.; Zhang, C.E.; Li, J.Y.; Wang, L.F.; et al. Metabolomics Coupled with Multivariate Data and Pathway Analysis on Potential Biomarkers in Cholestasis and Intervention Effect of Paeonia lactiflora Pall. *Front. Pharmacol.* **2016**, *7*, 14. [CrossRef]

85. Zhang, C.E.; Niu, M.; Li, R.Y.; Feng, W.W.; Ma, X.; Dong, Q.; Ma, Z.J.; Li, G.Q.; Meng, Y.K.; Wang, Y.; et al. Untargeted Metabolomics Reveals Dose-Response Characteristics for Effect of Rhubarb in a Rat Model of Cholestasis. *Front. Pharmacol.* **2016**, *7*, 85. [CrossRef]

86. Sun, H.; Zhang, A.H.; Zou, D.X.; Sun, W.J.; Wu, X.H.; Wang, X.J. Metabolomics coupled with pattern recognition and pathway analysis on potential biomarkers in liver injury and hepatoprotective effects of yinchenhao. *Appl. Biochem. Biotechnol.* **2014**, *173*, 857–869. [CrossRef]

87. Li, Y.F.; Wu, J.S.; Li, Y.Y.; Dai, Y.; Zheng, M.; Zeng, J.K.; Wang, G.F.; Wang, T.M.; Li, W.K.; Zhang, X.Y.; et al. Chicken bile powder protects against alpha-naphthylisothiocyanate-induced cholestatic liver injury in mice. *Oncotarget* **2017**, *8*, 97137–97152. [CrossRef]

88. Wu, J.S.; Li, Y.F.; Li, Y.Y.; Dai, Y.; Li, W.K.; Zheng, M.; Shi, Z.C.; Shi, R.; Wang, T.M.; Ma, B.L.; et al. Huangqi Decoction Alleviates Alpha-Naphthylisothiocyanate Induced Intrahepatic Cholestasis by Reversing Disordered Bile Acid and Glutathione Homeostasis in Mice. *Front. Pharmacol.* **2017**, *8*, 938. [CrossRef]

89. Han, H.; Xu, L.; Xiong, K.; Zhang, T.; Wang, Z. Exploration of Hepatoprotective Effect of Gentiopicroside on Alpha-Naphthylisothiocyanate-Induced Cholestatic Liver Injury in Rats by Comprehensive Proteomic and Metabolomic Signatures. *Cell Physiol. Biochem.* **2018**, *49*, 1304–1319. [CrossRef]

90. Zhu, G.; Feng, F. UPLC-MS-based metabonomic analysis of intervention effects of Da-Huang-Xiao-Shi decoction on ANIT-induced cholestasis. *J. Ethnopharmacol.* **2019**, *238*, 111860. [CrossRef]

91. Ma, X.; Idle, J.R.; Krausz, K.W.; Tan, D.X.; Ceraulo, L.; Gonzalez, F.J. Urinary metabolites and antioxidant products of exogenous melatonin in the mouse. *J. Pineal Res.* **2006**, *40*, 343–349. [CrossRef]

92. Ma, X.; Chen, C.; Krausz, K.W.; Idle, J.R.; Gonzalez, F.J. A metabolomic perspective of melatonin metabolism in the mouse. *Endocrinology* **2008**, *149*, 1869–1879. [CrossRef]

93. Yu, H.; Li, Y.; Xu, Z.; Wang, D.; Shi, S.; Deng, H.; Zeng, B.; Zheng, Z.; Sun, L.; Deng, X.; et al. Identification of potential biomarkers in cholestasis and the therapeutic effect of melatonin by metabolomics, multivariate data and pathway analyses. *Int J. Mol. Med.* **2018**, *42*, 2515–2526. [CrossRef]

94. Lin, S.; Wang, T.Y.; Xu, H.R.; Zhang, X.N.; Wang, Q.; Liu, R.; Li, Q.; Bi, K.S. A systemic combined nontargeted and targeted LC-MS based metabolomic strategy of plasma and liver on pathology exploration of alpha-naphthylisothiocyanate induced cholestatic liver injury in mice. *J. Pharm. Biomed. Anal.* **2019**, *171*, 180–192. [CrossRef]

95. Dai, M.; Hua, H.; Lin, H.; Xu, G.; Hu, X.; Li, F.; Gonzalez, F.J.; Liu, A.; Yang, J. Targeted Metabolomics Reveals a Protective Role for Basal PPARalpha in Cholestasis Induced by alpha-Naphthylisothiocyanate. *J. Proteome Res.* **2018**, *17*, 1500–1508. [CrossRef]

96. Wang, B.L.; Zhang, C.W.; Wang, L.; Tang, K.L.; Tanaka, N.; Gonzalez, F.J.; Xu, Y.; Fang, Z.Z. Lipidomics reveal aryl hydrocarbon receptor (Ahr)-regulated lipid metabolic pathway in alpha-naphthyl isothiocyanate (ANIT)-induced intrahepatic cholestasis. *Xenobiotica* **2019**, *49*, 591–601. [CrossRef]

97. Fu, K.; Wang, C.; Gao, Y.; Fan, S.; Zhang, H.; Sun, J.; Jiang, Y.; Liu, C.; Guan, L.; Liu, J.; et al. Metabolomics and Lipidomics Reveal the Effect of Hepatic Vps33b Deficiency on Bile Acids and Lipids Metabolism. *Front. Pharmacol.* **2019**, *10*, 276. [CrossRef]

98. Long, Y.; Dong, X.; Yuan, Y.; Huang, J.; Song, J.; Sun, Y.; Lu, Z.; Yang, L.; Yu, W. Metabolomics changes in a rat model of obstructive jaundice: Mapping to metabolism of amino acids, carbohydrates and lipids as well as oxidative stress. *J. Clin. Biochem. Nutr.* **2015**, *57*, 50–59. [CrossRef]

99. Wei, D.D.; Wang, J.S.; Duan, J.A.; Kong, L.Y. Metabolomic Assessment of Acute Cholestatic Injuries Induced by Thioacetamide and by Bile Duct Ligation, and the Protective Effects of Huang-Lian-Jie-Du-Decoction. *Front. Pharmacol.* **2018**, *9*, 458. [CrossRef]

100. Yang, R.; Zhao, Q.; Hu, D.D.; Xiao, X.R.; Huang, J.F.; Li, F. Metabolomic analysis of cholestatic liver damage in mice. *Food Chem. Toxicol.* **2018**, *120*, 253–260. [CrossRef]

101. Lian, J.S.; Liu, W.; Hao, S.R.; Chen, D.Y.; Wang, Y.Y.; Yang, J.L.; Jia, H.Y.; Huang, J.R. A serum metabolomic analysis for diagnosis and biomarker discovery of primary biliary cirrhosis and autoimmune hepatitis. *Hepatobiliary Pancreat Dis. Int.* **2015**, *14*, 413–421. [CrossRef]

102. Trottier, J.; Bialek, A.; Caron, P.; Straka, R.J.; Heathcote, J.; Milkiewicz, P.; Barbier, O. Metabolomic profiling of 17 bile acids in serum from patients with primary biliary cirrhosis and primary sclerosing cholangitis: A pilot study. *Dig. Liver Dis.* **2012**, *44*, 303–310. [CrossRef]

103. Bell, L.N.; Wulff, J.; Comerford, M.; Vuppalanchi, R.; Chalasani, N. Serum metabolic signatures of primary biliary cirrhosis and primary sclerosing cholangitis. *Liver Int.* **2015**, *35*, 263–274. [CrossRef]

104. Tang, Y.M.; Wang, J.P.; Bao, W.M.; Yang, J.H.; Ma, L.K.; Yang, J.; Chen, H.; Xu, Y.; Yang, L.H.; Li, W.; et al. Urine and serum metabolomic profiling reveals that bile acids and carnitine may be potential biomarkers of primary biliary cirrhosis. *Int. J. Mol. Med.* **2015**, *36*, 377–385. [CrossRef]

105. Vignoli, A.; Orlandini, B.; Tenori, L.; Biagini, M.R.; Milani, S.; Renzi, D.; Luchinat, C.; Calabro, A.S. Metabolic Signature of Primary Biliary Cholangitis and Its Comparison with Celiac Disease. *J. Proteome Res.* **2019**, *18*, 1228–1236. [CrossRef]

106. Ozkan, S.; Ceylan, Y.; Ozkan, O.V.; Yildirim, S. Review of a challenging clinical issue: Intrahepatic cholestasis of pregnancy. *World J. Gastroenterol.* **2015**, *21*, 7134–7141. [CrossRef]

107. Ma, L.; Zhang, X.; Pan, F.; Cui, Y.; Yang, T.; Deng, L.; Shao, Y.; Ding, M. Urinary metabolomic analysis of intrahepatic cholestasis of pregnancy based on high performance liquid chromatography/mass spectrometry. *Clin. Chim. Acta.* **2017**, *471*, 292–297. [CrossRef]

108. Cui, Y.; Xu, B.; Zhang, X.; He, Y.; Shao, Y.; Ding, M. Diagnostic and therapeutic profiles of serum bile acids in women with intrahepatic cholestasis of pregnancy-a pseudo-targeted metabolomics study. *Clin. Chim. Acta.* **2018**, *483*, 135–141. [CrossRef]

109. Wang, P.; Zhong, H.; Song, Y.; Yuan, P.; Li, Y.; Lin, S.; Zhang, X.; Li, J.; Che, L.; Feng, B.; et al. Targeted metabolomics analysis of maternal-placental-fetal metabolism in pregnant swine reveals links in fetal bile acid homeostasis and sulfation capacity. *Am. J. Physiol. Gastrointest. Liver Physiol.* **2019**, *317*, G8–G16. [CrossRef]

110. Chen, X.; Zhang, X.; Xu, B.; Cui, Y.; He, Y.; Yang, T.; Shao, Y.; Ding, M. The urinary bile acid profiling analysis of asymptomatic hypercholanemia of pregnancy: A pseudo-targeted metabolomics study. *Clin. Chim. Acta* **2019**, *497*, 67–75. [CrossRef]

111. De Seymour, J.V.; Tu, S.; He, X.; Zhang, H.; Han, T.L.; Baker, P.N.; Sulek, K. Metabolomic profiling of maternal hair suggests rapid development of intrahepatic cholestasis of pregnancy. *Metabolomics* **2018**, *14*, 79. [CrossRef]

112. Li, Y.; Zhang, X.; Chen, J.; Feng, C.; He, Y.; Shao, Y.; Ding, M. Targeted metabolomics of sulfated bile acids in urine for the diagnosis and grading of intrahepatic cholestasis of pregnancy. *Genes Dis.* **2018**, *5*, 358–366. [CrossRef]

113. Li, W.W.; Yang, Y.; Dai, Q.G.; Lin, L.L.; Xie, T.; He, L.L.; Tao, J.L.; Shan, J.J.; Wang, S.C. Non-invasive urinary metabolomic profiles discriminate biliary atresia from infantile hepatitis syndrome. *Metabolomics* **2018**, *14*, 90. [CrossRef]

114. Bataller, R.; Brenner, D.A. Liver fibrosis. *J. Clin. Investig.* **2005**, *115*, 209–218. [CrossRef]

115. Goodman, Z.D. Grading and staging systems for inflammation and fibrosis in chronic liver diseases. *J. Hepatol.* **2007**, *47*, 598–607. [CrossRef]

116. D'Amico, G.; Garcia-Tsao, G.; Pagliaro, L. Natural history and prognostic indicators of survival in cirrhosis: A systematic review of 118 studies. *J. Hepatol.* **2006**, *44*, 217–231. [CrossRef]

117. Fleming, K.M.; Aithal, G.P.; Card, T.R.; West, J. All-cause mortality in people with cirrhosis compared with the general population: A population-based cohort study. *Liver Int.* **2012**, *32*, 79–84. [CrossRef]

118. Chang, M.L.; Yang, S.S. Metabolic Signature of Hepatic Fibrosis: From Individual Pathways to Systems Biology. *Cells* **2019**, *8*, 1423. [CrossRef]

119. Tokushige, K.; Hashimoto, E.; Kodama, K.; Tobari, M.; Matsushita, N.; Kogiso, T.; Taniai, M.; Torii, N.; Shiratori, K.; Nishizaki, Y.; et al. Serum metabolomic profile and potential biomarkers for severity of fibrosis in nonalcoholic fatty liver disease. *J. Gastroenterol.* **2013**, *48*, 1392–1400. [CrossRef]

120. Fishman, J.; Schneider, J.; Hershcope, R.J.; Bradlow, H.L. Increased estrogen-16 alpha-hydroxylase activity in women with breast and endometrial cancer. *J. Steroid Biochem.* **1984**, *20*, 1077–1081. [CrossRef]

121. Batista, A.D.; Barros, C.J.P.; Costa, T.; de Godoy, M.M.G.; Silva, R.D.; Santos, J.C.; de Melo Lira, M.M.; Juca, N.T.; Lopes, E.P.A.; Silva, R.O. Proton nuclear magnetic resonance-based metabonomic models for non-invasive diagnosis of liver fibrosis in chronic hepatitis C: Optimizing the classification of intermediate fibrosis. *World J. Hepatol.* **2018**, *10*, 105–115. [CrossRef]

122. Abellona, U.M.R.; Taylor-Robinson, S.D. Comments on Gabbani, et al. Metabolomic analysis with (1)H NMR for non-invasive diagnosis of hepatic fibrosis degree in patients with chronic hepatitis C. *Dig. Liver Dis.* **2018**, *50*, 209–210. [CrossRef]

123. Wu, F.; Zheng, H.; Yang, Z.T.; Cheng, B.; Wu, J.X.; Liu, X.W.; Tang, C.L.; Lu, S.Y.; Chen, Z.N.; Song, F.M.; et al. Urinary metabonomics study of the hepatoprotective effects of total alkaloids from Corydalis saxicola Bunting on carbon tetrachloride-induced chronic hepatotoxicity in rats using (1)H NMR analysis. *J. Pharm. Biomed. Anal.* **2017**, *140*, 199–209. [CrossRef]

124. Liu, X.W.; Tang, C.L.; Zheng, H.; Wu, J.X.; Wu, F.; Mo, Y.Y.; Liu, X.; Zhu, H.J.; Yin, C.L.; Cheng, B.; et al. Investigation of the hepatoprotective effect of Corydalis saxicola Bunting on carbon tetrachloride-induced liver fibrosis in rats by (1)H-NMR-based metabonomics and network pharmacology approaches. *J. Pharm. Biomed. Anal.* **2018**, *159*, 252–261. [CrossRef]

125. Feng, X.; Li, M.H.; Xia, J.; Deng Ba, D.J.; Ruan, L.Y.; Xing, Y.X.; Chen, C.; Wang, J.S.; Zhong, G.J. Tibetan Medical Formula Shi-Wei-Gan-Ning-Pill Protects Against Carbon Tetrachloride-Induced Liver Fibrosis—An NMR-Based Metabolic Profiling. *Front. Pharmacol.* **2018**, *9*, 965. [CrossRef]

126. Li, M.H.; Feng, X.; Deng Ba, D.J.; Chen, C.; Ruan, L.Y.; Xing, Y.X.; Chen, L.Y.; Zhong, G.J.; Wang, J.S. Hepatoprotection of Herpetospermum caudigerum Wall. against CCl4-induced liver fibrosis on rats. *J. Ethnopharmacol.* **2019**, *229*, 1–14. [CrossRef]

127. Yin, P.; Wan, D.; Zhao, C.; Chen, J.; Zhao, X.; Wang, W.; Lu, X.; Yang, S.; Gu, J.; Xu, G. A metabonomic study of hepatitis B-induced liver cirrhosis and hepatocellular carcinoma by using RP-LC and HILIC coupled with mass spectrometry. *Mol. Biosyst.* **2009**, *5*, 868–876. [CrossRef]

128. Xue, R.; Dong, L.; Wu, H.; Liu, T.; Wang, J.; Shen, X. Gas chromatography/mass spectrometry screening of serum metabolomic biomarkers in hepatitis B virus infected cirrhosis patients. *Clin. Chem. Lab. Med.* **2009**, *47*, 305–310. [CrossRef]

129. Waldhier, M.C.; Almstetter, M.F.; Nurnberger, N.; Gruber, M.A.; Dettmer, K.; Oefner, P.J. Improved enantiomer resolution and quantification of free D-amino acids in serum and urine by comprehensive two-dimensional gas chromatography-time-of-flight mass spectrometry. *J. Chromatogr. A* **2011**, *1218*, 4537–4544. [CrossRef]

130. Bastings, J.; van Eijk, H.M.; Olde Damink, S.W.; Rensen, S.S. d-amino Acids in Health and Disease: A Focus on Cancer. *Nutrients* **2019**, *11*, 2205. [CrossRef]

131. Huang, H.J.; Zhang, A.Y.; Cao, H.C.; Lu, H.F.; Wang, B.H.; Xie, Q.; Xu, W.; Li, L.J. Metabolomic analyses of faeces reveals malabsorption in cirrhotic patients. *Dig. Liver Dis.* **2013**, *45*, 677–682. [CrossRef]

132. Liu, Z.; Zhang, Z.; Huang, M.; Sun, X.; Liu, B.; Guo, Q.; Chang, Q.; Duan, Z. Taurocholic acid is an active promoting factor, not just a biomarker of progression of liver cirrhosis: Evidence from a human metabolomic study and in vitro experiments. *BMC Gastroenterol.* **2018**, *18*, 112. [CrossRef]

133. Patterson, A.D.; Maurhofer, O.; Beyoglu, D.; Lanz, C.; Krausz, K.W.; Pabst, T.; Gonzalez, F.J.; Dufour, J.F.; Idle, J.R. Aberrant lipid metabolism in hepatocellular carcinoma revealed by plasma metabolomics and lipid profiling. *Cancer Res.* **2011**, *71*, 6590–6600. [CrossRef]

134. Osman, D.; Ali, O.; Obada, M.; El-Mezayen, H.; El-Said, H. Chromatographic determination of some biomarkers of liver cirrhosis and hepatocellular carcinoma in Egyptian patients. *Biomed. Chromatogr.* **2017**, *31*. [CrossRef]

135. Wang, B.; Chen, D.; Chen, Y.; Hu, Z.; Cao, M.; Xie, Q.; Chen, Y.; Xu, J.; Zheng, S.; Li, L. Metabonomic profiles discriminate hepatocellular carcinoma from liver cirrhosis by ultraperformance liquid chromatography-mass spectrometry. *J. Proteome Res.* **2012**, *11*, 1217–1227. [CrossRef]

136. Koller, A.; Aldwin, L.; Natelson, S. Hepatic synthesis of canavaninosuccinate from ureidohomoserine and aspartate, and its conversion to guanidinosuccinate. *Clin. Chem.* **1975**, *21*, 1777–1782. [CrossRef] [PubMed]

137. Chen, D.Q.; Cao, G.; Chen, H.; Liu, D.; Su, W.; Yu, X.Y.; Vaziri, N.D.; Liu, X.H.; Bai, X.; Zhang, L.; et al. Gene and protein expressions and metabolomics exhibit activated redox signaling and wnt/beta-catenin pathway are associated with metabolite dysfunction in patients with chronic kidney disease. *Redox Biol.* **2017**, *12*, 505–521. [CrossRef] [PubMed]

138. Mindikoglu, A.L.; Opekun, A.R.; Putluri, N.; Devaraj, S.; Sheikh-Hamad, D.; Vierling, J.M.; Goss, J.A.; Rana, A.; Sood, G.K.; Jalal, P.K.; et al. Unique metabolomic signature associated with hepatorenal dysfunction and mortality in cirrhosis. *Transl. Res.* **2018**, *195*, 25–47. [CrossRef]

139. Liu, Y.; Hong, Z.; Tan, G.; Dong, X.; Yang, G.; Zhao, L.; Chen, X.; Zhu, Z.; Lou, Z.; Qian, B.; et al. NMR and LC/MS-based global metabolomics to identify serum biomarkers differentiating hepatocellular carcinoma from liver cirrhosis. *Int J. Cancer* **2014**, *135*, 658–668. [CrossRef]

140. McPhail, M.J.W.; Shawcross, D.L.; Lewis, M.R.; Coltart, I.; Want, E.J.; Antoniades, C.G.; Veselkov, K.; Triantafyllou, E.; Patel, V.; Pop, O.; et al. Multivariate metabotyping of plasma predicts survival in patients with decompensated cirrhosis. *J. Hepatol.* **2016**, *64*, 1058–1067. [CrossRef]

141. Dai, W.; Yin, P.; Chen, P.; Kong, H.; Luo, P.; Xu, Z.; Lu, X.; Xu, G. Study of urinary steroid hormone disorders: Difference between hepatocellular carcinoma in early stage and cirrhosis. *Anal. Bioanal. Chem.* **2014**, *406*, 4325–4335. [CrossRef]

142. Gao, R.; Cheng, J.; Fan, C.; Shi, X.; Cao, Y.; Sun, B.; Ding, H.; Hu, C.; Dong, F.; Yan, X. Serum Metabolomics to Identify the Liver Disease-Specific Biomarkers for the Progression of Hepatitis to Hepatocellular Carcinoma. *Sci. Rep.* **2015**, *5*, 18175. [CrossRef]

143. Hou, Q.; Duan, Z.J. Metabonomic window into hepatitis B virus-related hepatic diseases. *World J. Hepatol.* **2016**, *8*, 1–8. [CrossRef]

144. Lu, Y.; Fang, J.; Zou, L.; Cui, L.; Liang, X.; Lim, S.G.; Dan, Y.Y.; Ong, C.N. Omega-6-derived oxylipin changes in serum of patients with hepatitis B virus-related liver diseases. *Metabolomics* **2018**, *14*, 26. [CrossRef]

145. Cabral, M.; Martin-Venegas, R.; Moreno, J.J. Differential cell growth/apoptosis behavior of 13-hydroxyoctadecadienoic acid enantiomers in a colorectal cancer cell line. *Am. J. Physiol. Gastrointest. Liver Physiol.* **2014**, *307*, G664–G671. [CrossRef]

146. Zhao, C.Q.; Chen, L.; Cai, H.; Yao, W.L.; Zhou, Q.; Zhu, H.M.; Gao, Y.; Liu, P.; Gou, X.J.; Zhang, H. Classification of Gan Dan Shi Re Pattern and Gan Shen Yin Xu Pattern in Patients with Hepatitis B Cirrhosis Using Metabonomics. *Evid. Based Complement. Altern. Med.* **2018**, *2018*, 2697468. [CrossRef] [PubMed]

147. Zhou, K.; Xie, G.; Wen, J.; Wang, J.; Pan, W.; Zhou, Y.; Xiao, Y.; Wang, Y.; Jia, W.; Cai, W. Histamine is correlated with liver fibrosis in biliary atresia. *Dig. Liver Dis.* **2016**, *48*, 921–926. [CrossRef] [PubMed]

148. Jimenez, B.; Montoliu, C.; MacIntyre, D.A.; Serra, M.A.; Wassel, A.; Jover, M.; Romero-Gomez, M.; Rodrigo, J.M.; Pineda-Lucena, A.; Felipo, V. Serum metabolic signature of minimal hepatic encephalopathy by (1)H-nuclear magnetic resonance. *J. Proteome Res.* **2010**, *9*, 5180–5187. [CrossRef]

149. Martinez-Granados, B.; Morales, J.M.; Rodrigo, J.M.; Del Olmo, J.; Serra, M.A.; Ferrandez, A.; Celda, B.; Monleon, D. Metabolic profile of chronic liver disease by NMR spectroscopy of human biopsies. *Int. J. Mol. Med.* **2011**, *27*, 111–117. [CrossRef]

150. Schofield, Z.; Reed, M.A.; Newsome, P.N.; Adams, D.H.; Gunther, U.L.; Lalor, P.F. Changes in human hepatic metabolism in steatosis and cirrhosis. *World J. Gastroenterol.* **2017**, *23*, 2685–2695. [CrossRef]

151. Gao, H.; Lu, Q.; Liu, X.; Cong, H.; Zhao, L.; Wang, H.; Lin, D. Application of 1H NMR-based metabonomics in the study of metabolic profiling of human hepatocellular carcinoma and liver cirrhosis. *Cancer Sci.* **2009**, *100*, 782–785. [CrossRef]

152. Amathieu, R.; Nahon, P.; Triba, M.; Bouchemal, N.; Trinchet, J.C.; Beaugrand, M.; Dhonneur, G.; Le Moyec, L. Metabolomic approach by 1H NMR spectroscopy of serum for the assessment of chronic liver failure in patients with cirrhosis. *J. Proteome Res.* **2011**, *10*, 3239–3245. [CrossRef]

153. Qi, S.W.; Tu, Z.G.; Peng, W.J.; Wang, L.X.; Ou-Yang, X.; Cai, A.J.; Dai, Y. (1)H NMR-based serum metabolic profiling in compensated and decompensated cirrhosis. *World J. Gastroenterol.* **2012**, *18*, 285–290. [CrossRef]

154. Corbin, I.R.; Ryner, L.N.; Singh, H.; Minuk, G.Y. Quantitative hepatic phosphorus-31 magnetic resonance spectroscopy in compensated and decompensated cirrhosis. *Am. J. Physiol. Gastrointest. Liver Physiol.* **2004**, *287*, G379–G384. [CrossRef]

155. Traussnigg, S.; Kienbacher, C.; Gajdosik, M.; Valkovic, L.; Halilbasic, E.; Stift, J.; Rechling, C.; Hofer, H.; Steindl-Munda, P.; Ferenci, P.; et al. Ultra-high-field magnetic resonance spectroscopy in non-alcoholic fatty liver disease: Novel mechanistic and diagnostic insights of energy metabolism in non-alcoholic steatohepatitis and advanced fibrosis. *Liver Int.* **2017**, *37*, 1544–1553. [CrossRef]

156. Iebba, V.; Guerrieri, F.; Di Gregorio, V.; Levrero, M.; Gagliardi, A.; Santangelo, F.; Sobolev, A.P.; Circi, S.; Giannelli, V.; Mannina, L.; et al. Combining amplicon sequencing and metabolomics in cirrhotic patients highlights distinctive microbiota features involved in bacterial translocation, systemic inflammation and hepatic encephalopathy. *Sci. Rep.* **2018**, *8*, 8210. [CrossRef]

157. Liu, Y.; Li, J.; Jin, Y.; Zhao, L.; Zhao, F.; Feng, J.; Li, A.; Wei, Y. Splenectomy Leads to Amelioration of Altered Gut Microbiota and Metabolome in Liver Cirrhosis Patients. *Front. Microbiol.* **2018**, *9*, 963. [CrossRef] [PubMed]

158. Shao, L.; Ling, Z.; Chen, D.; Liu, Y.; Yang, F.; Li, L. Disorganized Gut Microbiome Contributed to Liver Cirrhosis Progression: A Meta-Omics-Based Study. *Front. Microbiol.* **2018**, *9*, 3166. [CrossRef]

159. Cox, I.J.; Idilman, R.; Fagan, A.; Turan, D.; Ajayi, L.; Le Guennec, A.D.; Taylor-Robinson, S.D.; Karakaya, F.; Gavis, E.; Andrew Atkinson, R.; et al. Metabolomics and microbial composition increase insight into the impact of dietary differences in cirrhosis. *Liver Int.* **2019**. [CrossRef]

160. Amathieu, R.; Triba, M.N.; Nahon, P.; Bouchemal, N.; Kamoun, W.; Haouache, H.; Trinchet, J.C.; Savarin, P.; Le Moyec, L.; Dhonneur, G. Serum 1H-NMR metabolomic fingerprints of acute-on-chronic liver failure in intensive care unit patients with alcoholic cirrhosis. *PLoS ONE* **2014**, *9*, e89230. [CrossRef]

161. Dabos, K.J.; Parkinson, J.A.; Sadler, I.H.; Plevris, J.N.; Hayes, P.C. (1)H nuclear magnetic resonance spectroscopy-based metabonomic study in patients with cirrhosis and hepatic encephalopathy. *World J. Hepatol.* **2015**, *7*, 1701–1707. [CrossRef]

162. Weiss, N.; Barbier Saint Hilaire, P.; Colsch, B.; Isnard, F.; Attala, S.; Schaefer, A.; Amador, M.D.; Rudler, M.; Lamari, F.; Sedel, F.; et al. Cerebrospinal fluid metabolomics highlights dysregulation of energy metabolism in overt hepatic encephalopathy. *J. Hepatol.* **2016**, *65*, 1120–1130. [CrossRef]

163. Embade, N.; Marino, Z.; Diercks, T.; Cano, A.; Lens, S.; Cabrera, D.; Navasa, M.; Falcon-Perez, J.M.; Caballeria, J.; Castro, A.; et al. Metabolic Characterization of Advanced Liver Fibrosis in HCV Patients as Studied by Serum 1H-NMR Spectroscopy. *PLoS ONE* **2016**, *11*, e0155094. [CrossRef]

164. Gabbani, T.; Marsico, M.; Bernini, P.; Lorefice, E.; Grappone, C.; Biagini, M.R.; Milani, S.; Annese, V. Metabolomic analysis with (1)H-NMR for non-invasive diagnosis of hepatic fibrosis degree in patients with chronic hepatitis C. *Dig. Liver Dis.* **2017**, *49*, 1338–1344. [CrossRef]

165. Wei, D.D.; Wang, J.S.; Wang, P.R.; Li, M.H.; Yang, M.H.; Kong, L.Y. Toxic effects of chronic low-dose exposure of thioacetamide on rats based on NMR metabolic profiling. *J. Pharm. Biomed. Anal.* **2014**, *98*, 334–338. [CrossRef]

166. Zhang, H.; Wang, X.; Hu, P.; Zhou, W.; Zhang, M.; Liu, J.; Wang, Y.; Liu, P.; Luo, G. Serum Metabolomic Characterization of Liver Fibrosis in Rats and Anti-Fibrotic Effects of Yin-Chen-Hao-Tang. *Molecules* **2016**, *21*, 126. [CrossRef] [PubMed]

167. Song, Y.N.; Zhang, G.B.; Lu, Y.Y.; Chen, Q.L.; Yang, L.; Wang, Z.T.; Liu, P.; Su, S.B. Huangqi decoction alleviates dimethylnitrosamine-induced liver fibrosis: An analysis of bile acids metabolic mechanism. *J. Ethnopharmacol.* **2016**, *189*, 148–156. [CrossRef] [PubMed]

168. Yu, J.; He, J.Q.; Chen, D.Y.; Pan, Q.L.; Yang, J.F.; Cao, H.C.; Li, L.J. Dynamic changes of key metabolites during liver fibrosis in rats. *World J. Gastroenterol.* **2019**, *25*, 941–954. [CrossRef] [PubMed]

169. Zhang, K.; Zhang, Y.; Li, N.; Xing, F.; Zhao, J.; Yang, T.; Liu, C.; Feng, N. An herbal-compound-based combination therapy that relieves cirrhotic ascites by affecting the L-arginine/nitric oxide pathway: A metabolomics-based systematic study. *J. Ethnopharmacol.* **2019**, *241*, 112034. [CrossRef] [PubMed]

170. Wang, G.; Li, Z.; Li, H.; Li, L.; Li, J.; Yu, C. Metabolic Profile Changes of CCl(4)-Liver Fibrosis and Inhibitory Effects of Jiaqi Ganxian Granule. *Molecules* **2016**, *21*, 698. [CrossRef]

171. Chang, H.; Meng, H.Y.; Wang, Y.; Teng, Z.; Liu, S.M. [Inhibitory effect of Scutellariae Radix on hepatic fibrosis based on urinary metabonomic]. *Zhongguo Zhong Yao Za Zhi* **2018**, *43*, 2140–2146. [CrossRef]

172. Zheng, M.; Li, Y.Y.; Wang, G.F.; Jin, J.Y.; Wang, Y.H.; Wang, T.M.; Yang, L.; Liu, S.Y.; Wu, J.S.; Wang, Z.T.; et al. Protective effect of cultured bear bile powder against dimethylnitrosamine-induced hepatic fibrosis in rats. *Biomed. Pharmacother.* **2019**, *112*, 108701. [CrossRef]

173. EASL; EASD; EASO. EASL-EASD-EASO Clinical Practice Guidelines for the management of non-alcoholic fatty liver disease. *J. Hepatol.* **2016**, *64*, 1388–1402. [CrossRef]

174. Puri, P.; Daita, K.; Joyce, A.; Mirshahi, F.; Santhekadur, P.K.; Cazanave, S.; Luketic, V.A.; Siddiqui, M.S.; Boyett, S.; Min, H.K.; et al. The presence and severity of nonalcoholic steatohepatitis is associated with specific changes in circulating bile acids. *Hepatology* **2018**, *67*, 534–548. [CrossRef]

175. Fedchuk, L.; Nascimbeni, F.; Pais, R.; Charlotte, F.; Housset, C.; Ratziu, V.; Group, L.S. Performance and limitations of steatosis biomarkers in patients with nonalcoholic fatty liver disease. *Aliment. Pharmacol. Ther.* **2014**, *40*, 1209–1222. [CrossRef]

176. Mato, J.M.; Alonso, C.; Noureddin, M.; Lu, S.C. Biomarkers and subtypes of deranged lipid metabolism in non-alcoholic fatty liver disease. *World J. Gastroenterol.* **2019**, *25*, 3009–3020. [CrossRef] [PubMed]

177. Johnson, C.H.; Ivanisevic, J.; Siuzdak, G. Metabolomics: Beyond biomarkers and towards mechanisms. *Nat. Rev. Mol. Cell Biol.* **2016**, *17*, 451–459. [CrossRef]

178. Puri, P.; Wiest, M.M.; Cheung, O.; Mirshahi, F.; Sargeant, C.; Min, H.K.; Contos, M.J.; Sterling, R.K.; Fuchs, M.; Zhou, H.; et al. The plasma lipidomic signature of nonalcoholic steatohepatitis. *Hepatology* **2009**, *50*, 1827–1838. [CrossRef] [PubMed]

179. Barr, J.; Vazquez-Chantada, M.; Alonso, C.; Perez-Cormenzana, M.; Mayo, R.; Galan, A.; Caballeria, J.; Martin-Duce, A.; Tran, A.; Wagner, C.; et al. Liquid chromatography-mass spectrometry-based parallel metabolic profiling of human and mouse model serum reveals putative biomarkers associated with the progression of nonalcoholic fatty liver disease. *J. Proteome Res.* **2010**, *9*, 4501–4512. [CrossRef] [PubMed]

180. Kalhan, S.C.; Guo, L.; Edmison, J.; Dasarathy, S.; McCullough, A.J.; Hanson, R.W.; Milburn, M. Plasma metabolomic profile in nonalcoholic fatty liver disease. *Metabolism* **2011**, *60*, 404–413. [CrossRef] [PubMed]

181. Li, H.; Wang, L.; Yan, X.; Liu, Q.; Yu, C.; Wei, H.; Li, Y.; Zhang, X.; He, F.; Jiang, Y. A proton nuclear magnetic resonance metabonomics approach for biomarker discovery in nonalcoholic fatty liver disease. *J. Proteome Res.* **2011**, *10*, 2797–2806. [CrossRef]

182. Lehmann, R.; Franken, H.; Dammeier, S.; Rosenbaum, L.; Kantartzis, K.; Peter, A.; Zell, A.; Adam, P.; Li, J.; Xu, G.; et al. Circulating lysophosphatidylcholines are markers of a metabolically benign nonalcoholic fatty liver. *Diabetes Care* **2013**, *36*, 2331–2338. [CrossRef]

183. Ferslew, B.C.; Xie, G.; Johnston, C.K.; Su, M.; Stewart, P.W.; Jia, W.; Brouwer, K.L.; Barritt, A.S.t. Altered Bile Acid Metabolome in Patients with Nonalcoholic Steatohepatitis. *Dig. Dis. Sci.* **2015**, *60*, 3318–3328. [CrossRef]

184. Lake, A.D.; Novak, P.; Shipkova, P.; Aranibar, N.; Robertson, D.G.; Reily, M.D.; Lehman-McKeeman, L.D.; Vaillancourt, R.R.; Cherrington, N.J. Branched chain amino acid metabolism profiles in progressive human nonalcoholic fatty liver disease. *Amino. Acids* **2015**, *47*, 603–615. [CrossRef]

185. Loomba, R.; Quehenberger, O.; Armando, A.; Dennis, E.A. Polyunsaturated fatty acid metabolites as novel lipidomic biomarkers for noninvasive diagnosis of nonalcoholic steatohepatitis. *J. Lipid Res.* **2015**, *56*, 185–192. [CrossRef]

186. Mannisto, V.T.; Simonen, M.; Hyysalo, J.; Soininen, P.; Kangas, A.J.; Kaminska, D.; Matte, A.K.; Venesmaa, S.; Kakela, P.; Karja, V.; et al. Ketone body production is differentially altered in steatosis and non-alcoholic steatohepatitis in obese humans. *Liver Int.* **2015**, *35*, 1853–1861. [CrossRef] [PubMed]

187. Rodriguez-Gallego, E.; Guirro, M.; Riera-Borrull, M.; Hernandez-Aguilera, A.; Marine-Casado, R.; Fernandez-Arroyo, S.; Beltran-Debon, R.; Sabench, F.; Hernandez, M.; del Castillo, D.; et al. Mapping of the circulating metabolome reveals alpha-ketoglutarate as a predictor of morbid obesity-associated non-alcoholic fatty liver disease. *Int. J. Obes.* **2015**, *39*, 279–287. [CrossRef] [PubMed]

188. Zhou, Y.; Oresic, M.; Leivonen, M.; Gopalacharyulu, P.; Hyysalo, J.; Arola, J.; Verrijken, A.; Francque, S.; Van Gaal, L.; Hyotylainen, T.; et al. Noninvasive Detection of Nonalcoholic Steatohepatitis Using Clinical Markers and Circulating Levels of Lipids and Metabolites. *Clin. Gastroenterol. Hepatol.* **2016**, *14*, 1463–1472. [CrossRef] [PubMed]

189. Chiappini, F.; Coilly, A.; Kadar, H.; Gual, P.; Tran, A.; Desterke, C.; Samuel, D.; Duclos-Vallee, J.C.; Touboul, D.; Bertrand-Michel, J.; et al. Metabolism dysregulation induces a specific lipid signature of nonalcoholic steatohepatitis in patients. *Sci. Rep.* **2017**, *7*, 46658. [CrossRef] [PubMed]

190. Dong, S.; Zhan, Z.Y.; Cao, H.Y.; Wu, C.; Bian, Y.Q.; Li, J.Y.; Cheng, G.H.; Liu, P.; Sun, M.Y. Urinary metabolomics analysis identifies key biomarkers of different stages of nonalcoholic fatty liver disease. *World J. Gastroenterol.* **2017**, *23*, 2771–2784. [CrossRef]

191. O'Sullivan, J.F.; Morningstar, J.E.; Yang, Q.; Zheng, B.; Gao, Y.; Jeanfavre, S.; Scott, J.; Fernandez, C.; Zheng, H.; O'Connor, S.; et al. Dimethylguanidino valeric acid is a marker of liver fat and predicts diabetes. *J. Clin. Investig.* **2017**, *127*, 4394–4402. [CrossRef]

192. Qi, S.; Xu, D.; Li, Q.; Xie, N.; Xia, J.; Huo, Q.; Li, P.; Chen, Q.; Huang, S. Metabonomics screening of serum identifies pyroglutamate as a diagnostic biomarker for nonalcoholic steatohepatitis. *Clin. Chim. Acta* **2017**, *473*, 89–95. [CrossRef]

193. Keogh, A.; Senkardes, S.; Idle, J.R.; Kucukguzel, S.G.; Beyoglu, D. A Novel Anti-Hepatitis C Virus and Antiproliferative Agent Alters Metabolic Networks in HepG2 and Hep3B Cells. *Metabolites* **2017**, *7*, 23. [CrossRef]

194. Golla, S.; Golla, J.P.; Krausz, K.W.; Manna, S.K.; Simillion, C.; Beyoglu, D.; Idle, J.R.; Gonzalez, F.J. Metabolomic Analysis of Mice Exposed to Gamma Radiation Reveals a Systemic Understanding of Total-Body Exposure. *Radiat Res.* **2017**, *187*, 612–629. [CrossRef]

195. Wang, M.; Keogh, A.; Treves, S.; Idle, J.R.; Beyoglu, D. The metabolomic profile of gamma-irradiated human hepatoma and muscle cells reveals metabolic changes consistent with the Warburg effect. *PeerJ* **2016**, *4*, e1624. [CrossRef]

196. Yang, R.X.; Hu, C.X.; Sun, W.L.; Pan, Q.; Shen, F.; Yang, Z.; Su, Q.; Xu, G.W.; Fan, J.G. Serum Monounsaturated Triacylglycerol Predicts Steatohepatitis in Patients with Non-alcoholic Fatty Liver Disease and Chronic Hepatitis B. *Sci. Rep.* **2017**, *7*, 10517. [CrossRef] [PubMed]

197. Hoyles, L.; Fernandez-Real, J.M.; Federici, M.; Serino, M.; Abbott, J.; Charpentier, J.; Heymes, C.; Luque, J.L.; Anthony, E.; Barton, R.H.; et al. Molecular phenomics and metagenomics of hepatic steatosis in non-diabetic obese women. *Nat. Med.* **2018**, *24*, 1070–1080. [CrossRef] [PubMed]

198. Mayo, R.; Crespo, J.; Martinez-Arranz, I.; Banales, J.M.; Arias, M.; Minchole, I.; Aller de la Fuente, R.; Jimenez-Aguero, R.; Alonso, C.; de Luis, D.A.; et al. Metabolomic-based noninvasive serum test to diagnose nonalcoholic steatohepatitis: Results from discovery and validation cohorts. *Hepatol. Commun.* **2018**, *2*, 807–820. [CrossRef] [PubMed]

199. Perakakis, N.; Polyzos, S.A.; Yazdani, A.; Sala-Vila, A.; Kountouras, J.; Anastasilakis, A.D.; Mantzoros, C.S. Non-invasive diagnosis of non-alcoholic steatohepatitis and fibrosis with the use of omics and supervised learning: A proof of concept study. *Metabolism* **2019**, *101*, 154005. [CrossRef] [PubMed]

200. Pietzner, M.; Budde, K.; Homuth, G.; Kastenmuller, G.; Henning, A.K.; Artati, A.; Krumsiek, J.; Volzke, H.; Adamski, J.; Lerch, M.M.; et al. Hepatic Steatosis Is Associated With Adverse Molecular Signatures in Subjects Without Diabetes. *J. Clin. Endocrinol. Metab.* **2018**, *103*, 3856–3868. [CrossRef] [PubMed]

201. Romero-Ibarguengoitia, M.E.; Vadillo-Ortega, F.; Caballero, A.E.; Ibarra-Gonzalez, I.; Herrera-Rosas, A.; Serratos-Canales, M.F.; Leon-Hernandez, M.; Gonzalez-Chavez, A.; Mummidi, S.; Duggirala, R.; et al. Family history and obesity in youth, their effect on acylcarnitine/aminoacids metabolomics and non-alcoholic fatty liver disease (NAFLD). Structural equation modeling approach. *PLoS ONE* **2018**, *13*, e0193138. [CrossRef]

202. Boone, S.; Mook-Kanamori, D.; Rosendaal, F.; den Heijer, M.; Lamb, H.; de Roos, A.; le Cessie, S.; Willems van Dijk, K.; de Mutsert, R. Metabolomics: A search for biomarkers of visceral fat and liver fat content. *Metabolomics* **2019**, *15*, 139. [CrossRef]

203. Tan, Y.; Liu, X.; Zhou, K.; He, X.; Lu, C.; He, B.; Niu, X.; Xiao, C.; Xu, G.; Bian, Z.; et al. The Potential Biomarkers to Identify the Development of Steatosis in Hyperuricemia. *PLoS ONE* **2016**, *11*, e0149043. [CrossRef]

204. Von Schonfels, W.; Patsenker, E.; Fahrner, R.; Itzel, T.; Hinrichsen, H.; Brosch, M.; Erhart, W.; Gruodyte, A.; Vollnberg, B.; Richter, K.; et al. Metabolomic tissue signature in human non-alcoholic fatty liver disease identifies protective candidate metabolites. *Liver Int.* **2015**, *35*, 207–214. [CrossRef]

205. Alonso, C.; Fernandez-Ramos, D.; Varela-Rey, M.; Martinez-Arranz, I.; Navasa, N.; Van Liempd, S.M.; Lavin Trueba, J.L.; Mayo, R.; Ilisso, C.P.; de Juan, V.G.; et al. Metabolomic Identification of Subtypes of Nonalcoholic Steatohepatitis. *Gastroenterology* **2017**, *152*, 1449–1461. [CrossRef]

206. Chen, Y.; Li, C.; Liu, L.; Guo, F.; Li, S.; Huang, L.; Sun, C.; Feng, R. Serum metabonomics of NAFLD plus T2DM based on liquid chromatography-mass spectrometry. *Clin. Biochem.* **2016**, *49*, 962–966. [CrossRef] [PubMed]

207. Semmo, N.; Weber, T.; Idle, J.R.; Beyoglu, D. Metabolomics reveals that aldose reductase activity due to AKR1B10 is upregulated in hepatitis C virus infection. *J. Viral Hepat.* **2015**, *22*, 617–624. [CrossRef] [PubMed]

208. Liu, C.R.; Li, X.; Chan, P.L.; Zhuang, H.; Jia, J.D.; Wang, X.; Lo, Y.R.; Walsh, N. Prevalence of hepatitis C virus infection among key populations in China: A systematic review. *Int. J. Infect. Dis.* **2019**, *80*, 16–27. [CrossRef] [PubMed]

209. Alkhouri, N.; Cikach, F.; Eng, K.; Moses, J.; Patel, N.; Yan, C.; Hanouneh, I.; Grove, D.; Lopez, R.; Dweik, R. Analysis of breath volatile organic compounds as a noninvasive tool to diagnose nonalcoholic fatty liver disease in children. *Eur. J. Gastroenterol. Hepatol.* **2014**, *26*, 82–87. [CrossRef]

210. Reid, D.T.; McDonald, B.; Khalid, T.; Vo, T.; Schenck, L.P.; Surette, M.G.; Beck, P.L.; Reimer, R.A.; Probert, C.S.; Rioux, K.P.; et al. Unique microbial-derived volatile organic compounds in portal venous circulation in murine non-alcoholic fatty liver disease. *Biochim. Biophys. Acta* **2016**, *1862*, 1337–1344. [CrossRef]

211. Pastore, A.; Alisi, A.; di Giovamberardino, G.; Crudele, A.; Ceccarelli, S.; Panera, N.; Dionisi-Vici, C.; Nobili, V. Plasma levels of homocysteine and cysteine increased in pediatric NAFLD and strongly correlated with severity of liver damage. *Int. J. Mol. Sci.* **2014**, *15*, 21202–21214. [CrossRef]

212. Jin, R.; Banton, S.; Tran, V.T.; Konomi, J.V.; Li, S.; Jones, D.P.; Vos, M.B. Amino Acid Metabolism is Altered in Adolescents with Nonalcoholic Fatty Liver Disease-An Untargeted, High Resolution Metabolomics Study. *J. Pediatr.* **2016**, *172*, 14–19. [CrossRef]

213. Troisi, J.; Pierri, L.; Landolfi, A.; Marciano, F.; Bisogno, A.; Belmonte, F.; Palladino, C.; Guercio Nuzio, S.; Campiglia, P.; Vajro, P. Urinary Metabolomics in Pediatric Obesity and NAFLD Identifies Metabolic Pathways/Metabolites Related to Dietary Habits and Gut-Liver Axis Perturbations. *Nutrients* **2017**, *9*, 485. [CrossRef]

214. Goffredo, M.; Santoro, N.; Trico, D.; Giannini, C.; D'Adamo, E.; Zhao, H.; Peng, G.; Yu, X.; Lam, T.T.; Pierpont, B.; et al. A Branched-Chain Amino Acid-Related Metabolic Signature Characterizes Obese Adolescents with Non-Alcoholic Fatty Liver Disease. *Nutrients* **2017**, *9*, 642. [CrossRef]

215. Troisi, J.; Belmonte, F.; Bisogno, A.; Pierri, L.; Colucci, A.; Scala, G.; Cavallo, P.; Mandato, C.; Di Nuzzi, A.; Di Michele, L.; et al. Metabolomic Salivary Signature of Pediatric Obesity Related Liver Disease and Metabolic Syndrome. *Nutrients* **2019**, *11*, 274. [CrossRef]

216. Hartley, A.; Santos Ferreira, D.L.; Anderson, E.L.; Lawlor, D.A. Metabolic profiling of adolescent non-alcoholic fatty liver disease. *Wellcome Open Res.* **2018**, *3*, 166. [CrossRef]

217. Khusial, R.D.; Cioffi, C.E.; Caltharp, S.A.; Krasinskas, A.M.; Alazraki, A.; Knight-Scott, J.; Cleeton, R.; Castillo-Leon, E.; Jones, D.P.; Pierpont, B.; et al. Development of a Plasma Screening Panel for Pediatric Nonalcoholic Fatty Liver Disease Using Metabolomics. *Hepatol. Commun.* **2019**, *3*, 1311–1321. [CrossRef]

218. Tanaka, N.; Matsubara, T.; Krausz, K.W.; Patterson, A.D.; Gonzalez, F.J. Disruption of phospholipid and bile acid homeostasis in mice with nonalcoholic steatohepatitis. *Hepatology* **2012**, *56*, 118–129. [CrossRef]

219. Tanaka, N.; Takahashi, S.; Fang, Z.Z.; Matsubara, T.; Krausz, K.W.; Qu, A.; Gonzalez, F.J. Role of white adipose lipolysis in the development of NASH induced by methionine- and choline-deficient diet. *Biochim. Biophys. Acta* **2014**, *1841*, 1596–1607. [CrossRef] [PubMed]

220. Thomas, A.; Stevens, A.P.; Klein, M.S.; Hellerbrand, C.; Dettmer, K.; Gronwald, W.; Oefner, P.J.; Reinders, J. Early changes in the liver-soluble proteome from mice fed a nonalcoholic steatohepatitis inducing diet. *Proteomics* **2012**, *12*, 1437–1451. [CrossRef] [PubMed]

221. Depner, C.M.; Traber, M.G.; Bobe, G.; Kensicki, E.; Bohren, K.M.; Milne, G.; Jump, D.B. A metabolomic analysis of omega-3 fatty acid-mediated attenuation of western diet-induced nonalcoholic steatohepatitis in LDLR-/- mice. *PLoS ONE* **2013**, *8*, e83756. [CrossRef]

222. Lake, A.D.; Novak, P.; Shipkova, P.; Aranibar, N.; Robertson, D.; Reily, M.D.; Lu, Z.; Lehman-McKeeman, L.D.; Cherrington, N.J. Decreased hepatotoxic bile acid composition and altered synthesis in progressive human nonalcoholic fatty liver disease. *Toxicol. Appl. Pharmacol.* **2013**, *268*, 132–140. [CrossRef] [PubMed]

223. Chao, J.; Huo, T.I.; Cheng, H.Y.; Tsai, J.C.; Liao, J.W.; Lee, M.S.; Qin, X.M.; Hsieh, M.T.; Pao, L.H.; Peng, W.H. Gallic acid ameliorated impaired glucose and lipid homeostasis in high fat diet-induced NAFLD mice. *PLoS ONE* **2014**, *9*, e96969. [CrossRef] [PubMed]

224. Lai, Y.S.; Chen, W.C.; Kuo, T.C.; Ho, C.T.; Kuo, C.H.; Tseng, Y.J.; Lu, K.H.; Lin, S.H.; Panyod, S.; Sheen, L.Y. Mass-Spectrometry-Based Serum Metabolomics of a C57BL/6J Mouse Model of High-Fat-Diet-Induced Non-alcoholic Fatty Liver Disease Development. *J. Agric. Food Chem.* **2015**, *63*, 7873–7884. [CrossRef]

225. Tu, L.N.; Showalter, M.R.; Cajka, T.; Fan, S.; Pillai, V.V.; Fiehn, O.; Selvaraj, V. Metabolomic characteristics of cholesterol-induced non-obese nonalcoholic fatty liver disease in mice. *Sci. Rep.* **2017**, *7*, 6120. [CrossRef]

226. Chen, C.J.; Liao, W.L.; Chang, C.T.; Lin, Y.N.; Tsai, F.J. Identification of Urinary Metabolite Biomarkers of Type 2 Diabetes Nephropathy Using an Untargeted Metabolomic Approach. *J. Proteome Res.* **2018**, *17*, 3997–4007. [CrossRef] [PubMed]

227. Pandey, V.; Sultan, M.; Kashofer, K.; Ralser, M.; Amstislavskiy, V.; Starmann, J.; Osprian, I.; Grimm, C.; Hache, H.; Yaspo, M.L.; et al. Comparative analysis and modeling of the severity of steatohepatitis in DDC-treated mouse strains. *PLoS ONE* **2014**, *9*, e111006. [CrossRef] [PubMed]

228. Sanyal, A.J.; Pacana, T. A Lipidomic Readout of Disease Progression in A Diet-Induced Mouse Model of Nonalcoholic Fatty Liver Disease. *Trans. Am. Clin. Climatol. Assoc.* **2015**, *126*, 271–288. [PubMed]

229. Patterson, R.E.; Kalavalapalli, S.; Williams, C.M.; Nautiyal, M.; Mathew, J.T.; Martinez, J.; Reinhard, M.K.; McDougall, D.J.; Rocca, J.R.; Yost, R.A.; et al. Lipotoxicity in steatohepatitis occurs despite an increase in tricarboxylic acid cycle activity. *Am. J. Physiol. Endocrinol. Metab.* **2016**, *310*, E484–E494. [CrossRef]

230. Qian, M.; Hu, H.; Zhao, D.; Wang, S.; Pan, C.; Duan, X.; Gao, Y.; Liu, J.; Zhang, Y.; Yang, S.; et al. Coordinated changes of gut microbiome and lipidome differentiates nonalcoholic steatohepatitis (NASH) from isolated steatosis. *Liver Int.* **2019**. [CrossRef]

231. Kim, K.E.; Jung, Y.; Min, S.; Nam, M.; Heo, R.W.; Jeon, B.T.; Song, D.H.; Yi, C.O.; Jeong, E.A.; Kim, H.; et al. Caloric restriction of db/db mice reverts hepatic steatosis and body weight with divergent hepatic metabolism. *Sci. Rep.* **2016**, *6*, 30111. [CrossRef]

232. Gogiashvili, M.; Edlund, K.; Gianmoena, K.; Marchan, R.; Brik, A.; Andersson, J.T.; Lambert, J.; Madjar, K.; Hellwig, B.; Rahnenfuhrer, J.; et al. Metabolic profiling of ob/ob mouse fatty liver using HR-MAS (1)H-NMR combined with gene expression analysis reveals alterations in betaine metabolism and the transsulfuration pathway. *Anal. Bioanal. Chem.* **2017**, *409*, 1591–1606. [CrossRef]

233. Li, J.; Liu, Z.; Guo, M.; Xu, K.; Jiang, M.; Lu, A.; Gao, X. Metabolomics profiling to investigate the pharmacologic mechanisms of berberine for the treatment of high-fat diet-induced nonalcoholic steatohepatitis. *Evid. Based Complement. Altern. Med.* **2015**, *2015*, 897914. [CrossRef]

234. Wang, Y.; Niu, M.; Jia, G.L.; Li, R.S.; Zhang, Y.M.; Zhang, C.E.; Meng, Y.K.; Cui, H.R.; Ma, Z.J.; Li, D.H.; et al. Untargeted Metabolomics Reveals Intervention Effects of Total Turmeric Extract in a Rat Model of Nonalcoholic Fatty Liver Disease. *Evid. Based Complement. Altern. Med.* **2016**, *2016*, 8495953. [CrossRef]

235. Van Pelt, C.K.; Huang, M.C.; Tschanz, C.L.; Brenna, J.T. An octaene fatty acid, 4,7,10,13,16,19,22,25-octacosaoctaenoic acid (28:8n-3), found in marine oils. *J. Lipid Res.* **1999**, *40*, 1501–1505.

236. Lu, Y.; Chen, Y.; Wu, Y.; Hao, H.; Liang, W.; Liu, J.; Huang, R. Marine unsaturated fatty acids: Structures, bioactivities, biosynthesis and benefits. *RSC Adv.* **2019**, *9*, 35312–35327. [CrossRef]

237. Han, J.; Dzierlenga, A.L.; Lu, Z.; Billheimer, D.D.; Torabzadeh, E.; Lake, A.D.; Li, H.; Novak, P.; Shipkova, P.; Aranibar, N.; et al. Metabolomic profiling distinction of human nonalcoholic fatty liver disease progression from a common rat model. *Obesity (Silver Spring)* **2017**, *25*, 1069–1076. [CrossRef] [PubMed]

238. Liu, X.L.; Ming, Y.N.; Zhang, J.Y.; Chen, X.Y.; Zeng, M.D.; Mao, Y.M. Gene-metabolite network analysis in different nonalcoholic fatty liver disease phenotypes. *Exp. Mol. Med.* **2017**, *49*, e283. [CrossRef] [PubMed]

239. Maciejewska, D.; Palma, J.; Dec, K.; Skonieczna-Zydecka, K.; Gutowska, I.; Szczuko, M.; Jakubczyk, K.; Stachowska, E. Is the Fatty Acids Profile in Blood a Good Predictor of Liver Changes? Correlation of Fatty Acids Profile with Fatty Acids Content in the Liver. *Diagnostics* **2019**, *9*, 197. [CrossRef] [PubMed]

240. Tang, Y.; Zhang, J.; Li, J.; Lei, X.; Xu, D.; Wang, Y.; Li, C.; Li, X.; Mao, Y. Turnover of bile acids in liver, serum and caecal content by high-fat diet feeding affects hepatic steatosis in rats. *Biochim. Biophys. Acta Mol. Cell Biol. Lipids* **2019**, *1864*, 1293–1304. [CrossRef] [PubMed]

241. Papandreou, C.; Bullo, M.; Tinahones, F.J.; Martinez-Gonzalez, M.A.; Corella, D.; Fragkiadakis, G.A.; Lopez-Miranda, J.; Estruch, R.; Fito, M.; Salas-Salvado, J. Serum metabolites in non-alcoholic fatty-liver disease development or reversion; a targeted metabolomic approach within the PREDIMED trial. *Nutr. Metab.* **2017**, *14*, 58. [CrossRef]

242. Del Chierico, F.; Nobili, V.; Vernocchi, P.; Russo, A.; De Stefanis, C.; Gnani, D.; Furlanello, C.; Zandona, A.; Paci, P.; Capuani, G.; et al. Gut microbiota profiling of pediatric nonalcoholic fatty liver disease and obese patients unveiled by an integrated meta-omics-based approach. *Hepatology* **2017**, *65*, 451–464. [CrossRef]

243. Gawlik, A.; Shmoish, M.; Hartmann, M.F.; Wudy, S.A.; Olczak, Z.; Gruszczynska, K.; Hochberg, Z. Steroid metabolomic signature of liver disease in nonsyndromic childhood obesity. *Endocr. Connect.* **2019**, *8*, 764–771. [CrossRef]

244. Robertson, D.G. Metabonomics in toxicology: A review. *Toxicol. Sci.* **2005**, *85*, 809–822. [CrossRef]

245. Miao, H.; Zhao, Y.H.; Vaziri, N.D.; Tang, D.D.; Chen, H.; Chen, H.; Khazaeli, M.; Tarbiat-Boldaji, M.; Hatami, L.; Zhao, Y.Y. Lipidomics Biomarkers of Diet-Induced Hyperlipidemia and Its Treatment with Poria cocos. *J. Agric. Food Chem.* **2016**, *64*, 969–979. [CrossRef]

5

Targeted Analysis of 46 Bile Acids to Study the Effect of Acetaminophen in Rat by LC-MS/MS

Vivaldy Prinville, Leanne Ohlund and Lekha Sleno *

Department of Chemistry, Université du Québec à Montréal (UQAM), P.O. Box 8888 Downtown Station, Montreal, QC H3C 3P8, Canada; vivaldyp@hotmail.com (V.P.); ohlund@gmail.com (L.O.)
* Correspondence: sleno.lekha@uqam.ca

Abstract: Bile acids represent a large class of steroid acids synthesized in the liver and further metabolized by many bacterial and mammalian enzymes. Variations in bile acid levels can be used as a measure of liver function. There still exists, however, a need to study the variation of individual circulating bile acids in the context of hepatotoxity or liver disease. Acetaminophen (APAP), a drug commonly taken to relieve pain and decrease fever, is known to cause acute liver failure at high doses. We have developed a targeted liquid chromatography-tandem mass spectrometry method to monitor the effects of different doses of APAP on the bile acid plasma profile in a rat model. The analysis method was optimized to ensure chromatographic resolution of isomeric species using a mixture of 46 standard bile acids, and 14 isotopically-labeled internal standard (IS) compounds detected in multiple reaction monitoring (MRM) mode on a triple quadrupole mass spectrometer. Four doses of acetaminophen were studied, the highest of which shows signs of hepatotoxicity in rats. This targeted method revealed that high dose APAP has an important effect on bile acid profiles. Changes were seen in several unconjugated bile acids as well as glycine conjugates; however, no obvious changes were apparent for taurine-conjugated species.

Keywords: bile acids; metabolomics; rat plasma; tandem mass spectrometry; liquid chromatography; acetaminophen; hepatotoxicity

1. Introduction

Bile acids play many roles crucial for metabolism and liver health. They are formed from cholesterol through a series of enzymatic reactions and they represent the primary pathway for cholesterol catabolism [1]. In addition, bile acids emulsify fat from our diet and help absorb lipids and cholesterol [2]. Primary bile acids, such as cholic acid (CA) and chenodeoxycholic acid (CDCA) in humans and α-muricholic acid (α-MCA) and β-muricholic acid (β-MCA) in rodents, are synthesized in the liver. Before being secreted by the liver, bile acids can be conjugated to taurine or glycine amino acids. In the intestines, bile acids are unconjugated and converted into secondary bile acids, such as deoxycholic acid (DCA) and lithocholic acid. Most bile acids are reabsorbed in the liver, conjugated again, and excreted in the bile to complete the enterohepatic circulation [2,3].

An increased plasma concentration of bile acids is a sign of liver disease [4]. High concentrations are toxic, though the potential for toxicity depends on the bile acid profile. For example, it has been reported that chenodeoxycholic acid and lithocholic acid, as well as their conjugates, can damage hepatic cells and induce mitochondrial malfunction, oxidative stress, and apoptosis [5–8]. Bile acids can also damage cells within the colon [9,10]. The different physiological functions of bile acids and their implication in pathological processes highlight the importance of understanding circulating bile acid profiles in drug-induced hepatotoxicity.

Acetaminophen (APAP) is a drug commonly used to relieve pain and decrease fever. When taken in therapeutics doses, APAP is considered a very safe drug. With excessive doses, APAP can become highly toxic [11]. In North America, it is the main cause of acute liver failure, and often requires liver transplantation if too severe or not treated rapidly enough [12]. In extreme cases, APAP toxicity can cause death within 48 h. Previous studies have shown APAP interferes with bile acid synthesis [13–15].

Different LC-MS based methods to measure bile acids exist [16,17], but a gap still remains with regards to the wide range of bile acid derivatives that exist and their changing profiles with APAP dose. By studying the effect on individual bile acids, specific reactions related to bile acid metabolism can be assessed as being relevant to follow altered hepatic metabolism. The goal of this study was to develop an optimized and semi-quantitative method to evaluate the effects of APAP on numerous bile acids, including free and conjugated forms. Liquid chromatography coupled to tandem mass spectrometry is a powerful technique that offers many advantages for selective detection of individual bile acids, which are uniquely challenging due to the presence of many isomers. Bile acids can be difficult to analyze due to the similarities between the structures. In this study, we developed a rapid method to monitor 46 bile acids by LC-MS/MS on a triple quadrupole platform in multiple reaction monitoring (MRM) mode.

2. Results and Discussion

A targeted liquid chromatography-multiple reaction monitoring (LC-MRM) method was developed to monitor 46 bile acids in rat plasma following a simple sample preparation to evaluate the effect of increasing APAP dose. Bile acids were extracted by protein precipitation using methanol, following the addition of an isotopically labeled internal standard mix. A reverse-phase solid-core C18 column was employed to separate the 46 bile acids with excellent resolution and peak shape using acidified water and acetonitrile as mobile phase, within a 45 min gradient. As shown in Figure 1, all 46 bile acids in the standard mix were well resolved, including many bile acid isomers (e.g., UDCA, CDCA, and DCA). For example, LC-MRM chromatograms for α-TMCA, β-TMCA, and TCA in rat plasma show good resolution obtained and highlight the usefulness of this method to monitor these isomers. The list of bile acids assessed in this study was based on the availability of a standard mix as well as multiple isotopically-labeled bile acids for relative quantitation, through a generous gift from MRM Proteomics Inc. The separation of these internal standard (IS) compounds is shown in Figure 2.

LC-MRM analyses in negative ion mode yielded better results than in positive ion mode in terms of sensitivity (data not shown), though both were optimized. In positive mode, precursor ions were often associated to in-source water losses and had limited sensitivity as compared to negative mode. In negative mode, unconjugated bile acids were monitored with two transitions, the highest signal coming from monitoring the pseudo-MRM transition of precursor ion to precursor ion, since their fragmentation resulted in a complex mix of fragments, thus limiting sensitivity for more specific fragment ions [18]. For conjugated bile acids, fragment ions resulting from the taurine and glycine moieties were employed as product ions. For each bile acid, however, secondary transitions were monitored for confirmatory purposes. In rat plasma samples, 39 of the 46 bile acids were measurable, with peaks having signal-to-noise of at least 10 and retention time matching that of the standard mix. No peak was observed for GDHCA, TDHCA, IDCA, DHCA, TLCA, AILCA and ILCA in rat plasma samples. DHCA is a synthetic product of the oxidation of CA and is mainly converted into 3-α-hydroxylated-oxo bile acids [19]. It is therefore normal that the conjugated bile acids of DHCA (GDHCA and TDHCA) are not present in rat plasma either. Iso-bile acids (IDCA, AILCA and ILCA) are excreted in the feces of animals [20]. Of the 39 bile acids remaining, several had very small peaks that did not yield any statistically-significant changes between APAP doses, including GHCA, GLCA, GUDCA, NCA, NUDCA, DHLCA, LCA, di-oxo-LCA and 6,7 diketo-LCA.

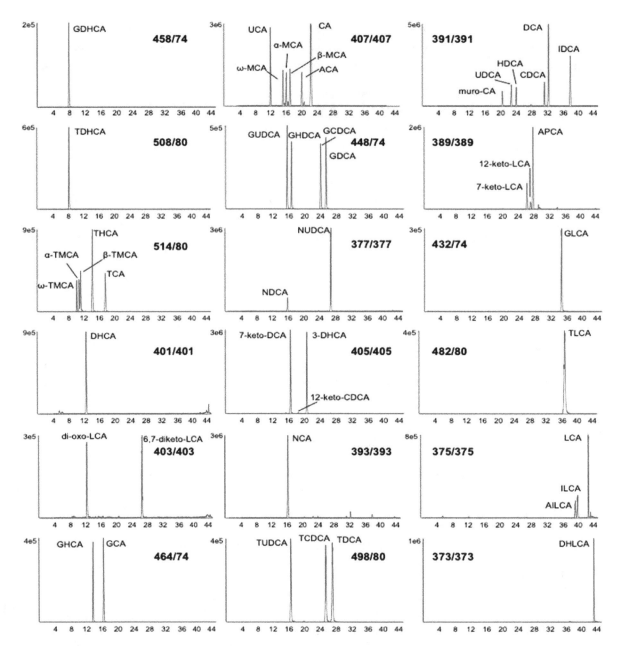

Figure 1. Representative LC-MRM chromatograms in negative mode of a standard mixture containing 46 bile acids (using the most sensitive transition for each bile acid, as shown). Acronyms for each bile acid species are listed in the Abbreviations (and Methods) section.

The highest APAP dose administered in this study significantly influenced the peaks corresponding to several bile acids (Figure 3). Table S1 shows the p-values and fold changes seen for each of these changing bile acids at each of the dosing levels compared to the lowest dose. This table also shows the integration data considering both MRM transitions monitored for each of these bile acids, and confirms that for all except two which were too small to properly integrate, these secondary transitions correlated well with the first (more sensitive) transition. Each MRM peak was also investigated for saturation effects. Although no linear ranges were determined directly, based on the peak heights of these bile acids, it was confirmed that we would be able to detect changes in terms of fold change (up or down). It is, however, very important to state here that fold changes of peak area ratios do not directly translate into concentration fold changes. These results are reported to determine which bile acids of the 46 from the standard mix were well observed in rat plasma samples and which were altered significantly with increased APAP dose. Thirteen bile acids of the 30 having significant signal-to-noise in our samples were shown to have statistically-relevant changes between the lowest and highest dose given in this study, with a p-value of lower than 0.05, six of which had p-values lower than 0.01. Increasing the APAP dose affected the concentration of some bile acids more than others. The bile acids with the most significant changes (with $p < 0.01$) were GCA, GDCA, 7-keto-DCA, APCA, CA and DCA. The graphs in Figure 3 show the peak area ratios at all four doses of APAP. The taurine conjugates monitored did not show any statistically relevant changes with APAP dose. An important effect was seen, however, for several conjugated glycine conjugates. All four glycine conjugates having adequate peak size (GCA, GCDCA, GDCA and GHDCA) were found to significantly increase between 75 and 600 mg/kg APAP. The three with less obvious quantitative changes were notably much smaller peaks in the rat plasma extracts. For example, the peak area ratio for GDCA was 10.1 times higher (with a p-value of 0.0024) with 600 mg/kg compared with 75 mg/kg APAP, while the corresponding taurine conjugate, TDCA, did not show any effect at the highest dose. Since the conjugation of bile acids is an important pathway for their secretion by the liver, our results indicate that APAP could influence the transfer pathway of bile acids from the liver to the bloodstream.

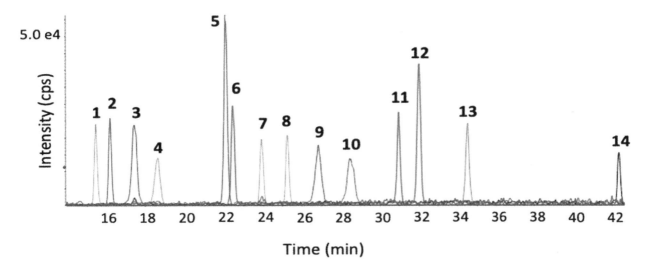

Figure 2. Representative LC-MRM chromatograms from a 20 µL injection of IS mix containing 0.013-0.1 µM final concentration of each IS compound. (1) d4-GUDCA (2) d4-GCA (3) d4-TUDCA (4) d4-TCA (5) d4-CA (6) d4-UDCA (7) d4-GCDCA (8) d4-GDCA (9) d4-TCDCA (10) d6-TDCA (11) d4-CDCA (12) d4-DCA (13) d4-GLCA (14) d4-LCA.

We found that for the two primary bile acids, CDCA and CA, only CA was found to have a statistically significant increase with APAP dose levels (fold change of 1.8 and p-value of 0.005 at highest dose). Peak area ratios for α-MCA, and ω-MCA had increased by 4.6-, and 7.4-fold (p-value of 0.0268, and 0.0322), respectively. Given that CDCA is transformed by 6β-hydroxylase in rat liver into α-MCA, β-MCA, and ω-MCA, it is likely that CDCA is mostly converted into different MCA isomers [21]. The peak area ratio of DCA increased 5.6-fold, (with a p-value of 0.0003). Interestingly, DCA has been reported to induce both early apoptosis and necrosis, thus affecting cell development [22]. The fold changes between different individual bile acids cannot be directly compared, of course, since the relative response and sensitivity of each compound by LC-MS/MS is unique. We are not assuming that a larger fold change from this data set gives a stronger change in actual concentration. This would need a follow-up study for absolute quantitation of individual bile acids, with calibration curves for each. This is quite difficult, however, considering we are not able to construct traditional calibration curves for endogenous metabolites in complex biological matrices, such as plasma, as is done for therapeutic drug monitoring.

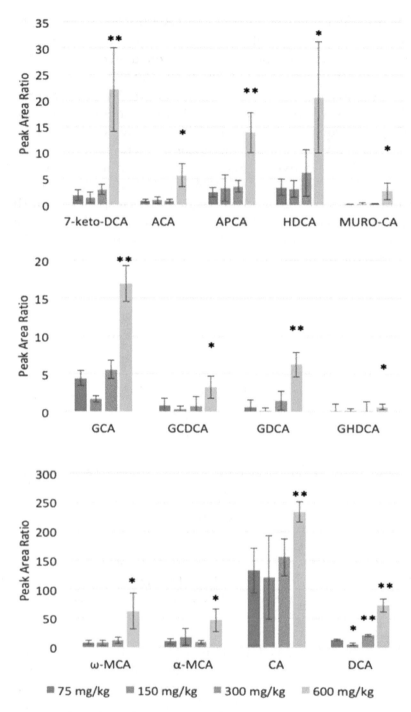

Figure 3. Peak area ratios for bile acids having significant changes between 75 mg/kg and 600 mg/kg APAP dosing, as measured in rat plasma after 24 h. * p-value < 0.05, ** p-value < 0.01.

The LC-MRM data was imported into metabolomics software (MarkerView™) to perform statistical analyses (Student's t-test, as shown previously) and also to visualize data presented within a principal component analysis (PCA). Figure 4 shows the PCA plot of the first two principal components (PC1 vs. PC2), with Pareto scaling to alleviate bias to highest peaks. This plot shows clearly that the highest dose of 600 mg/kg clusters separately to the three lower doses (75, 150, and 300 mg/kg), as was evident from the t-testing results of the individual bile acids. The PCA plot, which used all features from the LC-MRM data, following supervised peak integration, serves to show that the high dose had a marked effect compared to the three lower doses, instead of seeing a gradual shift between the four doses.

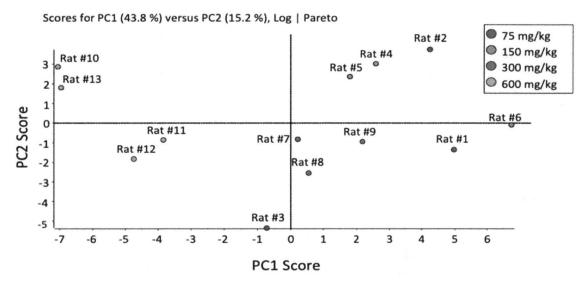

Figure 4. Unsupervised principal component analysis (PCA) of 39 bile acids detected in rat plasma samples (comparing four APAP dosing groups).

A higher throughput method could be devised to assess the specific bile acids perturbed by APAP in a follow-up study, for a more rapid assessment of changes in a clinical setting, for instance. It is important to note, however, that there exists many isomers of bile acids in biological samples and that even if we are interested in targeting a finite list of specific ones for a follow-up assay, we would still need to ensure proper separation of all these isomers. The study presented here focused specifically on evaluation the 46 bile acids available from a known standard mix. This method is not presented for the purpose of being a clinical assay, since it would likely not be high throughput enough considering the chromatographic separation needed to access all these different isomers. It also does not serve to accurately quantify each bile acid (in terms of concentration), rather it looks at relative amounts of bile acids (e.g., their profiles) in a biological matrix (rat plasma) to look for specific effects of APAP dose on individual bile acids. Therefore, this work should not be considered as a new validated method, as per US FDA guidelines. It would be interesting in a future study to validate a method for the bile acids specifically perturbed by high dose APAP. This is quite challenging in the case of endogenous metabolites since it would necessitate stable isotope standards for each metabolite to be quantified, as well as a suitable "blank" biological matrix to be used for preparing calibration curves for each analyte. Additionally, a non-targeted metabolomics approach using high-resolution tandem mass spectrometry would be able to access many more bile acid isomers, as well as sulfate and glucuronide metabolites, without the need for optimizing MS/MS parameters for MRM detection.

3. Materials and Methods

3.1. Materials

HPLC-grade acetonitrile (ACN) and methanol (MeOH), as well as LC-MS-grade formic acid were purchased from Sigma-Aldrich (Oakville, ON, Canada). Purified water was prepared in-house. MetaboloMetrics™ bile acids analysis kits were obtained from MRM Proteomics Inc. (Montreal, QC, Canada). Kits contained a mix of 46 bile acids and an IS mix of 14 deuterated isotope-labeled internal standards. Sprague-Dawley rats were dosed (IP) with 75, 150, 300, and 600 mg/kg APAP, in triplicate, and plasma was collected after 24 h at INRS Centre de Biologie Experimentale (Laval, QC, Canada), within standard ethical practices. The protocol was approved by the Ethics Committee of the INRS Centre de Biologie Experimentale under the ethical practices of the Canadian Council on Animal Care (project UQLK.14.02). These samples were collected in February 2014 and stored at −80 °C until proceeding with sample preparation.

- The standard mix containing 46 bile acids (each at 2.5 nmol), except for deoxycholic acid (5 nmol) and taurohyocholic acid (6.5 nmol) was provided as a dried sample (Tube A). The bile acids in the standard mix were as follows: glycodehydrocholic acid (GDHCA), taurodehydrocholic acid (TDHCA), tauro-ω-muricholic acid (ω-TMCA), tauro-α-muricholic acid (α-TMCA), tauro-β-muricholic acid (β-TMCA), taurohyocholic acid (THCA), taurocholic acid (TCA), dehydrocholic acid (DHCA), dioxolithocholic acid (di-oxo-LCA), 6,7-diketolithocholic acid (6,7-diketo-LCA), glycohyocholic acid (GHCA), glycocholic acid (GCA), ursocholic acid (UCA), ω-muricholic acid (ω-MCA), α-muricholic acid (α-MCA), β-muricholic acid (β-MCA), allocholic acid (ACA), cholic acid (CA), glycoursodeoxycholic acid (GUDCA), glycohyodeoxycholic acid (GHDCA), glycochenodeoxycholic acid (GCDCA), glycodeoxycholic acid (GDCA), nordeoxycholic acid (NDCA), norursodeoxycholic acid (NUDCA), 7-ketodeoxycholic acid (7-keto-DCA), 12-ketodeoxycholic acid (12-keto-DCA), 3-dehydrocholic acid (3-DHCA), norcholic acid (NCA), tauroursodeoxycholic acid (TUDCA), taurochenodeoxycholic acid (TCDCA), taurodeoxycholic acid (TDCA), murocholic acid (muro-CA), ursodeoxycholic acid (UDCA), hyodeoxycholic acid (HDCA), chenodeoxycholic acid (CDCA), deoxycholic acid (DCA), isodeoxycholic acid (IDCA), 7-ketolithocholic acid (7-keto-LCA), 12-ketolithocholic acid (12-keto-LCA), apocholic acid (APCA), glycolithocholic acid (GLCA), taurolithocholic acid (TLCA), alloisolithocholic acid (AILCA), isolithocholic acid (ILCA), lithocholic acid (LCA) and dehydrolithocholic acid (DHLCA).

- Isotopically labeled bile acids were provided as an IS mix for normalization purposes. The labeled bile acids were present at between 0.1–0.75 nmol, as a dried sample (Tube B). The labeled bile acids in the IS mix were as follows: glycoursodeoxycholic acid-d_4 (d_4-GUDCA), glycocholic acid-d_4 (d_4-GCA), tauroursodeoxycholic acid-d_4 (d_4-TUDCA), taurocholic acid-d_4 (d_4-TCA), cholic acid-d_4 (d_4-CA), ursodeoxycholic acid-d_4 (d_4-UDCA), glycochenodeoxycholic acid-d_4 (d_4-GCDCA), glycodeoxycholic acid-d_4 (d_4-5GDCA), taurochenodeoxycholic acid-d_4 (d_4-TCDCA), taurodeoxycholic acid-d_6 (d_6-TDCA), chenodeoxycholic acid-d_4 (d_4-CDCA), deoxycholic acid-d_4 (d_4-DCA), glycolithocholic acid-d_4 (d_4-GLCA) and lithocholic acid-d_4 (d_4-LCA).

3.2. Sample Preparation

For the standard mix preparation, 250 μL ACN was added to Tube A, followed by a 1:10 dilution with 40% ACN. This standard mix was injected (2 μL) with the LC-MRM method described (shown in Figure 1) for retention time matching of bile acids in samples. For the internal standard (IS) mix, 7.5 mL of 40% ACN was added to Tube B. Plasma samples (50 μL) were mixed with 50 μL of the reconstituted (Tube B) internal standard solution. The extraction of bile acids from rat plasma was then performed by adding 300 μL MeOH to precipitate proteins. Samples were vortexed and sonicated for 15 min, then centrifuged at 14,000 rpm for 8 min. Supernatants (300 μL) were transferred to new microtubes, dried under nitrogen and reconstituted with 150 μL 50% MeOH prior to analysis. Extracts were stored at −20 °C until LC-MS analysis.

3.3. LC-MS/MS

Extracted plasma and standards were separated on an Aeris™ PEPTIDE XB-C18 column (1.7 μm, 100 mm × 2.1 mm) (Phenomenex®, Torrance, CA, USA) using a Nexera ultra high performance liquid chromatography (UHPLC) system (Shimadzu, Columbia, MD, USA) at 50 °C with gradient elution using water and ACN, each containing 0.1% formic acid as mobile phase A and B, respectively, at a flow rate of 0.400 mL/min and injection volume of 15 μL. The gradient started at 10% B and was held for 1 min increased linearly to 25% for 2 min, to 35% over 17 min, to 50% over 20 min, to 60% over 2 min and 90% for 1 min, followed by a 10 min column re-equilibration time at starting conditions. MS data was collected using a QTRAP 5500 system (Sciex, Concord, ON, Canada). Electrospray ionization (ESI) in negative ion mode and multiple reaction monitoring (MRM) was used. The MRM parameters (first and second transitions with collision energies (CE)) for all 46 bile acids are listed in Table 1. Each transition was monitored throughout the chromatogram with a dwell time of 7 ms.

Because of the fragmentation behavior of the deprotonated unconjugated bile acids, the first transitions chosen for the unconjugated forms were simply precursor to precursor ions, as has been done in many previous reports on bile acid analysis [17,23–25]. This was necessary for ensuring the best sensitivity of detection for these unconjugated forms. For glycine conjugated bile acids, there was a specific and sensitive common fragment ion at m/z 74, corresponding to the deprotonated glycine moiety being lost. Similarly, taurine conjugates yielded a common fragment at m/z 80, corresponding to the HSO_3^- ion from the taurine group. The secondary transitions were used for confirmation. For those bile acids found to be altered significantly upon APAP dose, the secondary transition was also integrated and compared.

Table 1. Optimized MRM transitions and collision energies for 46 standard bile acids along with their respective retention times.

Bile Acid	RT (min)	1st Transition (CE)	2nd Transition (CE)	IS
GDHCA	7.9	458.2/74.0 (−66)	458.2/348.1 (−41)	CDCA-d$_4$
TDHCA	8.2	508.2/80.0 (−123)	508.2/124.1 (−67)	CDCA-d$_4$
T-ω-MCA	10.1	514.2/80.0 (−135)	514.2/107.0 (−82)	TCA-d$_4$
T-α-MCA	10.7	514.2/80.0 (−135)	514.2/107.0 (−82)	TCA-d$_4$
T-β-MCA	11.1	514.2/80.0 (−135)	514.2/124.0 (−65)	TCA-d$_4$
UCA	11.9	407.2/407.2 (−15)	407.2/343.1 (−46)	CA-d$_4$
di-oxo-LCA	12.3	403.2/403.2 (−18)	403.2/385.2 (−40)	CDCA-d$_4$
DHCA	12.4	401.2/401.2 (−18)	401.2/331.1 (−36)	CDCA-d$_4$
GHCA	13.6	464.2/74.0 (−82)	464.2/354.1 (−56)	GCA-d$_4$
THCA	14.1	514.2/80.0 (−135)	514.2/107.0 (−82)	TCA-d$_4$
ω-MCA	15.1	407.2/407.2 (−15)	407.2/371.1 (−43)	CA-d$_4$
GUDCA	15.5	448.2/74.0 (−83)	448.2/386.1 (−59)	GUDCA-d$_4$
NDCA	15.8	377.2/377.2 (−15)	377.2/331.1 (−46)	CDCA-d$_4$
α- MCA	16.0	407.2/407.2 (−15)	407.2/371.1 (−43)	CA-d$_4$
NCA	16.1	393.2/393.2 (−15)	393.2/375.1 (−45)	CDCA-d$_4$
GCA	16.2	464.2/74.0 (−82)	464.2/402.1 (−46)	GCA-d$_4$
7-keto-DCA	16.4	405.2/405.2 (−18)	405.2/289.1 (−51)	CDCA-d$_4$
TUDCA	16.4	498.2/80.0 (−130)	498.2/107 (−82)	TUDCA-d$_4$
GHDCA	16.6	448.2/74.0 (−83)	448.2/386.1 (−59)	GUDCA-d$_4$
β-MCA	16.9	407.2/407.2 (−15)	407.2/371.1 (−43)	CA-d$_4$
TCA	17.5	514.2/80.0 (−135)	514.2/124.0 (−65)	TCA-d$_4$
12-keto-CDCA	18.4	405.2/405.2 (−18)	405.2/387.1 (−45)	CDCA-d$_4$
ACA	19.9	407.2/407.2 (−15)	407.2/371.1 (−43)	CA-d$_4$
muro-CA	20.3	391.2/391.2 (−15)	391.2/343.1 (−53)	UDCA-d$_4$
3-DHCA	20.5	405.2/405.2 (−18)	405.2/289.1 (−51)	CDCA-d$_4$
CA	22.2	407.2/407.2 (−15)	407.2/343.1 (−46)	CA-d$_4$
UDCA	22.6	391.2/391.2 (−15)	391.2/373.2 (−48)	UDCA-d$_4$
HDCA	23.9	391.2/391.2 (−15)	391.2/373.2 (−48)	CDCA-d$_4$
GCDCA	24.0	448.2/74.0 (−83)	448.2/404.2 (−46)	GCDCA-d$_4$
TCDCA	25.3	498.2/80.0 (−130)	498.2/124 (−64)	TCDCA-d$_4$

Table 1. *Cont.*

Bile Acid	RT (min)	1st Transition (CE)	2nd Transition (CE)	IS
GDCA	25.3	448.2/74.0 (-83)	448.2/404.2 (-46)	GDCA-d$_4$
7-keto-LCA	26.1	389.2/389.2 (-18)	389.2/354.1 (-43)	LCA-d$_4$
6,7-diketo-LCA	26.5	403.2/403.2 (-18)	403.2/347.1 (-39)	LCA-d$_4$
NUDCA	26.7	377.2/377.2 (-15)	377.2/359.1 (-45)	CDCA-d$_4$
TDCA	27.0	498.2/80.0 (-130)	498.2/124 (-64)	TDCA-d$_6$
12-keto-LCA	27.1	389.2/389.2 (-18)	389.2/354.1 (-43)	LCA-d$_4$
APCA	27.6	389.2/389.2 (-18)	389.2/371.1 (-43)	CDCA-d$_4$
CDCA	31.1	391.2/391.2 (-15)	391.2/373.2 (-48)	CDCA-d$_4$
DCA	32.1	391.2/391.2 (-15)	391.2/343.1 (-53)	DCA-d$_4$
GLCA	34.6	432.2/74.0 (-66)	432.2/388.1 (-45)	GLCA-d$_4$
TLCA	36.6	482.2/80.0 (-135)	482.2/107 (-80)	LCA-d$_4$
IDCA	37.8	391.2/391.2 (-15)	391.2/345.1 (-45)	DCA-d$_4$
AILCA	39.1	375.2/375.2 (-15)	375.2/45 (-50)	LCA-d$_4$
ILCA	39.7	375.2/375.2 (-15)	375.2/45 (-50)	LCA-d$_4$
LCA	42.5	375.2/375.2 (-15)	375.2/45 (-50)	LCA-d$_4$
DHLCA	43.1	373.2/373.2 (-18)	373.2/45 (-50)	LCA-d$_4$

3.4. Statistical Analysis

A mixture of 14 deuterated bile acids was added to the plasma samples prior to metabolite extraction, for normalization of data as peak area ratios (analyte/IS) (see Table 2). For those bile acids without corresponding deuterated analogs, the closest eluting deuterated analog was used as IS, as noted in Table 1. Standards were used to confirm the identity of each bile acid, based on retention and MRM signal. Peak integration was performed using Multiquant™ 2.1 (Sciex). Statistical analyses were done using MarkerView™ 1.2.1 (Sciex). This software was used to perform Student's t-tests, yielding *p*-values and fold changes between different dosing groups, for each bile acid detected in rat plasma samples. Within Markerview software, principal component analysis was performed on the integrated LC-MRM data, without weighting and using Pareto scaling (unsupervised).

Table 2. Optimized MRM transitions and collision energies for 14 internal standards compounds, along with their respective retention times.

	RT (min)	Q1 (*m/z*)	Q3 (*m/z*)	CE (V)
GUDCA-d$_4$	15.5	452.3	74.0	-41
GCA-d$_4$	16.2	468.3	74.0	-45
TUDCA-d$_4$	17.4	502.3	80.0	-73
TCA-d$_4$	18.7	518.3	80.0	-80
CA-d$_4$	22.1	411.3	411.3	-15
UDCA-d$_4$	22.5	395.3	395.3	-15
GCDCA-d$_4$	23.8	452.3	74.0	-37
GDCA-d$_4$	25.3	452.3	74.0	-41
TCDCA-d$_4$	26.8	502.3	80.0	-80
TDCA-d$_6$	28.7	504.3	80.0	-80
CDCA-d$_4$	31	395.3	395.3	-15
DCA-d$_4$	32	395.3	395.3	-15
GLCA-d$_4$	34.5	436.3	74.0	-41
LCA-d$_4$	42.4	379.3	379.3	-15

4. Conclusions

In this study, we have developed a targeted metabolomics method to gain a better understanding of the effects of APAP on circulating bile acid profiles. A simple protein precipitation procedure in rat plasma was employed rapidly prepare samples for analysis. A standard mix of 46 bile acids was successfully resolved by LC-MRM, 39 of which were detected in rat plasma samples. These analyses highlighted significant changes in bile acid profiles with increasing APAP dose in rats. In general, these results indicate that APAP can have an important effect on the metabolism of bile acids. Depending on the dose level, exposure to high or repeated APAP doses has the potential to induce serious health problems, related to bile acid metabolism and excretion. The specificity of these biomarkers to APAP-related toxicity would still need to be investigated. Certain of these bile acids can also serve as biomarkers to establish the level of hepatotoxicity; however, more work would be needed to validate specific bile acid biomarkers for clinical use.

Supplementary Materials: Table S1: Comparison of p-values and fold-changes between the four doses of APAP administered in this study (using two MRM transitions for each peak) of known bile acids showing significant differences between the lowest and highest dose APAP.

Author Contributions: Conceptualization, L.S.; methodology, V.P., L.O., L.S.; formal analysis, V.P.; data curation, V.P.; writing—original draft preparation, V.P., L.S.; writing—review and editing, L.S.; supervision, L.S.; funding acquisition, L.S. All authors have read and agreed to the published version of the manuscript.

Acknowledgments: We would like to thank MRM Proteomics Inc. for the generous gift of the bile acid kit, containing the standard and IS mix.

Abbreviations

GDHCA	glycodehydrocholic acid
TDHCA	taurodehydrocholic acid
ω-TMCA	tauro-ω-muricholic acid
α-TMCA	tauro-α-muricholic acid
β-TMCA	tauro-β-muricholic acid
THCA	taurohyocholic acid
TCA	taurocholic acid
DHCA	dehydrocholic acid
di-oxo-LCA	dioxolithocholic acid
6,7-diketo-LCA	6,7-diketolithocholic acid
GHCA	glycohyocholic acid
GCA	glycocholic acid
UCA	ursocholic acid
ω-MCA	ω-muricholic acid
α-MCA	α-muricholic acid
β-MCA	β-muricholic acid
ACA	allocholic acid
CA	cholic acid
GUDCA	glycoursodeoxycholic acid
GHDCA	glycohyodeoxycholic acid
GCDCA	glycochenodeoxycholic acid
GDCA	glycodeoxycholic acid
NDCA	nordeoxycholic acid
NUDCA	norursodeoxycholic acid
7-keto-DCA	7-ketodeoxycholic acid
12-keto-DCA	12-ketodeoxycholic acid

3-DHCA	3-dehydrocholic acid
NCA	norcholic acid
TUDCA	tauroursodeoxycholic acid
TCDCA	taurochenodeoxycholic acid
TDCA	taurodeoxycholic acid
muro-CA	murocholic acid
UDCA	ursodeoxycholic acid
HDCA	hyodeoxycholic acid
CDCA	chenodeoxycholic acid
DCA	deoxycholic acid
IDCA	isodeoxycholic acid
7-keto-LCA	7-ketolithocholic acid
12-keto-LCA	12-ketolithocholic acid
APCA	apocholic acid
GLCA	glycolithocholic acid
TLCA	taurolithocholic acid
AILCA	alloisolithocholic acid
ILCA	isolithocholic acid
LCA	lithocholic acid
DHLCA	dehydrolithocholic acid

References

1. Russell, D.W. Fifty years of advances in bile acid synthesis and metabolism. *J. Lipid Res.* **2009**, *50*, S120–S125. [CrossRef] [PubMed]
2. Wilson, J.D. The role of bile acids in the overall regulation of steroid metabolism. *Arch. Intern. Med.* **1972**, *130*, 493–505. [CrossRef]
3. Boyer, J.L. Bile formation and secretion. *Compr. Physiol.* **2013**, *3*, 1035–1078. [CrossRef]
4. Hofmann, A.F. Bile Acids: The Good, the Bad, and the Ugly. *News Physiol. Sci.* **1999**, *14*, 24–29. [CrossRef] [PubMed]
5. Copple, B.L.; Jaeschke, H.; Klaassen, C.D. Oxidative stress and the pathogenesis of cholestasis. *Semin. Liver Dis.* **2010**, *30*, 195–204. [CrossRef] [PubMed]
6. Fang, Y.; Han, S.I.; Mitchell, C.; Gupta, S.; Studer, E.; Grant, S.; Hylemon, P.B.; Dent, P. Bile acids induce mitochondrial ROS, which promote activation of receptor tyrosine kinases and signaling pathways in rat hepatocytes. *Hepatology* **2004**, *40*, 961–971. [CrossRef] [PubMed]
7. Gupta, S.; Natarajan, R.; Payne, S.G.; Studer, E.J.; Spiegel, S.; Dent, P.; Hylemon, P.B. Deoxycholic acid activates the c-Jun N-terminal kinase pathway via FAS receptor activation in primary hepatocytes: Role of acidic sphingomyelinase-mediated ceramide generation in FAS receptor activation. *J. Biol. Chem.* **2004**, *279*, 5821–5828. [CrossRef] [PubMed]
8. Jaeschke, H.; Gores, G.J.; Cederbaum, A.I.; Hinson, J.A.; Pessayre, D.; Lemasters, J.J. Mechanisms of hepatotoxicity. *Toxicol. Sci.* **2002**, *65*, 166–176. [CrossRef]
9. Reddy, B.S.; Weisburger, J.H.; Wynder, E.L. Effects of high risk and low risk diets for colon carcinogenesis on fecal microflora and steroids in man. *J. Nutr.* **1975**, *105*, 878–884. [CrossRef]
10. Nagengast, F.M.; Grubben, M.J.A.L.; van Munster, I.P. Role of bile acids in colorectal carcinogenesis. *Eur. J. Cancer* **1995**, *31*, 1067–1070. [CrossRef]
11. Larson, A.M.; Polson, J.; Fontana, R.J.; Davern, T.J.; Lalani, E.; Hynan, L.S.; Reisch, J.S.; SchiØdt, F.V.; Ostapowicz, G.; Shakil, A.O.; et al. Acetaminophen-induced acute liver failure: Results of a United States multicenter, prospective study. *Hepatology* **2005**, *42*, 1364–1372. [CrossRef] [PubMed]
12. Lee, W.M. Acute liver failure in the United States. *Semin. Liver Dis.* **2003**, *23*, 217–226. [CrossRef]
13. Woolbright, B.L.; McGill, M.R.; Staggs, V.S.; Winefield, R.D.; Gholami, P.; Olyaee, M.; Sharpe, M.R.; Curry, S.C.; Lee, W.M.; Jaeschke, H.; et al. Glycodeoxycholic acid levels as prognostic biomarker in acetaminophen-induced acute liver failure patients. *Toxicol. Sci.* **2014**, *142*, 436–444. [CrossRef]

14. James, L.; Yan, K.; Pence, L.; Simpson, P.; Bhattacharyya, S.; Gill, P.; Letzig, L.; Kearns, G.; Beger, R. Comparison of Bile Acids and Acetaminophen Protein Adducts in Children and Adolescents with Acetaminophen Toxicity. *PLoS ONE* **2015**, *10*, e0131010. [CrossRef]

15. Bhushan, B.; Borude, P.; Edwards, G.; Walesky, C.; Cleveland, J.; Li, F.; Ma, X.; Apte, U. Role of bile acids in liver injury and regeneration following acetaminophen overdose. *Am. J. Pathol.* **2013**, *183*, 1518–1526. [CrossRef]

16. Scherer, M.; Gnewuch, C.; Schmitz, G.; Liebisch, G. Rapid quantification of bile acids and their conjugates in serum by liquid chromatography-tandem mass spectrometry. *J. Chromatogr. B* **2009**, *877*, 3920–3925. [CrossRef]

17. Suzuki, Y.; Kaneko, R.; Nomura, M.; Naito, H.; Kitamori, K.; Nakajima, T.; Ogawa, T.; Hattori, H.; Seno, H.; Ishii, A. Simple and rapid quantitation of 21 bile acids in rat serum and liver by UPLC-MS-MS: Effect of high fat diet on glycine conjugates of rat bile acids. *Nagoya J. Med. Sci.* **2013**, *75*, 57–72. [CrossRef]

18. Han, J.; Liu, Y.; Wang, R.; Yang, J.; Ling, V.; Borchers, C.H. Metabolic profiling of bile acids in human and mouse blood by LC-MS/MS in combination with phospholipid-depletion solid-phase extraction. *Anal. Chem.* **2015**, *87*, 1127–1136. [CrossRef]

19. Yousef, I.M.; Mignault, D.; Weber, A.M.; Tuchweber, B. Influence of dehydrocholic acid on the secretion of bile acids and biliary lipids in rats. *Digestion* **1990**, *45*, 40–51. [CrossRef] [PubMed]

20. Shefe, S.; Salen, G.; Hauser, S.; Dayal, B.; Batta, A.K. Metabolism of Iso-Bile Acids in the Rat. *J. Biol. Chem.* **1982**, *257*, 1401–1406.

21. Voigt, W.; Thomas, P.J.; Hsia, S.L. Enzymatic studies of bile acid metabolism. I. 6Beta-hydroxylation of chenodeoxycholic and taurochenodeoxycholic acids by microsomal preparations of rat liver. *J. Biol. Chem.* **1968**, *243*, 3493–3499. [PubMed]

22. Shiraki, K.; Ito, T.; Sugimoto, K.; Fuke, H.; Inoue, T.; Miyashita, K.; Yamanaka, T.; Suzuki, M.; Nabeshima, K.; Nakano, T.; et al. Different effects of bile acids, ursodeoxycholic acid and deoxycholic acid, on cell growth and cell death in human colonic adenocarcinoma cells. *Int. J. Mol. Med.* **2005**, *16*, 729–733. [PubMed]

23. Cai, X.; Liu, Y.; Zhou, X.; Navaneethan, U.; Shen, B.; Guo, B. An LC-ESI-MS method for the quantitative analysis of bile acids composition in fecal materials. *Biomed. Chromatogr.* **2012**, *26*, 101–108. [CrossRef] [PubMed]

24. Tagliacozzi, D.; Mozzi, A.F.; Casetta, B.; Bertucci, P.; Bernardini, S.; Di Ilio, C.; Urbani, A.; Federici, G. Quantitative analysis of bile acids in human plasma by liquid chromatography-electrospray tandem mass spectrometry: A simple and rapid one-step method. *Clin. Chem. Lab. Med.* **2003**, *41*, 1633–1641. [CrossRef]

25. Garcia-Canaveras, J.C.; Donato, M.T.; Castell, J.V.; Lahoz, A. Targeted profiling of circulating and hepatic bile acids in human, mouse, and rat using a UPLC-MRM-MS-validated method. *J. Lipid Res.* **2012**, *53*, 2231–2241. [CrossRef]

6

Important Considerations for Sample Collection in Metabolomics Studies with a Special Focus on Applications to Liver Functions

Lorraine Smith [1], **Joran Villaret-Cazadamont** [1], **Sandrine P. Claus** [2], **Cécile Canlet** [1], **Hervé Guillou** [1], **Nicolas J. Cabaton** [1] and **Sandrine Ellero-Simatos** [1,*]

[1] Toxalim (Research Center in Food Toxicology), Université de Toulouse, INRAE, ENVT, INP-Purpan, UPS, 31300 Toulouse, France; lorraine.smith@inrae.fr (L.S.); joran.villaret-cazadamont@inrae.fr (J.V.-C.); cecile.canlet@inrae.fr (C.C.); herve.guillou@inrae.fr (H.G.); nicolas.cabaton@inrae.fr (N.J.C.)

[2] LNC Therapeutics, 17 place de la Bourse, 33076 Bordeaux, France; sandrine.claus@lnc.bio

* Correspondence: sandrine.ellero-simatos@inrae.fr

Abstract: Metabolomics has found numerous applications in the study of liver metabolism in health and disease. Metabolomics studies can be conducted in a variety of biological matrices ranging from easily accessible biofluids such as urine, blood or feces, to organs, tissues or even cells. Sample collection and storage are critical steps for which standard operating procedures must be followed. Inappropriate sample collection or storage can indeed result in high variability, interferences with instrumentation or degradation of metabolites. In this review, we will first highlight important general factors that should be considered when planning sample collection in the study design of metabolomic studies, such as nutritional status and circadian rhythm. Then, we will discuss in more detail the specific procedures that have been described for optimal pre-analytical handling of the most commonly used matrices (urine, blood, feces, tissues and cells).

Keywords: metabolomics; standard operating procedures; urine; blood; feces; tissue; cells; liver function

---

1. Introduction

Metabolomics refers to the high-throughput quantification and characterization of small molecules (metabolites) in tissues or biofluids. Such biochemical profiles contain latent information relating to inherent parameters, such as the genotype, and environmental factors, including the diet, exposure to xenobiotics and gut microbiota. The liver is the heaviest organ in the human body, with a wide array of functions that can be divided into intermediary metabolism (including a central role in carbohydrate, lipid and nitrogen metabolism), immunological activity, secretion of bile, synthesis of various serum proteins, degradation of hormones, and detoxification of xenobiotics. Hepatic lipid catabolism plays a crucial role during fasting and/or prolonged exercise. Upon lowering of blood glucose, the liver increases glucose production by augmenting gluconeogenesis and glycogenolysis to maintain blood glucose levels; increases fatty acid oxidation and ketogenesis to provide extra-hepatic tissues with ketone bodies; and decreases lipogenesis to attenuate triglyceride storage. In the fed state, the opposite occurs and the liver increases glucose uptake to feed glycogenesis; limits lipid oxidation to favor lipogenesis and promotes saving of fatty acids in the form of triglycerides that are packaged in lipoproteins for remote storage in the white adipose tissue. Hence, the liver plays an essential role in the regulation of energy metabolism. Dysregulation of these metabolic pathways leads to metabolic diseases among which non-alcoholic fatty liver disease (NAFLD), which is diagnosed when more than 5% of hepatocytes are steatotic in patients who do not consume excessive alcohol. The disease severity ranges from simple steatosis to steatohepatitis, advanced fibrosis and cirrhosis. NAFLD epidemic represents a major public health burden [1] and remains an unmet medical need [2].

Metabolomics has found numerous applications in the study of liver functions in health and disease. Among others, these include: Non-invasive biomarker investigations to discriminate between the different stages of progression of NAFLD using non-invasive biofluids (urine and plasma) [3,4]; investigation of mechanisms underlying hepatic disease progression such as acute-on-chronic liver failure using serum metabolic profiling [5] or fibrosis [6]; characterization of the gut microbiota metabotypes in urine of NAFLD patients [4,7]; nutrimetabolomics studies to unravel hepatic pathways dysregulated directly in liver samples upon various nutritional challenges [8,9]; discovery of new metabolic functions for nuclear receptors, that are important regulators of liver physiology using direct hepatic metabolomics or other informative fluids such as urine and bile [10–13]; identification of patients at risk for idiosyncratic drug-induced liver injury (IDILI) before drug administration, a concept named "pharmaco-metabolomics", that was first demonstrated in urine of animal models [14] and is now extended to human biofluids (urine and serum) [15,16]; study of mechanisms of action for pharmaceutical drugs in urine and fecal samples [17] and environmental contaminants in HepG2 cells and animal biofluids and tissues [18,19].

There are many sources of variation in metabolomic studies, some of which are directly related to the pre-analytical handling steps. Pre-analytical questions are indeed a crucial part of metabolomics study designs since inadequate sample collection, pre-treatment or storage can significantly affect sample quality and result interpretation. The reliability of the metabolomics approach requires inactivation of ongoing metabolism, metabolite stabilization and maintenance of sample integrity. In consideration of this, it is useful to have standard operating procedures (SOP) for pre-analytical handling of samples before starting a metabolomic study. In this review, we discuss the influence of sample collection pre-analytical handling procedures and storage conditions on the metabolomic profiles of the biological matrices that are most commonly used to investigate liver functions, namely urine, blood, feces, tissues and cells. Of note, metabolic profiling of several other matrices such as bile and ascitic fluids can provide interesting information about liver functions [10,20,21] but will not be further discussed in this review given the paucity of data regarding sample collection and stability.

2. Overview of the Pre-Analytical Handling Procedures of the Most Commonly Used Biological Matrices in Metabolomics

2.1. Time of Collection

2.1.1. Considering Nutritional Status

The choice of time of collection is a crucial step for a successful metabolomics study and will depend on the research question under examination. Nutritional status of the experimental subjects greatly influences the circulating, urinary, fecal and tissue metabolomes and has to be carefully chosen. If one aims to identify a biomarker specifically associated with a food item, then acute postprandial urine will certainly be collected. Criteria for good biomarkers of habitual nutritional intake are metabolites that are metabolically inert and rapidly absorbed within 1.0–1.5 h of consumption in the upper gastrointestinal tract. Such markers are subsequently excreted 1.5–2.5 h later [22]. Plasma is more reflective of modulations in endogenous metabolism as a result of the food metabolome and it should be noted that perturbations of the plasma metabolic profile arise when homeostatic function is impaired. Therefore, fasting plasma samples are usually used to explore how systemic metabolism differs between populations with different dietary habits [23]. Of note, in rodents, 16-h fasting has been shown to affect 1/3 to 1/2 of monitored serum metabolites, with an increase in fatty and bile acids and a significant decrease in diet- and gut microbiota-derived metabolites [24]. Nutritional status also has a significant effect on the tissue metabolome. Especially in the liver, 77% of the hepatic metabolome has been shown to be sensitive to a nutritional high-fat-diet challenge at all times of day. Amino acids, xenobiotics and nucleotides were especially affected and decreased in HFD-fed mice at all time points [25]. Finally, the fecal (or cecal) metabolome is increasingly considered as a functional readout of the gut microbiome and can be used as an intermediate phenotype mediating host–microbiome interactions [4,26]. Although the microbial metabolome still represents an analytical challenge and many microbial metabolites still remains unknown, it is known that the fecal metabolome is highly sensitive to nutritional challenges [27,28] and influences the host hepatic metabolism [4,29,30].

2.1.2. Considering Circadian Rhythm

Circadian rhythms govern a large variety of behavioral, physiological and metabolic processes [31]. Recent advances reveal that a very large fraction of mammalian metabolism undergoes circadian oscillations. Many metabolic pathways are under circadian control and, in turn, may feedback to the clock system to assist in circadian timekeeping [32]. Transcriptomics studies have extensively illustrated a substantial fraction of the genome controlled by the molecular clock [33]. Metabolomics studies have also highlighted the circadian oscillations of metabolites in humans independently of sleep or feeding [34]. In mice, more than 40% of the serum metabolome and 45% of the liver metabolome have been shown to be sensitive to time, with both matrices providing different and complementary information. For example, more than 30% of the serum lipids were not found in the liver and more than half of them oscillated across the circadian cycle, while only 30% of the hepatic lipids oscillated [25]. Moreover, a high-fat challenge induced a loss of serum metabolite rythmicity, compared with the liver [25]. Therefore, when collecting samples for a metabolomics study, one should be aware that a tissue-specific and time-dependent disruption of metabolic homeostasis exists independently of feeding, but also in response to altered nutrition. Time of collection therefore needs to be carefully chosen, and if sample collection is spread between several days, time of collection should be homogenous between the collection days [35].

2.2. Common Sources of Variation in Pre-Analytical Handling of Main Biological Matrices

Specific SOPs have been described for collection, preparation and storage of metabolomics samples and will be described along the specificity of each biological matrix in the following sections. Several features of the pre-analytical steps are however shared between the different matrices. First, the numbers, weights or volumes of the samples are important points to anticipate before collection. Second, during collection, samples have to be kept at the lowest temperature possible, and immediate snap freezing is recommended in order to quench any rapid degradation activity such as oxidation of labile metabolites as well as enzymatic reactions.

Third, aliquoting the samples should also be considered whenever possible. This important step will avoid repeated freeze–thaw cycles that lead to progressive loss in sample quality. Finally, long term storage at −80 °C or less is recommended before analysis. These general recommendations, as well as matrix-specific pre-analytical factors that influence the results of metabolomics studies are summarized in Figure 1.

2.3. Urine

Urine is a biofluid commonly used for both human and animal metabolomics studies because sample collection is non-invasive. The simplicity of the collection allows multiple collections for kinetic studies and ensures reliability of the analysis. Urinary profiles contain signals derived from both endogenous and environmental sources, including diet and gut microbiota metabolic activity, and can therefore provide an overall measure of the metabolic phenotype. It is a collection of waste and biological by-products that reflects a large panel of metabolic processes that may have occurred over time and provides the researcher with a historical overview of the global metabolic events. In addition, it may contain cells (erythrocytes, leucocytes, urothelial cells, and epithelial cells), bacteria, fungi and non-cellular components including urates and mucus filaments [36]. Thus, it is a non-inert fluid and residual cellular or enzymatic activities could significantly change the metabolic composition of the samples. It is, therefore, necessary to remove cells and bacteria and/or to quench the ongoing enzymatic or metabolic activities in urine samples.

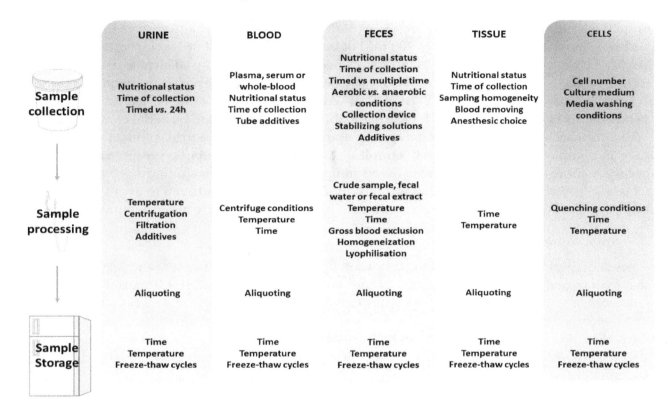

Figure 1. Summary of pre-analytical factors that can affect metabolite profiles in various matrices.

2.3.1. Timed vs. 24-Hour Collection

The first main consideration in urine collection is to choose the appropriate sampling time: 24-h collection or timed collection. It has been shown that there is a large variability depending of the collecting time (day vs. night, morning vs. afternoon) caused by the circadian rhythm regulating the energy metabolism and the gut microbiota metabolism and also due to a difference in physical activity and feeding state [37]. Therefore, 24-h sampling will be preferred if one aims at eliminating the day-time variability in metabolic profiles. Another advantage of 24-h sampling might be that it minimizes variation in urine concentrations compared to timed samples. Indeed, unlike blood where metabolite concentration is tightly maintained, urine concentration can vary drastically from sample to sample, thereby influencing the urine metabolome. In a recent review, Stevens et al. propose that pre-analytical normalization of urine (for e.g., to osmolarity) may improve the reliability of metabolomics analyses [38]. However, 24-h sampling is not always feasible, especially in humans. In rodents, specific individual metabolic cages or use of hydrophobic sand are required, in which mice are isolated and therefore mildly stressed [39,40]. 24-h sampling might also not be appropriate. For example, a timed sampling is needed to study a time-related trend and a kinetic sampling can be done to monitor the evolution of a targeted compound or the overall effect on the metabolism after drug or nutrient intake. In timed sampling, the time of collection is a very important point to ensure the reproducibility and quality of the study.

2.3.2. Sample Collection

The most commonly used preservation methods are filtration, centrifugation or addition of bacteriostatics. Saude et al. showed that spinning urine samples at 112 g for 10 min was less effective in conserving the metabolome composition than filtration through a 0.22 μm filter [41]. Bernini et al. have shown that a mild pre-centrifugation (between 1000 and 3000 g) combined with filtration is the safest way to avoid contamination of the metabolic profiles attributed to bacterial removal without leading to an additional contamination due to cell damages or breaking (higher centrifugation speed induced partial breaking of cells and lower centrifugation was not effective to eliminate bacteria) [36]. Boric acid and sodium azide (NaN_3) are the two most commonly used antimicrobial preservatives. It has been shown that the addition of 200 mM of boric acid or 10 mM of NaN_3 for 24-h samples or 2–20 mM of boric acid or 0.1–1 mM of NaN_3 for a timed sample are equally efficient to prevent bacterial overgrowth [42]. Nevertheless, boric acid is rarely used, as it induces formation of chemical complexes with endogenous metabolites [43]. Bernini et al. compared the use of NaN_3 to a 0.2 μm filtration, and showed the latter to be superior for sample stability over time due to bacterial removal [36].

To summarize, filtration showed superior ability to preserve the urinary metabolites during storage in comparison with unfiltered samples. Moreover, the metabolic profiles of centrifuged samples are more stable than non-centrifuged samples after one week storage at −80 °C, with this effect being less severe in samples that are rapidly frozen in liquid nitrogen to avoid cell breaking. A mild pre-centrifugation plus a filtration seems to be the best method to avoid sample degradation.

2.3.3. Sample Storage

For short-term storage, Gika et al. have shown that the storage of urine samples at 4 °C for up to 48 h maintained the metabolic integrity of the samples [44]. However, it is important to minimize sample storage at 4 °C as it has been shown that samples stored for more than 9 months will present an altered metabolome when compared to samples stored at −20 °C [45]. For long-term storage, metabolic profiles of urine samples stored at either −20 or −80 °C for 6 months did not show any significant differences [44]. This study, however, did not confirm whether or not the stored samples were identical to the original samples.

Freeze–thaw cycles have been shown to significantly modify the urine sample composition. Urine samples stored at −80 °C and thawed twice a week for 4 weeks (8 freeze–thaw cycles) indeed displayed a reduced metabolic stability in comparison to non-thawed ones stored at the same temperature. Metabolites deriving from bacterial metabolism (acetate, benzoate, succinate) increased [41]. Trivedi et al. showed that urinary metabolic profiles could be maintained only up to 3 freeze–thaw cycles using HILIC (Hydrophilic interaction liquid chromatography) mass-spectrometry [45].

2.4. Blood

Collecting blood is slightly more invasive than collecting urine, and the metabolic profiles of blood fractions provide a different, but complementary, metabolic information compared to the ones obtained with urine. Blood metabolic profiles are dynamic and vary continuously in response to changes in gene expression or changes induced by exogenous metabolites such as those provided by nutrients or drugs. Blood metabolic profiling is therefore widely used to study the dynamic variations of the endogenous metabolism in response to drug or food intake. Disruption in plasma metabolic profiles arises when homeostatic function is impaired. Serum and plasma are the most commonly used matrices, but other matrices do exist, such as platelet-free plasma (PFP), platelet-rich plasma (PRP) and whole blood, this latter receiving a growing interest.

Blood consists of two main components: plasma, which is a clear extracellular fluid containing clotting factors, proteins, glucose, minerals, and gases; and cellular elements, which are made up of blood cells (white blood cells, red blood cells) and platelets. Serum is the liquid fraction of whole blood, obtained by allowing the sample to clot naturally followed by a centrifugation step. The resulting supernatant is serum free of cells and of clotting factors such as the fibrinogen proteins. Plasma is prepared by collecting the whole blood into anticoagulant-treated tubes followed by a centrifugation step at 4 °C to separate blood cells. The supernatant designated as plasma is then immediately transferred into a clean tube. Plasma is a mixture of platelets, proteins, nutrients, hormones and gases. In some studies, further identification was given by naming it platelet-poor plasma (PPP) in opposition to platelet-free plasma or platelet-rich plasma by adding one or more additional centrifugation steps.

Depending on the aim of the experiment, for example, if one wants to take into consideration the influence of growth factors or cytokines released by the platelets, the platelet content of the sample has to be carefully accounted for. Various manual, semi-automatic, and fully automated commercial systems have become available to prepare PFP, PPP and PRP [46].

2.4.1. Sample Collection

Several studies have addressed a direct comparison of plasma vs. serum and have been recently reviewed [38]. The conclusions of this review highlight that both matrices are appropriate for blood metabolomics with minor differences between them.

The metabolomics analysis of serum is known to present a higher sensitivity of metabolites compared to plasma due to the lack of big particles. However, its processing time has the disadvantage of introducing variations due to enzymatic conversion and degradation processes, and to influence the metabolite composition [47]. Moreover, the reproducibility of serum is not as good as that of the whole blood because hemolysis can occur during collection or processing, leading to the presence of free hemoglobulin in the samples that influences the metabolic profiles [48].

In comparison, there is a better reproducibility in plasma due to the absence of the blood-clotting step. Moreover, it has been suggested that the absence of platelets and the lower protein content could be beneficial to small molecule analysis, because of a reduced competition [49]. For plasma preparation, the choice of anti-coagulant addition is critical and needs to be carefully accounted for before sample collection. Several anticoagulant collection tubes are available. The three most common additives are: heparin, ethylene diamine tetra acetic acid (EDTA) and citrate. They have often been compared with opposing conclusions depending on the analytical platform used. Actually, additives found in collection tubes can affect the ionization process during the MS run, thereby suppressing metabolite ionization and/or introducing interfering peaks. Bari et al. have compared heparin, EDTA and citrate anticoagulants using an untargeted UPLC-MS analysis. They noticed subtle metabolite differences between the different plasma preparations mainly due to ion suppression or enhancement caused by citrate and EDTA. Heparin did not cause interferences and was therefore recommended by the authors [50]. On the contrary, Yin et al. analyzed heparin, citrate, and EDTA collection tubes using a non-targeted LC-MS approach and they noticed that heparin led to chemical noise in the mass spectra. Citrate and heparin showed few additional signals. They recommended avoiding heparin, preferring EDTA [48]. As for NMR analysis, heparin is usually recommended, as EDTA, citrate and other stabilizers give additional signals in the NMR spectra [51]. The choice of collection tube for plasma preparation is therefore critical, should be consistent throughout the experiment and should be adapted according to the analytical platform used for subsequent analysis.

2.4.2. Sample Preparation

After collection, samples should be quickly stored on ice. The time between collection and cell separation should be long enough to allow complete clot formation but short enough to avoid compositional changes. In general, it is recommended that the time before separation of blood cells should not exceed 30 min to minimize further metabolism or active and passive transport of analytes between the intra- and extracellular compartments. As for urine, whenever possible, samples should be stored as aliquots, allowing the use of fresh samples for each experiment and avoiding the introduction of bias due to repeated freeze–thaw cycles.

2.4.3. Sample Storage

It is well established that serum and plasma contain high levels of enzymes, that are efficiently active at 37 °C. A reduced temperature decreases enzymatic activity, but it should be noted that this activity is not completely inhibited until temperatures below −56 °C are reached [52]. Lipids and lipoproteins are especially sensitive due to lipase activity [35]. Small changes have been observed in the plasma metabolic profiles after one-month storage at −20 °C [35,53], while storage at −80 °C for 4 years had minimal effects [54,55].

Data regarding the number of freeze–thaw cycles acceptable are variable [42,44,46]. Unfractionated serum samples can be stored frozen for later quantitative lipid analysis as minor effects occur on quantitative lipid composition for most of the biologically relevant lipid species in humans, even with one to three freeze–thaw cycles. At the opposite freezing prior to lipoprotein fractionation significantly introduce a large variability in high-density lipoprotein and low-density lipoprotein cholesterol as well as in very low-density lipoprotein free fatty acids compared with fresh samples: density-based fractionation should preferably be undertaken in fresh serum [39].

2.5. Feces

Feces represents a growing interest in metabolomics studies, as fecal metabolic profiles reflect the metabolic interplay between the host and its gut microbiota [56]. The fecal metabolome has been shown to largely reflect gut microbiota composition in humans (explaining on average 67.7% of its variance), and is considered to be a functional readout of the microbiome [26]. Despite the rising popularity of fecal metabolomics, the methods for collecting, preparing and analyzing fecal samples are still far from being standardized. In a recent review, Karu et al. provided the state of knowledge with regards to the protocols and technologies in human fecal metabolite analysis [57]. They also present a comprehensive database that contains over 6000 identified human fecal metabolites, thereby highlighting the potential richness of the information contained in the metabolomics analysis of fecal samples. While the first metabolomics study of human feces used headspace GC-MS to study volatile organic compounds (VOCs) [58,59], it is now recognized that the majority of fecal metabolites are non-volatile [57].

The largest part of stool is made up of water (60–80%, depending on fiber intake), while the dry matter contains bacteria (both alive and dead, representing 25–54% of biomass) derived from the gastro-intestinal microbiota, colonic epithelial cells, macromolecules, undigested food residues, and thousands of metabolites including sugars, organic acids and amino acids, that constitute the fecal metabolome [60]. The latter includes both compounds derived from the metabolic activity of the gut microbiota and various host endogenous metabolites such as signaling peptides or bile acids [61].

2.5.1. Sample Selection

Timed vs. multiple-timed sampling: Much information contained within the fecal metabolome derives from dietary inputs and biochemical events that have occurred during their digestion. Thus, there is inherent variability in fecal samples depending upon feeding state and bowel activity. Both the gut microbiota composition and metabolic activity have been shown to be highly circadian [62,63]. Therefore, as for urine, it can be expected that timed collection vs. 24-h collection will provide different information. In animal studies, both timed [64] and 24-h [65] fecal sampling are commonly used for specific biochemical assays such as sterol and bile acid profiling; however, to our knowledge, no direct and systemic comparison of timed vs. 24-h fecal metabolome has been performed yet. In humans, it might not be feasible or relevant to collect 24-h samples. However, it was shown that the ^{1}H-NMR-based fecal metabolic profiles from single time samples greatly varied within one individual (day to day variation), and multiple day sampling and pooling has been proposed to minimize errors arising from day to day variation [66].

Presence of blood in stools: Gut bleeding is a clinically prevalent phenomenon associated with many gastro-intestinal diseases. The impact of blood in stool on the fecal metabolome has been shown to be minimal if the level of contamination is low (occult blood). However, gross (visible) blood in the fecal sample significantly contaminates the fecal metabolome [67]. Therefore, Karu et al. recommend visually inspecting samples and considering excluding the fecal samples or portions of fecal samples with gross blood [57].

2.5.2. Sample Collection

Feces collection presents the advantage of being non-invasive. In animals, fecal samples can be directly obtained from the intestine after euthanasia or collected from alive subject and pooled if necessary. Twenty-four hour feces can easily be obtained using metabolic cages; however, a mild but significant increase in fecal output was observed when housing rats in metabolic cages [39]. In humans, fecal samples can be directly collected in a falcon tube, in a plastic container, in a sterile bag [68,69], or in special anaerobic pouch systems [70]. Stabilizing solutions such as nucleotide stabilizers present in some stool collection kits should be avoided because they interfere with subsequent metabolomic analysis. Similarly, if stool samples are to be collected prior to colonoscopy, Bezabeh et al. recommend collection before patients start taking the solutions used for colonoscopy [71]. Indeed, most of these solutions contain polyethylene glycol, which produces strong interfering signals in the ^{1}H-NMR spectrum.

Sample type and amount have to be decided beforehand and standardized. Samples for metabolomics study can be intact (crude) feces (usually for analysis of VOC), fecal water (the water fraction of an intact feces, obtained by ultracentrifugation of the stool), or a fecal aqueous extract (obtained after the addition of an aqueous buffer or of water to the stool, followed by homogenization and centrifugation). Fecal water generates a different metabolic coverage from feces and GC-MS analysis from crude feces samples yielded detection of more peaks than analysis of fecal water samples [67]. Stool samples are highly heterogeneous, and the topological position from the fecal sample has been shown to influence the fecal metabolome [72]. Therefore, it is sometimes recommended to collect as much sample as possible and to homogenize it before preparing aliquots, enabling a non-selective and more reproducible method [57,71]. The metabolic stability of aqueous extracts was shown to be higher than that of crude feces samples and it was recommended that fresh samples should be refrigerated and aqueous extraction conducted ideally within 1 h (and not longer than 24 h) after collection before aliquoting and freezing [57,72].

Exposure to aerobic conditions and room temperature might quickly change the fecal metabolome due to microbial fermentation. Some researchers therefore place their fecal samples in an anaerobic chamber within 10 min of collection [73]. Couch et al. investigated the differences between home-based self-collection (ex vivo) samples and lab-based endoscopic collection (in vivo) samples in healthy subjects [74]. Using GC-MS, they found modest differences in the overall chemical distribution with a slight bias toward oxidized metabolites in the ex vivo samples. Further investigation revealed significant differences in the VOC metabolomes between the two groups. The effect of post-collection storage is much more drastic in fecal samples than in any other biological matrix, and most researchers store their fecal samples at 4 °C or lower immediately after collection. Fecal metabolites have indeed been shown to be highly unstable upon several storage conditions. For example, using GC-MS analysis, Phua et al. showed that, over 268 analytes, only 28% remained stable when crude feces were stored for one day at 4 °C, and this declined to 10% at room temperature (29 °C) [67]. Immediate cooling of fecal samples is not always feasible, especially when human feces are collected at home or in clinics. Using LC-MS, Loftfield et al. compared several methods allowing preserving sample quality and demonstrated that crude fecal samples collected in 95% ethanol were stable for up to 96 h at room temperature [75]. Interestingly, these ethanol-preserved samples exhibited a metabolic profile more akin to fresh samples compared to immediately frozen-feces. This protocol represents an interesting alternative when immediate freezing of samples is not possible.

Water content in feces is variable (60–85% in human) and this can sometimes create a bias to compare experimental groups. Immediately after collection, or before metabolites extraction, it is possible to lyophilize or freeze dry the samples to remove the water present in the feces. This improves sample weight precision, reduces bias due to the volume of solvent and/or derivation reagents added to samples during the metabolite extraction steps and allows quantitative metabolite data to be given in units per dry matter weight. This latter point is especially important for meta-analysis of metabolomics results and to establish reference levels for clinical use. While working with dried samples is less laborious, more reproducible and prevents bacterial growth, it also results in a loss of detected metabolites, especially VOCs. Indeed, the effect of lyophilization has been compared with the use of fresh sample and results in a decrease in short chain fatty acids [76,77]. Therefore, Karu et al. suggest that, unless volatile compounds are specifically targeted for quantification, fecal samples should be dried and weighed prior to storage or analysis. However, some researchers recommend not using it to minimize the number of preparation steps and guarantee quantifiable levels of short-chain fatty acids among others.

2.5.3. Sample Storage

While the analysis of fresh fecal samples is therefore recommended, the use of frozen samples could be more convenient. Two NMR studies investigated the effects of freezing on crude feces and/or aqueous fecal extracts and showed higher levels of several amino acids (namely branched-chain and aromatic amino acids) and glucose upon a single freeze–thaw cycle [72,76]. This observation has been confirmed using GC-MS analysis. Phua et al. indeed observed that only 33% of the initial metabolites remained after one cycle, and 18% after two and three cycles [67]. In the same study, the metabolites also exhibited a poor stability at -80 °C, with only 24% of stable metabolites after 1 and 6 weeks of storage. The identity of the impacted metabolites was not given.

To summarize, although the immediate processing of fresh fecal samples is recommended, the use of frozen samples is often much more convenient. According to the last recommendations [57] and our present review, it seems that good practices would require fecal samples to be homogenized and aliquoted prior to freezing, while minimizing handling time at the lowest temperature possible. Very importantly, freeze–thaw cycle and storage duration should be minimized.

2.6. Tissue

Most metabolomics studies are based on non-invasive or minimally invasive sample types, such as blood, urine and feces. However, tissue analyses are also important, as the tissue represents the first place where the metabolic changes owing to a disease take place. Metabolomic studies have been conducted on almost every tissue (liver, intestine, muscle, adipose tissues from various locations, whole brain or selected brain areas, etc.). Most tissues are not homogenous. For example the liver has five different lobes, and within them the portal and periportal vascular regions are known to display different levels of some enzymatic systems such as those involved in glycolysis and gluconeogenesis [78–80]. Even when the tissue is composed of the same cell types, regional differences in composition may still exist. Such factors may result in increased biological variability, which should be taken into account during sampling [81].

2.6.1. Sample Collection

There are several critical points to be aware of during the handling step of tissues to avoid bias due to the collection procedure. The first important consideration is to ensure sample collection homogeneity throughout the experiment by always collecting samples from the same region to avoid bias due to biological variability. Whenever possible, it is also advisable that the same person collects the tissue samples throughout the experiment to minimize variability. Furthermore, to avoid contamination with blood metabolites, it is possible to wash the samples with cold deionized water or PBS after collection [82]. In some cases, saline in D_2O or PBS is injected into the organ-associated artery before the collection to remove residual blood in organs [83]. One should also be aware that contaminant signals can result from the anesthetic used during the experiment, or even from surgical instrument cleaning solutions, especially ethanol that produces additional signals in the ^{1}H-NMR spectra, thereby masking signals from endogenous metabolites.

2.6.2. Sample Storage

To obtain useful global metabolic profiles, sampling must be performed as rapidly as possible and samples should be either processed immediately or snap-frozen in liquid nitrogen to minimize further metabolism [84]. A good practice is to cut each sample into small pieces and to freeze the organs as rapidly as possible. For large prospective biobanking studies, this might not always be feasible and tissue samples might undergo several cycles of "storage-near-retrieval" due to storage constraints of adjacent samples for example. Testing different scenarios of storage–retrieval cycles in human liver tissues demonstrated that storage temperature affected metabolite concentrations only little, while there was a linear dependence on the number of temperature change cycles [85]. Metabolic changes induced by thawing were shown to be almost identical for all organs, with a marked increase in overall metabolite levels caused by increased protein and cell degradation [86].

2.7. Cells

Metabolomics analysis of cultured cells has emerged as an important technology for studying cellular biochemistry that provides an instantaneous snapshot of ongoing cellular metabolism. The major bottlenecks associated with metabolomics cell samples preparation workflow are efficient sampling, quenching and metabolites extraction in order to preserve the internal metabolite signatures [87].

2.7.1. Sample Preparation

Metabolomics analyses have been performed on a broad range of adherent cell numbers, ranging from 1×10^4 up to 4×10^7 cells [88]. Depending of the cells and the technology used to process the cell extractions, the seeding number must be optimized in order to get enough signal in NMR and/or MS, to be able to detect small metabolites that are present at low concentration but that still may be important for biological purposes, especially when global metabolomics is performed. Regarding the hepatic HepG2 cells for instance, tests have been performed to optimize the number of cells needed to obtain NMR metabolic fingerprints allowing to detect and identify the metabolite content in the cells. The number of 10^6 cells was selected, as this seeding allowed the detection of the subtle modulations occurring after exposing the cells to xenobiotics such as estradiol or bisphenol A [18]. For cell extracts, it is usually recommended to work in very low volumes and concentrate the extract in a maximum of 50 uL. Microvolumes are easily handled using MS-based metabolomics or can be transferred to NMR microtubes or capillary tubes for analysis.

Culture media composition is also important to consider as some media contain interfering anions such as Cl^-, SO_4^-, and PO_4^-, and depending on cultivated cells, amino acids, Good's buffers, organic acids, and complex biological mixtures such as fetal bovine serum. These components can cause substantial electrospray ionization suppression, additional signals in ^{1}H-NMR spectra or contaminate the intracellular metabolite pool [88]. With regard to NMR-based metabolomics, culture media that contain HEPES should be avoided or carefully removed, since HEPES gives many broad additional signals. For these reasons, cells have to be separated from the medium before analysis. The washing step is therefore very important and should be performed with caution to effectively remove all the extracellular media components. Kapoore et al. (2017) performed five different washing protocols on the breast cancer cell line MDA-MB-231, using either PBS or distilled water. Based on a few metabolites detected by GC-MS, these authors suggested that in their conditions, a single washing step with PBS followed by quenching using 60% methanol supplemented with 70 mM HEPES (−50 °C) was the best condition for minimizing intracellular metabolites leakage. More recently, three-dimensional multicellular tumor spheroids have been used to perform metabolomics analysis. The washing steps consisted of a rapid washing of the spheroids directly on the cultivation plate only once using PBS [89].

Another crucial point for reducing the variability and improving the quality of sample preparation is to quench the cells before the extraction. This procedure aims at stopping cellular metabolism to prevent the turnover of metabolites, maintaining the metabolite concentrations at their physiological levels. Thus, the quenching method should immediately stop all cellular enzymatic activities or cellular changes in metabolite concentrations, without changing the cell environment, since metabolites are very sensitive to any variation of their environment. As for the other points mentioned above, several protocols have been tested and used by scientists and were improved over time. Previously, metabolic quenching and extraction were performed using drastic culture conditions changes (acidic condition, high temperature) to inactivate all enzymatic activities, but taking into account the loss of heat-sensitive and pH-sensitive compounds [90]. Some papers reported quenching protocol using liquid nitrogen, for metabolomics studies, after detaching cells by trypsination [91]. In this case, cells are quenched and extracted at the same time [92]. This method substantially modifies the intra-cellular metabolic profiles because trypsin can induce cell stress, structural and protein disruption during cell detachment and consequently metabolite leakage [93]. Another method has been proposed to isolate the cells using filtration [88]. However, both filtration and centrifugation expose cells to a mechanical stress that can also modify the metabolic profiles. Recently, another method has been proposed to better preserve cell metabolism: after carefully removing the medium, cells are washed with PBS or deionized water at room temperature or at 37 °C. Finally, the cellular metabolism is quenched by adding liquid nitrogen or ice-cold methanol into the dishes. Cells can be stored at −80 °C or scraped with a cell lifter to be directly extracted. The solvents used for the quenching and metabolite extraction step is one critical step to anticipate, depending of which type of metabolites are targeted. It is admitted that up to now the choice of solvent was adapted to specific metabolite extractions. Usually, a mix of different proportions of solvents is used to quench, extract the cells and collect the metabolites. Mainly, methanol or acetonitrile are used as organic solvents, supplemented by water or acidified water [94]. Different ratios of organic solvents and water have been documented, such as methanol:water 50:50 (*v/v*) to perform global metabolomics [93] or acetonitrile:water 70:30 (*v/v*) to perform targeted amine profiling [95]. Some protocols include only a cold mix freshly prepared of acetonile and deionized water to seek polar metabolites [96]. The choice of methanol, acetonitrile and water, even at different ratios, is efficient to recover a large panel of metabolite families such as amino acids, organic acids, nucleotides precursors, sugars ad sugar alcohols [97]. Potassium hydroxide or perchloric acid have also been used, but the results were less reproducible and less efficient for extracting nucleotides, sugars, sugar phosphates and organic acids. These authors concluded that acidic and alkaline extractions did not suit the requirements for a global metabolome analysis [97]. Research is ongoing to optimize conditions in order to get as many metabolites as possible from the same sample extracts using appropriate mix of solvents.

2.7.2. Sample Storage

After quenching and metabolite extraction, cell extracts are usually snap frozen in liquid nitrogen and quickly stored at −80 °C until further analysis to prevent metabolite degradation. Similarly to animal tissues, freeze–thaw cycles must be avoided and the thawing step should be performed on ice to increase gradually the temperature of the samples.

3. Conclusions

Metabolomics offers detailed insights into the metabolic phenotype of the liver and each of the associated organs and biofluids (including the gut microbiota). It is, therefore, nowadays one of the most promising tools in systems biology in hepatology, and is expected to help especially in non-invasive biomarker discovery and identification of biological pathways operating in the liver in physiology and pathology. Metabolomics studies have therefore been performed in a variety of biological matrices to study liver functions. Depending on the research question, several points have to be carefully considered before analytical handling of the samples, including: type and time of sampling, sampling conditions, quenching of ongoing metabolism, use of preservatives, aliquoting and storage conditions. SOPs vary according to the biological matrices used but aim to enhance metabolite recovery and stability to optimize metabolic pathways investigations in liver functions. This raises the question of international consensus protocols and international committees working on continuous improvement of standardized pre-analytical issues.

Author Contributions: Writing—original draft preparation, L.S., J.V.-C., N.J.C. and S.E.-S.; writing—review and editing, S.P.C., C.C., H.G., N.J.C. and S.E.-S.; supervision, H.G., N.J.C. and S.E.-S.; project administration, H.G., N.J.C. and S.E.-S.; funding acquisition, H.G. and S.E.-S. All authors have read and agreed to the published version of the manuscript."

References

1. Estes, C.; Razavi, H.; Loomba, R.; Younossi, Z.; Sanyal, A.J. Modeling the epidemic of nonalcoholic fatty liver disease demonstrates an exponential increase in burden of disease. *Hepatology* **2018**, *67*, 123–133. [CrossRef] [PubMed]

2. Sanyal, A.J. Past, present and future perspectives in nonalcoholic fatty liver disease. *Nat. Rev. Gastroenterol. Hepatol.* **2019**, *16*, 377–386. [CrossRef]

3. Kalhan, S.C.; Guo, L.; Edmison, J.; Dasarathy, S.; McCullough, A.J.; Hanson, R.W.; Milburn, M. Plasma metabolomic profile in nonalcoholic fatty liver disease. *Metab Clin. Exp.* **2011**, *60*, 404–413. [CrossRef] [PubMed]

4. Hoyles, L.; Fernández-Real, J.-M.; Federici, M.; Serino, M.; Abbott, J.; Charpentier, J.; Heymes, C.; Luque, J.L.; Anthony, E.; Barton, R.H.; et al. Molecular phenomics and metagenomics of hepatic steatosis in non-diabetic obese women. *Nat. Med.* **2018**, *24*, 1070–1080. [CrossRef] [PubMed]

5. Moreau, R.; Clària, J.; Aguilar, F.; Fenaille, F.; Lozano, J.; Junot, C.; Colsch, B.; Caraceni, P.; Trebicka, J.; Pavesi, M.; et al. Blood metabolomics uncovers inflammation-associated mitochondrial dysfunction as a potential mechanism underlying ACLF. *J. Hepatol.* **2019**. [CrossRef] [PubMed]

6. Chang, M.-L.; Yang, S.-S. Metabolic Signature of Hepatic Fibrosis: From Individual Pathways to Systems Biology. *Cells* **2019**, *8*, 1423. [CrossRef]

7. Dumas, M.-E.; Barton, R.H.; Toye, A.; Cloarec, O.; Blancher, C.; Rothwell, A.; Fearnside, J.; Tatoud, R.; Blanc, V.; Lindon, J.C.; et al. Metabolic profiling reveals a contribution of gut microbiota to fatty liver phenotype in insulin-resistant mice. *PNAS* **2006**, *103*, 12511–12516. [CrossRef]

8. Soltis, A.R.; Kennedy, N.J.; Xin, X.; Zhou, F.; Ficarro, S.B.; Yap, Y.S.; Matthews, B.J.; Lauffenburger, D.A.; White, F.M.; Marto, J.A.; et al. Hepatic Dysfunction Caused by Consumption of a High-Fat Diet. *Cell Rep.* **2017**, *21*, 3317–3328. [CrossRef]

9. Torre Della, S.; Mitro, N.; Meda, C.; Lolli, F.; Pedretti, S.; Barcella, M.; Ottobrini, L.; Metzger, D.; Caruso, D.; Maggi, A. Short-Term Fasting Reveals Amino Acid Metabolism as a Major Sex-Discriminating Factor in the Liver. *Cell Metab.* **2018**, *28*, 256–267. [CrossRef]

10. Li, F.; Patterson, A.D.; Krausz, K.W.; Tanaka, N.; Gonzalez, F.J. Metabolomics reveals an essential role for peroxisome proliferator-activated receptor α in bile acid homeostasis. *J. Lipid Res.* **2012**, *53*, 1625–1635. [CrossRef]

11. Cho, J.-Y.; Kang, D.W.; Ma, X.; Ahn, S.-H.; Krausz, K.W.; Luecke, H.; Idle, J.R.; Gonzalez, F.J. Metabolomics reveals a novel vitamin E metabolite and attenuated vitamin E metabolism upon PXR activation. *J. Lipid Res.* **2009**, *50*, 924–937. [CrossRef] [PubMed]

12. Montagner, A.; Korecka, A.; Polizzi, A.; Lippi, Y.; Blum, Y.; Canlet, C.; Tremblay-Franco, M.; Gautier-Stein, A.; Burcelin, R.; Yen, Y.-C.; et al. Hepatic circadian clock oscillators and nuclear receptors integrate microbiome-derived signals. *Sci. Rep.* **2016**, *6*, 20127. [CrossRef]

13. Lukowicz, C.; Ellero-Simatos, S.; Régnier, M.; Oliviero, F.; Lasserre, F.; Polizzi, A.; Montagner, A.; Smati, S.; Boudou, F.; Lenfant, F.; et al. Dimorphic metabolic and endocrine disorders in mice lacking the constitutive androstane receptor. *Sci. Rep.* **2019**, *9*, 20169. [CrossRef] [PubMed]

14. Clayton, T.A.; Lindon, J.C.; Cloarec, O.; Antti, H.; Charuel, C.; Hanton, G.; Provost, J.-P.; Le Net, J.-L.; Baker, D.; Walley, R.J.; et al. Pharmaco-metabonomic phenotyping and personalized drug treatment. *Nature* **2006**, *440*, 1073–1077. [CrossRef] [PubMed]

15. Clayton, T.A.; Baker, D.; Lindon, J.C.; Everett, J.R.; Nicholson, J.K. Pharmacometabonomic identification of a significant host-microbiome metabolic interaction affecting human drug metabolism. *Proc. Natl. Acad. Sci. USA* **2009**, *106*, 14728–14733. [CrossRef] [PubMed]

16. Zhang, L.; Niu, M.; Wei, A.-W.; Tang, J.-F.; Tu, C.; Bai, Z.-F.; Zou, Z.-S.; Xiao, X.-H.; Liu, Y.-P.; Wang, J.-B. Risk profiling using metabolomic characteristics for susceptible individuals of drug-induced liver injury caused by Polygonum multiflorum. *Arch. Toxicol.* **2019**, *295*, 113. [CrossRef]

17. Yip, L.Y.; Aw, C.C.; Lee, S.H.; Hong, Y.S.; Ku, H.C.; Xu, W.H.; Chan, J.M.X.; Cheong, E.J.Y.; Chng, K.R.; Ng, A.H.Q.; et al. The liver-gut microbiota axis modulates hepatotoxicity of tacrine in the rat. *Hepatology* **2018**, *67*, 282–295. [CrossRef]

18. Cabaton, N.J.; Poupin, N.; Canlet, C.; Tremblay-Franco, M.; Audebert, M.; Cravedi, J.-P.; Riu, A.; Jourdan, F.; Zalko, D. An Untargeted Metabolomics Approach to Investigate the Metabolic Modulations of HepG2 Cells Exposed to Low Doses of Bisphenol A and 17β-Estradiol. *Front. Endocrinol.* **2018**, *9*, 571. [CrossRef]

19. Lukowicz, C.; Ellero-Simatos, S.; Régnier, M.; Polizzi, A.; Lasserre, F.; Montagner, A.; Lippi, Y.; Jamin, E.L.; Martin, J.-F.; Naylies, C.; et al. Metabolic Effects of a Chronic Dietary Exposure to a Low-Dose Pesticide Cocktail in Mice: Sexual Dimorphism and Role of the Constitutive Androstane Receptor. *Environ. Health Perspect.* **2018**, *126*, 067007. [CrossRef]

20. Weiss, J.M.; Davies, L.C.; Karwan, M.; Ileva, L.; Ozaki, M.K.; Cheng, R.Y.; Ridnour, L.A.; Annunziata, C.M.; Wink, D.A.; McVicar, D.W. Itaconic acid mediates crosstalk between macrophage metabolism and peritoneal tumors. *J. Clin. Invest.* **2018**, *128*, 3794–3805. [CrossRef]

21. Su, L.; Mao, J.; Hao, M.; Lu, T.; Mao, C.; Ji, D.; Tong, H.; Fei, C. Integrated Plasma and Bile Metabolomics Based on an UHPLC-Q/TOF-MS and Network Pharmacology Approach to Explore the Potential Mechanism of Schisandra chinensis-Protection From Acute Alcoholic Liver Injury. *Front. Pharmacol.* **2019**, *10*, 1543. [CrossRef] [PubMed]

22. Claus, S.P.; Swann, J.R. Nutrimetabonomics: Applications for nutritional sciences, with specific reference to gut microbial interactions. *Annu. Rev. Food Sci. Technol.* **2013**, *4*, 381–399. [CrossRef] [PubMed]

23. Ivey, K.L.; Rimm, E.B.; Kraft, P.; Clish, C.B.; Cassidy, A.; Hodgson, J.; Croft, K.; Wolpin, B.; Liang, L. Identifying the metabolomic fingerprint of high and low flavonoid consumers. *J. Nutr. Sci.* **2017**, *6*, e34. [CrossRef]

24. Robertson, D.G.; Ruepp, S.U.; Stryker, S.A.; Hnatyshyn, S.Y.; Shipkova, P.A.; Aranibar, N.; Mcnaney, C.A.; Fiehn, O.; Reily, M.D. Metabolomic and transcriptomic changes induced by overnight (16 h) fasting in male and female Sprague-Dawley rats. *Chem. Res. Toxicol.* **2011**, *24*, 481–487. [CrossRef] [PubMed]

25. Abbondante, S.; Eckel-Mahan, K.L.; Ceglia, N.J.; Baldi, P.; Sassone-Corsi, P. Comparative Circadian Metabolomics Reveal Differential Effects of Nutritional Challenge in the Serum and Liver. *J. Biol. Chem.* **2016**, *291*, 2812–2828. [CrossRef] [PubMed]

26. Zierer, J.; Jackson, M.A.; Kastenmüller, G.; Mangino, M.; Long, T.; Telenti, A.; Mohney, R.P.; Small, K.S.; Bell, J.T.; Steves, C.J.; et al. The fecal metabolome as a functional readout of the gut microbiome. *Nat. Genet.* **2018**, *50*, 790–795. [CrossRef]

27. Beaumont, M.; Portune, K.J.; Steuer, N.; Lan, A.; Cerrudo, V.; Audebert, M.; Dumont, F.; Mancano, G.; Khodorova, N.; Andriamihaja, M.; et al. Quantity and source of dietary protein influence metabolite production by gut microbiota and rectal mucosa gene expression: A randomized, parallel, double-blind trial in overweight humans. *Am. J. Clin. Nutr.* **2017**, *106*, 1005–1019. [CrossRef]

28. Zhang, X.; Grosfeld, A.; Williams, E.; Vasiliauskas, D.; Barretto, S.; Smith, L.; Mariadassou, M.; Philippe, C.; Devime, F.; Melchior, C.; et al. Fructose malabsorption induces cholecystokinin expression in the ileum and cecum by changing microbiota composition and metabolism. *FASEB J.* **2019**, *33*, 7126–7142. [CrossRef]

29. Choi, W.; Namkung, J.; Hwang, I.; Kim, H.; Lim, A.; Park, H.J.; Lee, H.W.; Han, K.-H.; Park, S.; Jeong, J.-S.; et al. Serotonin signals through a gut-liver axis to regulate hepatic steatosis. *Nat. Commun.* **2018**, *9*, 4824. [CrossRef]

30. Koh, A.; Molinaro, A.; Ståhlman, M.; Khan, M.T.; Schmidt, C.; Mannerås-Holm, L.; Wu, H.; Carreras, A.; Jeong, H.; Olofsson, L.E.; et al. Microbially Produced Imidazole Propionate Impairs Insulin Signaling through mTORC1. *Cell* **2018**, *175*, 947–961. [CrossRef]

31. Huang, W.; Ramsey, K.M.; Marcheva, B.; Bass, J. Circadian rhythms, sleep, and metabolism. *J. Clin. Invest.* **2011**, *121*, 2133–2141. [CrossRef] [PubMed]

32. Ramsey, K.M.; Yoshino, J.; Brace, C.S.; Abrassart, D.; Kobayashi, Y.; Marcheva, B.; Hong, H.-K.; Chong, J.L.; Buhr, E.D.; Lee, C.; et al. Circadian clock feedback cycle through NAMPT-mediated NAD+ biosynthesis. *Science* **2009**, *324*, 651–654. [CrossRef] [PubMed]

33. Hughes, M.E.; DiTacchio, L.; Hayes, K.R.; Vollmers, C.; Pulivarthy, S.; Baggs, J.E.; Panda, S.; Hogenesch, J.B. Harmonics of circadian gene transcription in mammals. *PLoS Genet.* **2009**, *5*, e1000442. [CrossRef] [PubMed]

34. Dallmann, R.; Viola, A.U.; Tarokh, L.; Cajochen, C.; Brown, S.A. The human circadian metabolome. *Proc. Natl. Acad. Sci. USA* **2012**, *109*, 2625–2629. [CrossRef]

35. Deprez, S.; Sweatman, B.C.; Connor, S.C.; Haselden, J.N.; Waterfield, C.J. Optimisation of collection, storage and preparation of rat plasma for 1H NMR spectroscopic analysis in toxicology studies to determine inherent variation in biochemical profiles. *J. Pharm. Biomed. Anal.* **2002**, *30*, 1297–1310. [CrossRef]

36. Bernini, P.; Bertini, I.; Luchinat, C.; Nincheri, P.; Staderini, S.; Turano, P. Standard operating procedures for pre-analytical handling of blood and urine for metabolomic studies and biobanks. *J. Biomol. NMR* **2011**, *49*, 231–243. [CrossRef]

37. Slupsky, C.M.; Rankin, K.N.; Wagner, J.; Fu, H.; Chang, D.; Weljie, A.M.; Saude, E.J.; Lix, B.; Adamko, D.J.; Shah, S.; et al. Investigations of the effects of gender, diurnal variation, and age in human urinary metabolomic profiles. *Anal. Chem.* **2007**, *79*, 6995–7004. [CrossRef]

38. Stevens, V.L.; Hoover, E.; Wang, Y.; Zanetti, K.A. Pre-Analytical Factors that Affect Metabolite Stability in Human Urine, Plasma, and Serum: A Review. *Metabolites* **2019**, *9*, 156. [CrossRef]

39. Eriksson, E.; Royo, F.; Lyberg, K.; Carlsson, H.-E.; Hau, J. Effect of metabolic cage housing on immunoglobulin A and corticosterone excretion in faeces and urine of young male rats. *Exp. Physiol.* **2004**, *89*, 427–433. [CrossRef]

40. Hoffman, J.F.; Fan, A.X.; Neuendorf, E.H.; Vergara, V.B.; Kalinich, J.F. Hydrophobic Sand Versus Metabolic Cages: A Comparison of Urine Collection Methods for Rats (Rattus norvegicus). *J. Am. Assoc. Lab. Anim. Sci.* **2018**, *57*, 51–57.

41. Saude, E.J.; Sykes, B.D. Urine stability for metabolomic studies: Effects of preparation and storage. *Metabolomics* **2007**, *3*, 19–27. [CrossRef]

42. Thongboonkerd, V.; Saetun, P. Bacterial overgrowth affects urinary proteome analysis: Recommendation for centrifugation, temperature, duration, and the use of preservatives during sample collection. *J. Proteome Res.* **2007**, *6*, 4173–4181. [CrossRef] [PubMed]

43. Fernández-Peralbo, M.A.; Luque de Castro, M.D. Preparation of urine samples prior to targeted or untargeted metabolomics mass-spectrometry analysis. *TrAC Trends Anal. Chem.* **2012**, *41*, 75–85. [CrossRef]

44. Gika, H.G.; Theodoridis, G.A.; Wilson, I.D. Liquid chromatography and ultra-performance liquid chromatography–mass spectrometry fingerprinting of human urine: Sample stability under different handling and storage conditions for metabonomics studies. *J. Chromatogr. A* **2008**, *1189*, 314–322. [CrossRef] [PubMed]

45. Trivedi, D.K.; Jones, H.; Shah, A.J.; Iles, R.K. Development of Zwitterionic Hydrophilic Liquid Chromatography (ZIC®HILIC-MS) metabolomics method for Shotgun analysis of human urine. *J. Chromatogr. Sep. Tech.* **2012**, *3*. [CrossRef]

46. Rachita Dhurat, M.S. Principles and Methods of Preparation of Platelet-Rich Plasma: A Review and Author's Perspective. *J. Cutan. Aesthetic Surg.* **2014**, *7*, 189–197. [CrossRef]

47. Teahan, O.; Gamble, S.; Holmes, E.; Waxman, J.; Nicholson, J.K.; Charlotte Bevan, A.; Keun, H.C. Impact of Analytical Bias in Metabonomic Studies of Human Blood Serum and Plasma. *Anal. Chem.* **2006**, *78*, 4307–4318. [CrossRef]

48. Yin, P.; Lehmann, R.; Xu, G. Effects of pre-analytical processes on blood samples used in metabolomics studies. *Anal. Bioanal. Chem.* **2015**, *407*, 4879–4892. [CrossRef]

49. Denery, J.R.; Nunes, A.A.K.; Dickerson, T.J. Characterization of differences between blood sample matrices in untargeted metabolomics. *Anal. Chem.* **2011**, *83*, 1040–1047. [CrossRef]

50. Barri, T.; Dragsted, L.O. UPLC-ESI-QTOF/MS and multivariate data analysis for blood plasma and serum metabolomics: Effect of experimental artefacts and anticoagulant. *Anal. Chim. Acta* **2013**, *768*, 118–128. [CrossRef]

51. Beckonert, O.; Keun, H.C.; Ebbels, T.M.D.; Bundy, J.; Holmes, E.; Lindon, J.C.; Nicholson, J.K. Metabolic profiling, metabolomic and metabonomic procedures for NMR spectroscopy of urine, plasma, serum and tissue extracts. *Nat. Protoc.* **2007**, *2*, 2692–2703. [CrossRef] [PubMed]

52. Dunn, W.B.; Broadhurst, D.; Begley, P.; Zelena, E.; Francis-McIntyre, S.; Anderson, N.; Brown, M.; Knowles, J.D.; Halsall, A.; Haselden, J.N.; et al. Human Serum Metabolome (HUSERMET) Consortium Procedures for large-scale metabolic profiling of serum and plasma using gas chromatography and liquid chromatography coupled to mass spectrometry. *Nat. Protoc.* **2011**, *6*, 1060–1083. [CrossRef] [PubMed]

53. Pinto, J.; Domingues, M.R.M.; Galhano, E.; Pita, C.; Almeida, M.D.C.; Carreira, I.M.; Gil, A.M. Human plasma stability during handling and storage: Impact on NMR metabolomics. *Analyst* **2014**, *139*, 1168–1177. [CrossRef] [PubMed]

54. Mitchell, B.L.; Yasui, Y.; Li, C.I.; Fitzpatrick, A.L.; Lampe, P.D. Impact of freeze-thaw cycles and storage time on plasma samples used in mass spectrometry based biomarker discovery projects. *Cancer Inform* **2005**, *1*, 98–104. [CrossRef] [PubMed]

55. Hernandes, V.V.; Barbas, C.; Dudzik, D. A review of blood sample handling and pre-processing for metabolomics studies. *Electrophoresis* **2017**, *38*, 2232–2241. [CrossRef]

56. Schroeder, B.O.; Bäckhed, F. Signals from the gut microbiota to distant organs in physiology and disease. *Nat. Med.* **2016**, *22*, 1079–1089. [CrossRef]

57. Karu, N.; Deng, L.; Slae, M.; Guo, A.C.; Sajed, T.; Huynh, H.; Wine, E.; Wishart, D.S. A review on human fecal metabolomics: Methods, applications and the human fecal metabolome database. *Anal. Chim. Acta* **2018**, *1030*, 1–24. [CrossRef]

58. Probert, C.S.J.; Jones, P.R.H.; Ratcliffe, N.M. A novel method for rapidly diagnosing the causes of diarrhoea. *Gut* **2004**, *53*, 58–61. [CrossRef]

59. Garner, C.E.; Smith, S.; de Lacy Costello, B.; White, P.; Spencer, R.; Probert, C.S.J.; Ratcliffe, N.M. Volatile organic compounds from feces and their potential for diagnosis of gastrointestinal disease. *FASEB J.* **2007**, *21*, 1675–1688. [CrossRef]

60. Rose, C.; Parker, A.; Jefferson, B.; Cartmell, E. The Characterization of Feces and Urine: A Review of the Literature to Inform Advanced Treatment Technology. *Crit. Rev. Environ. Sci. Technol.* **2015**, *45*, 1827–1879. [CrossRef]

61. Matysik, S.; Le Roy, C.I.; Liebisch, G.; Claus, S.P. Metabolomics of fecal samples: A practical consideration. *Trends Food Sci. Technol.* **2016**, *57*, 244–255. [CrossRef]

62. Liang, X.; Bushman, F.D.; FitzGerald, G.A. Rhythmicity of the intestinal microbiota is regulated by gender and the host circadian clock. *Proc. Natl. Acad. Sci. USA* **2015**, *112*, 10479–10484. [CrossRef] [PubMed]

63. Leone, V.; Gibbons, S.M.; Martinez, K.; Hutchison, A.L.; Huang, E.Y.; Cham, C.M.; Pierre, J.F.; Heneghan, A.F.; Nadimpalli, A.; Hubert, N.; et al. Effects of diurnal variation of gut microbes and high-fat feeding on host circadian clock function and metabolism. *Cell Host Microbe* **2015**, *17*, 681–689. [CrossRef] [PubMed]

64. Duparc, T.; Plovier, H.; Marrachelli, V.G.; Van Hul, M.; Essaghir, A.; Ståhlman, M.; Matamoros, S.; Geurts, L.; Pardo-Tendero, M.M.; Druart, C.; et al. Hepatocyte MyD88 affects bile acids, gut microbiota and metabolome contributing to regulate glucose and lipid metabolism. *Gut* **2016**, *66*, 620–632. [CrossRef]

65. Sberna, A.L.; Assem, M.; Gautier, T.; Grober, J.; Guiu, B.; Jeannin, A.; Pais de Barros, J.-P.; Athias, A.; Lagrost, L.; Masson, D. Constitutive androstane receptor activation stimulates faecal bile acid excretion and reverse cholesterol transport in mice. *J. Hepatol.* **2011**, *55*, 154–161. [CrossRef] [PubMed]

66. Lamichhane, S.; Sundekilde, U.K.; Blædel, T.; Dalsgaard, T.K.; Larsen, L.H.; Dragsted, L.O.; Astrup, A.; Bertram, H.C. Optimizing sampling strategies for NMR-based metabolomics of human feces: Pooled vs. unpooled analyses. *Anal. Methods* **2017**, *9*, 4476–4480. [CrossRef]

67. Phua, L.C.; Koh, P.K.; Cheah, P.Y.; Ho, H.K.; Chan, E.C.Y. Global gas chromatography/time-of-flight mass spectrometry (GC/TOFMS)-based metabonomic profiling of lyophilized human feces. *J. Chromatogr. B* **2013**, *937*, 103–113. [CrossRef]

68. Lamichhane, S.; Yde, C.C.; Schmedes, M.S.; Jensen, H.M.; Meier, S.; Bertram, H.C. Strategy for Nuclear-Magnetic-Resonance-Based Metabolomics of Human Feces. *Anal. Chem.* **2015**, *87*, 5930–5937. [CrossRef]

69. Le Gall, G.; Noor, S.O.; Ridgway, K.; Scovell, L.; Jamieson, C.; Johnson, I.T.; Colquhoun, I.J.; Kemsley, E.K.; Narbad, A. Metabolomics of fecal extracts detects altered metabolic activity of gut microbiota in ulcerative colitis and irritable bowel syndrome. *J. Proteome Res.* **2011**, *10*, 4208–4218. [CrossRef]

70. Armstrong, C.W.; McGregor, N.R.; Lewis, D.P.; Butt, H.L.; Gooley, P.R. The association of fecal microbiota and fecal, blood serum and urine metabolites in myalgic encephalomyelitis/chronic fatigue syndrome. *Metabolomics* **2016**, *13*, 8. [CrossRef]

71. Bezabeh, T.; Somorjai, R.L.; Smith, I.C.P. MR metabolomics of fecal extracts: Applications in the study of bowel diseases. *Magn. Reson. Chem.* **2009**, *47*, S54–S61. [CrossRef] [PubMed]

72. Gratton, J.; Phetcharaburanin, J.; Mullish, B.H.; Williams, H.R.T.; Thursz, M.; Nicholson, J.K.; Holmes, E.; Marchesi, J.R.; Li, J.V. Optimized Sample Handling Strategy for Metabolic Profiling of Human Feces. *Anal. Chem.* **2016**, *88*, 4661–4668. [CrossRef] [PubMed]

73. Yen, S.; McDonald, J.A.K.; Schroeter, K.; Oliphant, K.; Sokolenko, S.; Blondeel, E.J.M.; Allen-Vercoe, E.; Aucoin, M.G. Metabolomic Analysis of Human Fecal Microbiota: A Comparison of Feces-Derived Communities and Defined Mixed Communities. *J. Proteome Res.* **2015**, *14*, 1472–1482. [CrossRef]

74. Couch, R.D.; Navarro, K.; Sikaroodi, M.; Gillevet, P.; Forsyth, C.B.; Mutlu, E.; Engen, P.A.; Keshavarzian, A. The Approach to Sample Acquisition and Its Impact on the Derived Human Fecal Microbiome and VOC Metabolome. *PLoS ONE* **2013**, *8*, e81163. [CrossRef]

75. Loftfield, E.; Vogtmann, E.; Sampson, J.N.; Moore, S.C.; Nelson, H.; Knight, R.; Chia, N.; Sinha, R. Comparison of Collection Methods for Fecal Samples for Discovery Metabolomics in Epidemiologic Studies. *Cancer Epidemiol. Biomark. Prev.* **2016**, *25*, 1483–1490. [CrossRef]

76. Saric, J.; Wang, Y.; Li, J.; Coen, M.; Utzinger, J.; Marchesi, J.R.; Keiser, J.; Veselkov, K.; Lindon, J.C.; Nicholson, J.K.; et al. Species variation in the fecal metabolome gives insight into differential gastrointestinal function. *J. Proteome Res.* **2008**, *7*, 352–360. [CrossRef] [PubMed]

77. Moosmang, S.; Pitscheider, M.; Sturm, S.; Seger, C.; Tilg, H.; Halabalaki, M.; Stuppner, H. Metabolomic analysis-Addressing NMR and LC-MS related problems in human feces sample preparation. *Clin. Chim. Acta* **2017**, *489*, 169–176. [CrossRef] [PubMed]

78. Jungermann, K.; Katz, N. Functional specialization of different hepatocyte populations. *Physiol. Rev.* **1989**, *69*, 708–764. [CrossRef]

79. Braeuning, A.; Ittrich, C.; Köhle, C.; Hailfinger, S.; Bonin, M.; Buchmann, A.; Schwarz, M. Differential gene expression in periportal and perivenous mouse hepatocytes. *FEBS J.* **2006**, *273*, 5051–5061. [CrossRef]

80. Isse, K.; Lesniak, A.; Grama, K.; Maier, J.; Specht, S.; Castillo-Rama, M.; Lunz, J.; Roysam, B.; Michalopoulos, G.; Demetris, A.J. Preexisting epithelial diversity in normal human livers: A tissue-tethered cytometric analysis in portal/periportal epithelial cells. *Hepatology* **2013**, *57*, 1632–1643. [CrossRef] [PubMed]

81. Want, E.J.; Masson, P.; Michopoulos, F.; Wilson, I.D.; Theodoridis, G.; Plumb, R.S.; Shockcor, J.; Loftus, N.; Holmes, E.; Nicholson, J.K. Global metabolic profiling of animal and human tissues via UPLC-MS. *Nat. Protoc.* **2013**, *8*, 17–32. [CrossRef]

82. Hu, Z.-P.; Browne, E.R.; Liu, T.; Angel, T.E.; Ho, P.C.; Chan, E.C.Y. Metabonomic profiling of TASTPM transgenic Alzheimer's disease mouse model. *J. Proteome Res.* **2012**, *11*, 5903–5913. [CrossRef]

83. Garrod, S.; Humpfer, E.; Spraul, M.; Connor, S.C.; Polley, S.; Connelly, J.; Lindon, J.C.; Nicholson, J.K.; Holmes, E. High-resolution magic angle spinning 1H NMR spectroscopic studies on intact rat renal cortex and medulla. *Magn. Reson. Med.* **1999**, *41*, 1108–1118. [CrossRef]

84. Zhou, L.; Zhang, W.; Xie, W.; Chen, H.; Yu, W.; Li, H.; Shen, G. Tributyl phosphate impairs the urea cycle and alters liver pathology and metabolism in mice after short-term exposure based on a metabonomics study. *Sci. Total Environ.* **2017**, *603-604*, 77–85. [CrossRef] [PubMed]

85. Abuja, P.M.; Ehrhart, F.; Schoen, U.; Schmidt, T.; Stracke, F.; Dallmann, G.; Friedrich, T.; Zimmermann, H.; Zatloukal, K. Alterations in Human Liver Metabolome during Prolonged Cryostorage. *J. Proteome Res.* **2015**, *14*, 2758–2768. [CrossRef] [PubMed]

86. Torell, F.; Bennett, K.; Cereghini, S.; Rännar, S.; Lundstedt-Enkel, K.; Moritz, T.; Haumaitre, C.; Trygg, J.; Lundstedt, T. Tissue sample stability: Thawing effect on multi-organ samples. *Metabolomics* **2015**, *12*, 19. [CrossRef]

87. Kapoore, R.V.; Coyle, R.; Staton, C.A.; Brown, N.J.; Vaidyanathan, S. Influence of washing and quenching in profiling the metabolome of adherent mammalian cells: A case study with the metastatic breast cancer cell line MDA-MB-231. *Analyst* **2017**, *142*, 2038–2049. [CrossRef]

88. Lorenz, M.A.; Burant, C.F.; Kennedy, R.T. Reducing time and increasing sensitivity in sample preparation for adherent mammalian cell metabolomics. *Anal. Chem.* **2011**, *83*, 3406–3414. [CrossRef]

89. Rusz, M.; Rampler, E.; Keppler, B.K.; Jakupec, M.A.; Koellensperger, G. Single Spheroid Metabolomics: Optimizing Sample Preparation of Three-Dimensional Multicellular Tumor Spheroids. *Metabolites* **2019**, *9*, 304. [CrossRef]

90. Shryock, J.C.; Rubio, R.; Berne, R.M. Extraction of adenine nucleotides from cultured endothelial cells. *Anal. Biochem.* **1986**, *159*, 73–81. [CrossRef]

91. Kořínek, M.; Šístek, V.; Mládková, J.; Mikeš, P.; Jiráček, J.; Selicharová, I. Quantification of homocysteine-related metabolites and the role of betaine–homocysteine S-methyltransferase in HepG2 cells. *Biomed. Chromatogr.* **2013**, *27*, 111–121. [CrossRef] [PubMed]

92. Ibáñez, C.; Simó, C.; Valdés, A.; Campone, L.; Piccinelli, A.L.; García-Cañas, V.; Cifuentes, A. Metabolomics of adherent mammalian cells by capillary electrophoresis-mass spectrometry: HT-29 cells as case study. *J. Pharm. Biomed. Anal.* **2015**, *110*, 83–92. [CrossRef] [PubMed]

93. Dettmer, K.; Nürnberger, N.; Kaspar, H.; Gruber, M.A.; Almstetter, M.F.; Oefner, P.J. Metabolite extraction from adherently growing mammalian cells for metabolomics studies: Optimization of harvesting and extraction protocols. *Anal. Bioanal. Chem.* **2011**, *399*, 1127–1139. [CrossRef] [PubMed]

94. León, Z.; García-Cañaveras, J.C.; Donato, M.T.; Lahoz, A. Mammalian cell metabolomics: Experimental design and sample preparation. *Electrophoresis* **2013**, *34*, 2762–2775. [CrossRef]

95. Yuan, W.; Anderson, K.W.; Li, S.; Edwards, J.L. Subsecond absolute quantitation of amine metabolites using isobaric tags for discovery of pathway activation in mammalian cells. *Anal. Chem.* **2012**, *84*, 2892–2899. [CrossRef]

96. Poupin, N.; Corlu, A.; Cabaton, N.J.; Dubois-Pot-Schneider, H.; Canlet, C.; Person, E.; Bruel, S.; Frainay, C.; Vinson, F.; Maurier, F.; et al. Large-Scale Modeling Approach Reveals Functional Metabolic Shifts during Hepatic Differentiation. *J. Proteome Res.* **2019**, *18*, 204–216. [CrossRef]

97. Villas-Bôas, S.G.; Højer-Pedersen, J.; Akesson, M.; Smedsgaard, J.; Nielsen, J. Global metabolite analysis of yeast: Evaluation of sample preparation methods. *Yeast* **2005**, *22*, 1155–1169. [CrossRef]

7

A Lipidomic Analysis of Docosahexaenoic Acid (22:6, ω3) Mediated Attenuation of Western Diet Induced Nonalcoholic Steatohepatitis in Male *Ldlr* $^{-/-}$ Mice

Manuel García-Jaramillo [1,2,3], **Kelli A. Lytle** [1,3,†], **Melinda H. Spooner** [1,3] **and Donald B. Jump** [1,3,*]

[1] Nutrition Program, School of Biological and Population Health Sciences, Oregon State University, Corvallis, OR 97331, USA; Manuel.g.jaramillo@oregonstate.edu (M.G.-J.); Kelli.Lytle@mayo.edu (K.A.L.); Spoonerm@oregonstate.edu (M.H.S.)
[2] Department of Chemistry, Oregon State University, Corvallis, OR 97331, USA
[3] The Linus Pauling Institute, Oregon State University, Corvallis, OR 97331, USA
* Correspondence: Donald.Jump@oregonstate.edu
† Current affiliation: Endocrine Research Unit, Mayo Clinic, Rochester, MN 55902, USA.

Abstract: Nonalcoholic fatty liver disease (NAFLD) is a major public health problem worldwide. NAFLD ranges in severity from benign steatosis to nonalcoholic steatohepatitis (NASH), cirrhosis, and primary hepatocellular cancer (HCC). Obesity and type 2 diabetes mellitus (T2DM) are strongly associated with NAFLD, and the western diet (WD) is a major contributor to the onset and progression of these chronic diseases. Our aim was to use a lipidomic approach to identify potential lipid mediators of diet-induced NASH. We previously used a preclinical mouse (low density lipoprotein receptor null mouse, *Ldlr* $^{-/-}$) model to assess transcriptomic mechanisms linked to WD-induced NASH and docosahexaenoic acid (DHA, 22:6, ω3)-mediated remission of NASH. This report used livers from the previous study to carry out ultra-high-performance liquid chromatography coupled with tandem mass spectrometry (LC-MS/MS) and high-performance liquid chromatography coupled with dynamic multi-reaction monitoring (HPLC-dMRM) to assess the impact of the WD and DHA on hepatic membrane lipid and oxylipin composition, respectively. Feeding mice the WD increased hepatic saturated and monounsaturated fatty acids and arachidonic acid (ARA, 20:4, ω6) in membrane lipids and suppressed ω3 polyunsaturated fatty acids (PUFA) in membrane lipids and ω3 PUFA-derived anti-inflammatory oxylipins. Supplementing the WD with DHA lowered hepatic ARA in membrane lipids and ARA-derived oxylipins and significantly increased hepatic DHA and its metabolites in membrane lipids, as well as C_{20-22} ω3 PUFA-derived oxylipins. NASH markers of inflammation and fibrosis were inversely associated with hepatic C_{20-22} ω3 PUFA-derived Cyp2C- and Cyp2J-generated anti-inflammatory oxylipins (false discovery rate adjusted p-value; $q \leq 0.026$). Our findings suggest that dietary DHA promoted partial remission of WD-induced NASH, at least in part, by lowering hepatic pro-inflammatory oxylipins derived from ARA and increasing hepatic anti-inflammatory oxylipins derived from C_{20-22} ω3 PUFA.

Keywords: nonalcoholic fatty liver disease; nonalcoholic steatohepatitis; arachidonic acid; docosahexaenoic acid; inflammation; fibrosis; lipidomics; mass spectrometry

1. Introduction

Nonalcoholic fatty liver disease (NAFLD) is the most common chronic fatty liver disease worldwide [1–3] and is defined as excessive neutral lipid deposition in the liver in individuals who consume little or no alcohol [4,5]. Obesity and type 2 diabetes mellitus (T2DM) are strongly associated with NAFLD [3,6–8]. In fact, 60% of patients with a BMI > 30 display evidence of liver steatosis [9]. Based on estimates from the Centers for Disease Control, ~93 million adults [10] and ~14 million children [11] in the US are obese. As such, both obese children and adults are at risk of developing NAFLD [12]. Lifestyle, diet, genetics, and endocrine status contribute to the onset of NAFLD and its progression to nonalcoholic steatohepatitis (NASH), cirrhosis, and primary hepatocellular cancer (HCC) [7,13]. Moreover, NAFLD is a risk factor for cardiovascular disease [14–16]. The top four risk factors for NAFLD are obesity, T2DM, dyslipidemia, and metabolic syndrome [17,18].

The progression of benign steatosis to NASH is a multicellular and multi-hit process [19–23] that is associated with excessive lipid accumulation in hepatocytes leading to insulin resistance and hepatic injury involving endoplasmic reticulum stress, oxidative stress, and inflammation [24]. Hepatic injury leads to cell death and fibrosis [25–27]. The best strategies to prevent NAFLD and stop its progression from benign steatosis to NASH remain ill-defined [28–31]. While current strategies focus on lifestyle management (exercise and diet) [28,32–43], patient noncompliance remains a major concern when using lifestyle interventions to improve health outcomes [44–46]. Although targeted pharmacological agents are in development to treat NAFLD [46–48], adverse drug effects arising from off-target mechanisms often occur. To date, the Food and Drug Administration has not approved any specific therapies for NASH [49]. The absence of specific treatment strategies makes NAFLD a major public health concern [30].

While the clinical features of NAFLD are well described, the impact of diet, such as the western diet, on hepatic physiology and lipid metabolism remains poorly defined. Accordingly, we developed a preclinical NASH model using the low density lipoprotein (LDL)-receptor null ($Ldlr^{-/-}$) mouse and the western diet (WD). This model recapitulates human NASH in male and female mice [50–52]. Mice fed the WD become obese and the liver presents all the hallmarks of NASH, i.e., hepatosteatosis, leukocyte accumulation in the liver, centrilobular fibrosis, and increased expression of HCC markers.

A key outcome of our research established that the WD lowers hepatic content of C_{18-22} polyunsaturated fatty acids (PUFA, both ω3 and ω6). The WD is moderately high in saturated (SFA) and monounsaturated (MUFA) fatty acids, simple sugar and cholesterol, but low in essential fatty acids, e.g., linoleic acid (LA, 18:2,ω6) and α-linolenic acid (ALA, 18:3,ω3) [50,53,54]. Interestingly, clinical studies have shown that NASH patients have low hepatic C_{18-22} PUFA when compared to patients with benign steatosis [55–57]. Moreover, PUFA and ω3 PUFA, specifically, affect whole body lipid metabolism by decreasing blood triglycerides, suppressing fatty acid synthesis, and promoting fatty acid oxidation. In contrast, dietary ω6 PUFAs are precursors to bioactive pro-inflammatory oxylipins [58,59]. As such, changes in the relative abundance of hepatic SFA, MUFA, PUFA, and the type of PUFA, i.e., ω3 versus ω6 PUFA, has the potential to affect whole body and liver health.

To reinforce the role of dietary PUFA in NAFLD development, we established that supplementing the WD with docosahexaenoic acid (DHA, 22:6,ω3) at 2% total calories restored hepatic C_{20-22} ω3 PUFA, lowered arachidonic acid (ARA, 20:4,ω6), a precursor to harmful pro-inflammatory ARA-derived oxylipins, and lowered histologic and transcriptomic markers of inflammation, oxidative stress, and fibrosis [52]. More recently, we used a lipidomic approach to assess the impact of the WD on hepatic membrane lipids and oxylipins in female $Ldlr^{-/-}$ mice [60]. These studies established that feeding mice the WD significantly changed the acyl chain composition of multiple hepatic membrane lipid classes and ω3 and ω6 PUFA-derived oxylipins. Specifically, the WD increased the hepatic membrane content of SFA and MUFA, as well as ARA and ARA-derived oxylipins. The hepatic abundance of ω3 PUFA-derived oxylipins, however, was low in mice fed the WD. This oxylipin profile was associated with increased hepatic markers of inflammation, oxidative stress, fibrosis, apoptosis, autophagy, notch and hedgehog signaling, and hepatic cancer [60].

Fatty acids and their derivatives are well-established regulators of cell function. The principal targets for this action include regulation of membrane lipid composition, oxylipin type and abundance, and regulation of cell signaling originating from the plasma membrane, as well as targeting nuclear receptors [59,61]. The rationale for using DHA to combat NASH is based on the well-established role of C_{20-22} ω3 PUFA in the control of blood triglycerides and hepatic fatty acid synthesis and oxidation [62].

Moreover, C_{20-22} ω3 PUFA interfere with ARA-derived oxylipin production and function [58]. Finally, clinical studies support the use of ω3 PUFA dietary supplementation to treat NAFLD [12,47]. Recent meta-analyses of clinical trials using C_{20-22} ω3 PUFA dietary supplementation indicate significant improvement in several metabolic outcomes, including lowering plasma triglycerides and hepatic fat content [12,47]. The most consistent improvement in liver health is seen with dietary DHA [12] or the combination of DHA and eicosapentaenoic acid (EPA, 20:5, ω3), e.g., Lovaza™, GlaxoSmithKline [63]. EPA treatment alone, however, has proven ineffective in improving liver health in NAFLD patients [50,64].

In this report, we used liver samples from our previous study which documented the capacity of DHA to block NASH progression (Figure 1) [52]. This study included detailed gas chromatographic (GC) analysis of diet effects on hepatic lipids as well as extensive transcriptomic analysis of hepatic markers of inflammation and fibrosis. Herein, we expanded our lipidomic analysis by using ultra-high-performance liquid chromatography coupled with tandem mass spectrometry (UPLC-MS/MS) and high-performance liquid chromatography coupled with dynamic multi-reaction monitoring (HPLC-dMRM), as described [60]. Our aim was to document how the WD and DHA altered hepatic membrane lipid and non-esterified oxylipin composition in a preclinical NASH model. We then used a statistical approach to determine how these diet-induced changes in hepatic lipids correlated with changes in hepatic markers of inflammation and fibrosis.

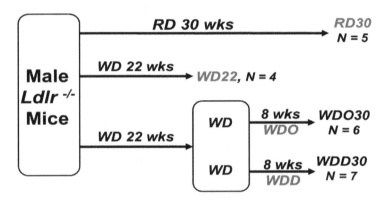

Figure 1. Study design for docosahexaenoic acid (DHA)-mediated nonalcoholic steatohepatitis (NASH) remission in male *Ldlr* $^{-/-}$ mice. Liver samples used in this lipidomic analysis were obtained from our previously published study assessing the capacity of DHA to promote NASH remission [52]. Briefly, mice at 10 wks of age were fed a chow diet (Purina Pico Lab diet 5053) and served as a reference diet (RD) group. The RD group was maintained on the RD for the duration of the study, i.e., 30 weeks (wks; RD30, number of animals (N) = 5). Mice were also fed the western diet (WD) (Research Diets, D12079B) for 22 wks. At 22 wks, a group of WD-fed mice were euthanized for recovery of blood and liver. This group (WD22, N = 5) served as a baseline for disease progression. The remaining WD-fed mice were switched to a WD supplemented with either olive oil (WDO30, N = 6) or DHASCO (WDD30, N = 7) and euthanized 8 weeks (8 wks) later. See Materials and Methods for more details.

2. Results

2.1. Impact of the Western Diet (WD) on Membrane Lipids

The study designed included 4 groups of male *Ldlr* $^{-/-}$ mice as described in Figure 1. A control group consisted of mice maintained on a reference diet (RD) for 30 weeks. The remaining mice were fed the WD for 22 weeks. At 22 weeks, WD-fed mice were split into three groups. One group was euthanized and served as the baseline group (WD22) for NASH progression analysis. The remaining mice were fed the WD supplemented with either olive oil (WDO) or DHASCO (WDD) for 8 weeks (see Materials and Methods). The WDO and WDD diets were matched for calories as fat. The dose of DHA used in these studies was equivalent to a human taking 4 g of Lovaza™ (GlaxoSmithKline)/day to treat hypertriglyceridemia [65]. After 8 weeks on the WDO and WDD diets, mice were euthanized for blood and liver collection. The group identifications for these mice are WDO30 and WDD30, respectively.

Total hepatic lipids were extracted and fractionated using the UPLC-MS/MS approach described in Materials and Methods.

Our UPLC-MS/MS analysis identified 13 classes of membrane lipids (Figure 2). To assess the impact of diet on these lipids, we quantified the cumulative saturation index (CSI). The CSI reflects the amount of lipid within a lipid class and the level of saturation of the fatty acyl chains within each lipid class. Figure 2A represents the CSI across all major membrane lipids in mice maintained on the RD for 30 weeks (RD30). The highest CSI was in the lipid classes including phosphatidyl choline (PC) and phosphatidyl ethanolamine (PE) and the lowest in lysophosphatidyl serine (lyso PS).

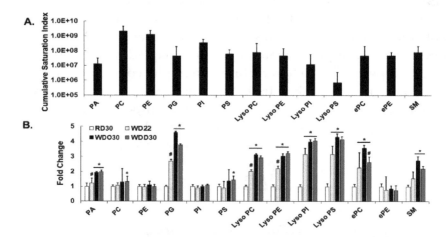

Figure 2. Diet effects on membrane lipids. (**A**): Cumulative saturation index of lipids in each lipid class. The saturation index (SI) was calculated as follows: one minus (number of double bonds) divided by (number of fatty acyl carbons minus one). The cumulative saturation index was calculated by multiplying the SI by the peak intensity of each lipid species and summing all lipids within each lipid class. (**B**): Effect of diet on the cumulative saturation index for each lipid class. Results are presented as fold change, mean ± standard error of the mean (SEM); *, $q < 0.05$ vs. RD30; #, $q < 0.05$ vs. WDO30; [q-value is the false discovery rate (FDR) adjusted p-value].

The impact of the WD and DHA on CSI is shown in Figure 2B. Since the WD is enriched in SFA and MUFA, we expected a significant increase in the CSI. Accordingly, feeding mice the WD increased the CSI in phosphatidic acid (PA), phosphatidyl glycerol (PG), phosphatidyl serine (PS), all lysophospholipids [(lysophosphatidyl choline (lyso PC), lysophosphatidyl ethanolamine PE (lyso PE), phosphatidyl inositol (lyso PI), phosphatidyl serine (lyso PS)], ether phosphatidyl choline (ePC), and sphingomyelin (SM), but not in PC, PE, phosphatidyl inositol (PI), or ether phosphatidyl ethanolamine (ePE). PA is a precursor to multiple membrane lipids, while PG is a precursor to cardiolipins. Surprisingly, including DHA in the WD significantly lowered the CSI (by 20%) in only one lipid class, ePC. Yet, a detailed examination of all lipid species within each lipid class revealed assimilation of DHA and its metabolites (20:5, ω3; 22:5, ω3) in all lipid classes, except SM (Table S1: diet effects on all lipids). While the WD significantly increased the CSI as a result of increased dietary SFA and MUFA content, DHA and its metabolites had little impact on the overall CSI of most lipid classes.

We next used a statistical approach to establish differences between treatment groups. Accordingly, all lipid data from the UPLC-MS/MS and HPLC-dMRM analysis plus our previous GC analysis [52] was subject to a principal component analysis (PCA) (Figure 3). While four groups were included in our study, the PCA revealed only three clusters. Two clusters (WD22 and WDO30) overlapped indicating that these groups differed little in terms of lipid composition. The lipid composition of the WD22 and WDO30 groups clearly differed from the reference diet group (RD30). Interestingly, the WDD30 group does not overlap with either the RD30 or WD22 and WD30 clusters, reflecting its unique lipid composition. This outcome indicates that 8 wks of DHA treatment does not restore hepatic membrane lipid acyl chain composition to that seen in the RD30 group.

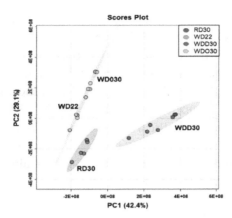

Figure 3. Principal component analysis of diet effects on hepatic lipids. All lipid data collected for this study and our previous study [52] was used in this analysis. The data included fatty acid methyl esters reported previously [52] and all membrane lipid and oxylipin data obtained by UPLC-MS/MS and HPLC-dMRM analysis, respectively. The principal component analysis was carried out using the statistical package in Metabolanalyst 4.0 [66].

Further analysis identified the top 25 highly significant differences ($q \leq 3.0 \times 10^{-7}$) in lipid composition amongst the four groups (Figure 4 and Table S2: Lipids significantly affected by diet). A key result of this analysis was that the WD increased 20:4, ω6 and its metabolites in multiple membrane lipids (PC 38:4, PG 42.8; PE 40:5, lyso PC 20:3; lyso PC 22:4; lyso PE 20:3), but lowered oxylipins derived from linoleic acid (18:2, ω6), i.e., 12,13-DiHOME. This finding replicates our previous results documenting the effects of the WD on hepatic lipids derived from WD-fed female *Ldlr* $^{-/-}$ mice [60].

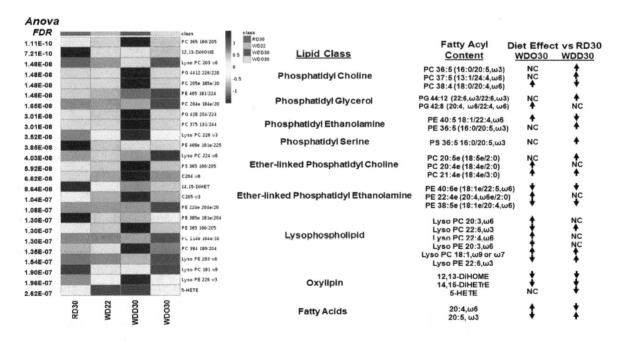

Figure 4. Heat map illustrating diet effects on the top 25 lipid features. As in Figure 3 all lipid data was used to perform an ANOVA (one-way) and a heat map was constructed using the statistical package in Metabolanalyst features [66]. The top 25 highly significant lipid features are illustrated in the heat map. The *q*-value for each lipid is on the left side of the heat map. Columns at the right list specific lipids within each lipid class that were on the heat map. Arrows indicate the effect of the diet WDO30 and WDD30 when compared to the RD30 group (increase, decrease, no change (NC)) (WD supplemented with either olive oil (WDO) or DHASCO (WDD)).

Addition of DHA to the WD not only increased the abundance of DHA and its metabolites in hepatic phospholipids (PC 36:5, PG 44:12, PS 36.5, lyso PC 22:6, lyso PE 22:6), but also decreased levels of specific membrane lipids containing 20:4,ω6 and its metabolites (PC 38:4, PE 40:5, PE 38.5). Such effects of dietary ω3 PUFA on membrane lipid composition are not new. What is new, however, is the impact of WD and DHA on a broad range of hepatic lipids, including phosphoglycerol lipids (PC, PE, PG, PI, PS), ether lipids (ePC, ePE), lysophospholipids (lyso-PC, -PE, -PI, -PS), and sphingolipids. The sphingolipids were the only lipid class significantly affected by WD and DHA, but found to contain no C_{20-22} PUFA (both ω3 and ω6) (Table S1: Diet effects on all lipids). As such, DHA mediated effects on SM acyl chain content likely involves DHA regulation of hepatic abundance of SFA and MUFA, as well as the incorporation of these fatty acyls into SM.

2.2. Diet Effects on Hepatic Non-Esterified Oxylipins

Intrahepatic non-esterified oxylipins arise from phospholipase-mediated excision of fatty acyls from membrane lipids. These non-esterified fatty acids serve as substrates for cell-specific pathways generating oxylipins that, in turn, serve as regulatory ligands for G-protein receptors (GPR) and nuclear receptors [61,66]. Herein, we examined the effect of the WD and DHA on hepatic oxylipins derived from LA, ARA, EPA, and DHA (Figures 5 and 6) and the expression of enzymes involved in oxylipin metabolism (Figure 7); results are summarized in Figure 8.

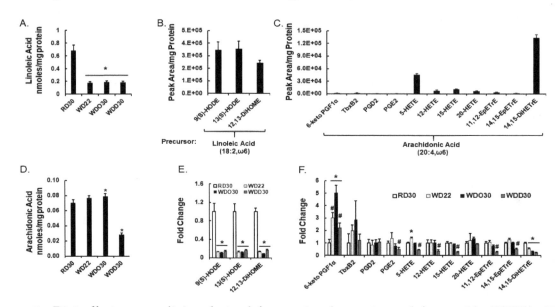

Figure 5. Diet effects on oxylipins derived from ω6 polyunsaturated fatty acids (PUFA). (**A,D**): Hepatic content of linoleic acid (LA; 18:2, ω6) and arachidonic acid (ARA; 20:4, ω6) as determined by gas chromatographic (GC) analysis. Results are presented as nmoles/mg protein, mean ± SEM. Oxylipins derived from LA (**B**) and ARA (**C**) were quantified, by HPLC-dMRM as described in the Materials and Methods Section. Liver samples were derived from the RD group and oxylipin levels are presented as the peak area/mg protein, mean ± SEM. Effects of diet on specific oxylipins are presented in (Panels E,F) as Fold Change, mean ± SEM. (Panels **E,F**) present LA- and ARA-derived oxylipins, respectively. *, $q < 0.05$ vs. RD30; #, $q < 0.05$ vs. WDO30. 9(S)-HODE, 9(S) hydroxyl octadecadienoic acid; 13(S)-HODE, 13(S) hydroxyl octadecadienoic acid; 12,13-DiHOME, 12,13-dihydroxy octadecenoic acid; 6-keto PGF1α, 6-keto prostaglandin F1α; TbxB2, thromboxane B2; PGD2, prostaglandin D2; PGE2, prostaglandin E2, 5-HETE, 5-hydroxyeicosatrienoic acid; 12-HETE, 12-hydroxyeicosatrienoic acid; 15-HETE, 15-hydroxyeicosatrienoic acid; 20-HETE, 20-hydroxyeicosatrienoic acid; 11,12-EpETrE, 11,12 epoxyeicosatrienoic acid; 14,15-EpETrE, 14,15 epoxyeicosatrienoic acid; 14,15-diHETrE, 14,15-dihydroxyeicosatrienoic acid.

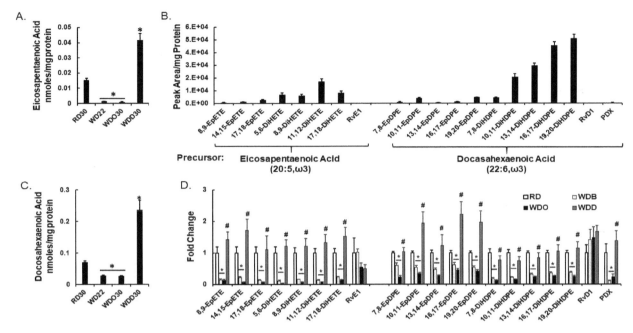

Figure 6. Diet effects on oxylipins derived from ω3 PUFA. Hepatic content of eicosapentaenoic acid (EPA; 20:5, ω3) (Panel **A**) and docosahexaenoic (DHA; 22:6, ω3) (Panel **C**). Hepatic EPA and DHA were quantified as described in the Materials and Methods Section and presented as the mean ± SEM of nmoles/mg hepatic protein.   (Panels **B,D**): Effects of diet on EPA and DHA derived oxylipins, respectively.   Results are presented as Peak area/mg protein (Panel **B**) and Fold Change, mean ± SEM (Panel **D**). *, $q < 0.05$ vs. RD30; #, $q < 0.05$ vs. WDO30. 8,9-EpETE, 8,9-epoxyeicosatetraenoic acid; 14,15-EpETE, 14,15-epoxyeicosatetraenoic acid; 17,18-EpETE, 17,18-epoxyeicosatetraenoic acid; 5,6-DiHETE, 5,6-dihydroxyeicosatetraenoic acid; 8,9-DiHETE, 8,9-dihydroxyeicosatetraenoic acid; 11,12-DiHETE, 11,12-dihydroxyeicosatetraenoic acid; 17,18-DiHETE, 17,18-dihydroxyeicosatetraenoic acid; RvE1, resolvin E1; 7,8-EpDPE, 7,8-epoxydocosapentaenoic acid; 10,11-EpDPE, 10,11-epoxydocosapentaenoic acid; 13,14-EpDPE, 13,14-epoxydocosapentaenoic acid; 16,17-EpDPE, 16,17-epoxydocosapentaenoic acid; 19,20-EpDPE, 19,20-epoxydocosapentaenoic acid; 7,8-DiHDPE, 7,8-dihydroxydocosapentaenoic acid; 10,11-DiHDPE, 10,11-dihydroxydocosapentaenoic acid; 13,14-DiHDPE, 13,14-dihydroxydocosapentaenoic acid; 16,17-DiHDPE, 16,17-dihydroxydocosapentaenoic acid; 19,20-DiHDPE, 19,20-dihydroxydocosapentaenoic acid; RvD1, resolvin D1; PDX, protectin DX.

We previously reported that feeding female *Ldlr*⁻/⁻ mice fed the WD decreased hepatic oxylipins derived from linoleic acid (LA, 18:2, ω6), but increased hepatic oxylipins derived from arachidonic acid (ARA, 20:4, ω6) [60]. As illustrated in Figure 5, the WD and WDO diets had similar effects on hepatic oxylipins in male *Ldlr*⁻/⁻ mice as seen in female mice [60]. Our oxylipin analysis identified 14 ω6 PUFA-derived oxylipins; three from LA and 11 from ARA (Figure 5). Three oxylipins, 12,13-DiHOME; 14,15-DiHETE; and 5-HETE ranked in the top 25 highly significantly lipids affected by the WD (Figure 4). The dihydroxy fatty acid, 12,13-DiHOME, is one of three LA-derived oxylipins, and 14,15-DiHETE is one of eleven ARA-derived oxylipins identified in our analysis (Figures 5 and 8). These dihydroxy oxylipins are generated by the action of a soluble epoxide hydrolase (Ephx2) action on epoxy fatty acids, i.e., 12,13-EpHOME and 14,15-EpETrE, respectively. The LA and ARA derived epoxides are generated by hepatic epoxygenases (Cyp2C; Cyp2J). Highly abundant ω6 PUFA-derived oxylipins include 9(S)-HODE, 13(S)HODE, 12,13-DiHOME, 5-HETE, and 12,15-DiHETrE, while low abundance oxylipins include 6-keto PGF1α, TBXB2, PGD2, PGE2, and HETEs (12-, 15-, 20-HETE) and 14,15-EpETrE. WD or WDO feeding increased hepatic ARA and significantly increased 6-keto PGF1α and TBX2B, but had little effect on other 20:4, ω6 derived oxylipins (Figure 5C,D).

We identified eight and 12 oxylipins derived from EPA and DHA, respectively, in male mice fed the RD, i.e., RD30 group (Figures 6 and 8). Feeding female *Ldlr*⁻/⁻ mice the WD lowered hepatic levels of all ω3 PUFA-derived oxylipins [60]. Male *Ldlr* $^{-/-}$ mice fed the WD or WDO resulted in significantly lower levels of all hepatic ω3-PUFA-derived oxylipins (Figure 6). The decline in these oxylipins paralleled the WD-mediated decline in hepatic EPA and DHA (Figure 6A,C).

Supplementing the WD with DHA, i.e., WDD30 group, had no effect on hepatic LA or LA-derived oxylipin abundance. The WDD, however, significantly lowered hepatic ARA and all ARA-derived oxylipins, except PGD2 and 20-HETE (Figure 5D,F). The decline in hepatic 20:4, ω6-derived oxylipins paralleled the DHA-mediated suppression of hepatic 20:4, ω6 content (Figure 5D). Clearly, the WD has a potent effect on hepatic oxylipin type and abundance. Supplementing the WD with DHA had an equally potent effect on hepatic ω3 PUFA-derived oxylipins by reversing the WD effect on ARA-derived and C$_{20-22}$ ω3 PUFA-derived oxylipins.

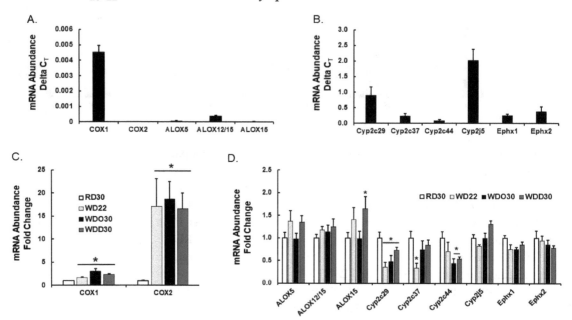

Figure 7. Diet effects on hepatic enzymes involved in oxylipin metabolism. Hepatic RNA was extracted, converted to cDNA and used to quantify transcript abundance using qRTPCR as previously described [52]. The primers used to measure each transcript were previously described [51,60]. Cyclophilin was used as the reference gene. (Top panels **A,B**): Relative abundance of transcripts encoding enzymes involved in hepatic oxylipin metabolism. Results are presented as delta C_T, mean ± SEM. (Lower panels **C,D**): Diet effects on hepatic transcripts encoding enzymes involved in oxylipin metabolism. Results are presented as Fold Change, mean ± SEM; *, $q < 0.05$ vs. RD30. COX, cyclooxygenase; ALOX, arachidonic lipoxygenase; CYP, cytochrome P450, Ephx1, microsomal epoxide hydrolase; Ephx2, soluble epoxide hydrolase.

We next examined the diet effects on hepatic enzymes involved in generating hepatic oxylipins (Figure 7). Cyclooxygenases (Cox1, Cox2) and arachidonic acid lipoxygenases (Alox5, Alox12/15, Alox15) are expressed at low levels in mouse liver (Figure 7A), whereas enzymes generating fatty epoxides (Cyp2C29, Cyp2C37, Cyp2C44, Cyp2J5) and dihydroxy fatty acids (Ephx1, Ephx2) are highly expressed in liver (Figure 7B). The differential expression of these enzymes likely reflects cell specific expression in the liver. For example, Cox1 and Cox2 are expressed in liver, but not in hepatic parenchymal cells, i.e., hepatocytes. These enzymes are likely expressed in resident macrophage (Kupffer cells) and infiltrating leukocytes. Hepatocytes, however, express receptors for Cox products, e.g., EP4, and respond to changes in oxylipins through paracrine mechanisms [67].

Feeding mice the WD and WDO resulted in the induction of both Cox1 and Cox2, but the WD and WDO diets had no significant effects on the Alox subtypes (5-, 12/15-, 15-Alox) (Figure 7). Supplementing the WD with DHA did not attenuate Cox1 or Cox 2 expression. If Cox 1 and Cox 2 expression parallels Cox 1 and 2 activity, then the decline in Cox-products, e.g., prostacyclin (PGI2, precursor of 6-keto PGF1α), PGE2, and thromboxane A2 (precursor of TBXB2) cannot be explained by a suppression of enzyme expression. As such, our data suggest that the DHA-mediated decline in Cox products may be due, at least in part, to the DHA-mediated suppression of hepatic ARA levels, particularly in membrane lipids (Figures 4 and 5). Cyp2c29, Cyp2c37 and Cyp2c44 expression was suppressed ~50% by the WD. Only Cyp2c29 expression was partially restored by the addition of DHA to the diet. Neither WDO nor WDD affected the expression of Cyp2J or Ephx subtypes.

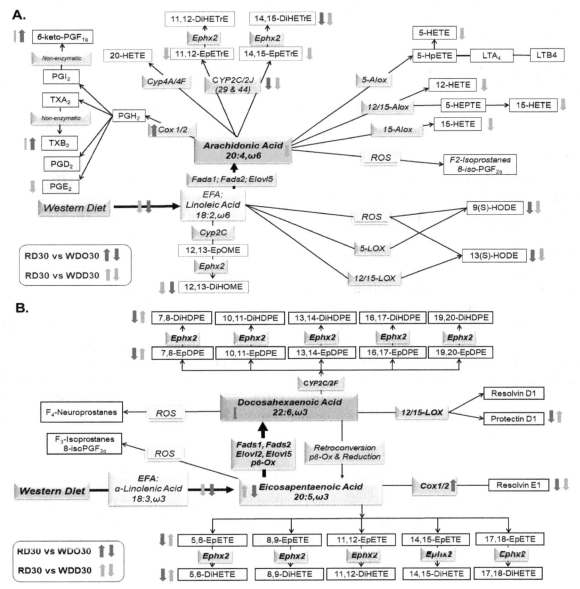

Figure 8. Summary of WD and DHA effects on hepatic oxylipins derived from ω6 PUFA (**A**) and ω3 PUFA (**B**). The diagrams illustrate the pathway for the conversion of dietary essential fatty acids to C_{18-22} PUFA and the conversion of PUFA to oxylipins. The pathways are modified from pathways published by Gabbs et al. [61]. Oxylipins highlighted in blue represent oxylipins that were quantified by LC/MS or gas chromatography (Figures 5 and 6). Enzymes involved in oxylipin metabolism are in gray boxes (Figure 7). Red and green arrows are used to represent the effects (increase; decrease) of the WDO versus RD30 (red arrows) and WDD30 versus RD30 (green arrows) on hepatic abundance of fatty acids, oxylipins, and transcripts involved in PUFA and oxylipins metabolism. Thin and thick arrows represent a weak and strong response to diet, respectively. EFA: essential fatty acids; ROS, reactive oxygen species. *Fads*, fatty acid desaturase; *Elovl*, fatty acid elongase; pβOx, peroxisomal β-oxidation; COX, cyclooxygenase; *ALOX*, arachidonic lipoxygenase; CYP, cytochrome P450, *Ephx1*, microsomal epoxide hydrolase; *Ephx2*, soluble epoxide hydrolase.

2.3. Associations between Hepatic Lipids and NASH Markers of Inflammation and Fibrosis

We previously reported that the WD promoted hepatic inflammation and fibrosis, while addition of DHA to the WD blocked disease progression by attenuating expression of inflammation and fibrosis markers [52]. Herein, we asked if changes in specific transcriptomic markers of inflammation and fibrosis were associated with changes in membrane lipids and oxylipins. Accordingly, we used an unbiased statistical approach, i.e., Pattern Hunter in Metabolanalyst 4.0 [66], to identify associations between diet-induced changes in membrane lipids, oxylipins, and NASH pathology, i.e., inflammation and fibrosis (Tables 1 and 2). The transcriptomic data for this analysis was from our previous study [52], the same study used for the current lipidomic analysis. Results are presented as the top 10 positive and negative associations between specific lipids and markers of inflammation (Table 1: osteopontin (*Opn*), monocyte chemoattractant protein 1 (*Mcp1*), cell differentiation 68 (*CD68*)) and fibrosis (Table 2: collagen 1A1 (*Col1A2*), tissue inhibitor metalloprotease 1 (*Timp1*) and lysyl oxidase (*Lox*)).

2.3.1. Inflammation

Lipids positively associated with *Opn* expression include phosphatidyl glycerol (PG) containing MUFA and PUFA ($\omega 6 > \omega 3$) while 50% of the lipids negatively associated with *Opn* expression were $\omega 3$ PUFA-derived oxylipins (Table 1). In contrast, lipids positively associated with *Mcp1* and *CD68* include no PG, but several ether lipids (e.g., PC 16:0e; PC 18:1e) containing predominantly MUFA and short and long chain SFAs. Lipids negatively associated with *Mcp1* and *CD68* expression include oxylipins (12,13-DiHOME, 14,15-DiHETrE) and membrane phospholipids (PA, PE, PI) containing C_{18-22} $\omega 3$ and $\omega 6$ PUFA. These association studies indicate that elevated expression of inflammation markers was associated with increased membrane abundance of C_{18-20} MUFA and C_{20-22} $\omega 6$ PUFA, while attenuated expression of these markers was associated with increased membrane content of C_{18-22} $\omega 3$ and $\omega 6$ PUFA and hepatic levels of $\omega 3$ and $\omega 6$ PUFA derived oxylipins. The epoxygenase and epoxide hydrolase pathways (Cyp2C, Cyp2J and Ephx2) rather than the Cox/Alox and oxidative stress pathways generate the majority of these oxylipins. In addition, lipids associated (positively and negatively) with *Opn* expression are clearly distinct from the lipids associated with *Mcp1* and *CD68* expression, suggesting different membrane-associated mechanisms involved in the expression of these inflammation markers.

2.3.2. Fibrosis

Lipids positively and negatively associated with the expression of *Col1A2* and *Timp1* are nearly identical; and include membrane lipids (lyso PA, lyso PE, lyso PC, SM) containing C_{14-16} SFA, C_{18} MUFA, and C_{18-22} $\omega 6$ PUFA, but no $\omega 3$ PUFA. Lipids negatively associated with *Col1A2* and *Timp1* expression include DHA derived oxylipins (7, 8-DiHDPE; 10, 11-DiHDPE) and membrane lipids (PA, PC, PE, PI) containing C_{16-22} MUFA and C_{18-20} $\omega 6$ PUFA. Interestingly, lipids positively and negatively associated with Lox expression are remarkably similar to those associated with *Opn* expression. PG containing MUFA and C_{20-22} $\omega 6$ PUFA are positively associated with *Lox* expression, while 60% of the lipids negatively associated with Lox expression are oxylipins derived from ARA and EPA. This outcome may reflect common membrane-associated mechanisms associated with *Lox* and *Opn* expression.

Table 1. Top 10 hepatic lipids positively and negatively associated with hepatic gene expression markers of inflammation [1].

Gene	Opn			Mcp1			CD68		
Association	Lipid	CC[2]	q-Value[3]	Lipid	CC	q-Value	Lipid	CC	q-Value
Positive	PG 38:4 18:1/20:3,ω6	0.74	5.9×10^{-4}	Lyso PC 18:1	0.86	8.6×10^{-6}	Lyso PC 18:1	0.78	5.3×10^{-4}
Positive	Lyso PC 22:4,ω6	0.74	6.4×10^{-4}	PC 17:0e 14:0e/3:0	0.85	1.3×10^{-5}	SM d36:2 d14:0/22:2	0.78	5.4×10^{-4}
Positive	Lyso PE 22:4,ω6	0.74	6.6×10^{-4}	PC 16:0e 14:0e/2:0	0.84	2.3×10^{-5}	Lyso PC 20:3,ω6	0.77	6.4×10^{-4}
Positive	PG 36:4 16:0/20:4,ω6	0.73	8.4×10^{-4}	SM d35:1 d14:0/21:1	0.82	3.8×10^{-5}	PS 42:3 26:0/16:3	0.76	6.9×10^{-4}
Positive	PG 38:5 18:1/20:4,ω6	0.72	9.9×10^{-4}	PA 36:2 18:1/18:1	0.82	4.3×10^{-5}	PC 17:0e 14:0e/3:0	0.76	7.7×10^{-4}
Positive	20:1,ω9	0.72	1.1×10^{-3}	PC 21:3e 18:3e/3:0	0.81	6.6×10^{-5}	PC 21:3e 18:3e/3:0	0.74	1.0×10^{-3}
Positive	PG 38:2 18:1/20:1	0.71	1.2×10^{-3}	PC 18:1e 16:1e/2:0	0.81	6.7×10^{-5}	SM d34:0 d14:0/20:0	0.74	1.1×10^{-3}
Positive	PG 36:2 18:1/18:1	0.71	1.3×10^{-3}	PE 20:1e 14:1e/6:0	0.80	7.8×10^{-5}	PC 18:1e 16:1e/2:0	0.72	1.4×10^{-3}
Positive	PG 42:9 20:3,ω6/22:6,ω3	0.71	1.3×10^{-3}	PC 19:1e 14:1e/5:0	0.80	8.6×10^{-5}	PC 16:0e 14:0e/2:0	0.72	1.4×10^{-3}
Positive	Lyso PE 20:3,ω6	0.70	1.4×10^{-3}	SM d34:1 d14:0/20:1	0.80	9.2×10^{-5}	PE 20:1e 14:1e/6:0	0.72	1.6×10^{-3}
Negative	PA 34:3 16:1,ω7/18:2,ω6	-0.69	1.9×10^{-3}	12,13-DiHOME	-0.78	1.3×10^{-4}	PI 36:2 18:1/18:1	-0.77	6.4×10^{-4}
Negative	7,8-DiHDPE	-0.62	6.9×10^{-3}	18:3,ω3	-0.76	2.9×10^{-4}	PE 34:2 16:0/18:2,ω6	-0.76	6.9×10^{-4}
Negative	13,14-DiHDPE	-0.62	6.9×10^{-3}	PI 36:2 18:1/18:1	-0.76	2.9×10^{-4}	PI 36:4 16:0/20:4,ω6	-0.76	7.7×10^{-4}
Negative	7,8-EpDPE	-0.62	6.9×10^{-3}	PE 40:6e 18:1e/22:5,ω3	-0.74	4.9×10^{-4}	PI 36:3 16:0/20:3,ω6	-0.74	1.0×10^{-3}
Negative	PE 34:2 16:0/18:2,ω6	-0.62	7.2×10^{-3}	PI 36:4 16:0/20:4,ω6	-0.73	6.0×10^{-4}	PE 34:3e 16:1e/18:2,ω3	-0.74	1.2×10^{-3}
Negative	10,11-DiHDPE	-0.62	7.2×10^{-3}	PE 34:2 16:0/18:2,ω6	-0.73	6.2×10^{-4}	12,13-DiHOME	-0.73	1.4×10^{-3}
Negative	Lyso PE 18:2,ω6	-0.62	7.4×10^{-3}	18:2,ω6	-0.73	6.3×10^{-4}	PE 36:2 18:0/18:2,ω6	-0.72	1.4×10^{-3}
Negative	PI 36:3 16:0/20:3,ω6	-0.61	8.9×10^{-3}	PA 34:3 16:1,ω7/18:2,ω6	-0.72	6.8×10^{-4}	PE 36:2 18:1/18:1	-0.72	1.5×10^{-3}
Negative	PC 35:2 13:1/22:1	-0.59	1.1×10^{-2}	14,15-DiHETrE	-0.72	6.9×10^{-4}	PE 40:6e 18:1e/22:5,ω3	-0.71	1.8×10^{-3}
Negative	5,6-DiHETE	-0.59	1.1×10^{-2}	13(S)-HODE	-0.71	1.1×10^{-3}	18:3,ω3	-0.71	1.8×10^{-3}

[1] Associations between NASH inflammation markers and lipids were determined using the statistical package "Pattern Hunter in Metabolanalyst [66]. [2] CC, correlation coefficient; [3] q-value, see Statistical Analysis, Materials and methods.

Table 2. Associations between hepatic gene expression markers of fibrosis and lipids [1].

GENE	Col1A2			Timp1			Lox		
Association	Lipid	CC[2]	q-Value[3]	Lipid	CC	q-Value	Lipid	CC	q-Value
Positive	20:1,ω9	0.81	4.2×10^{-5}	20:1,ω9	0.81	5.6×10^{-5}	Lyso PC 22:4,ω6	0.84	1.2×10^{-5}
Positive	18:1,ω9	0.81	4.9×10^{-5}	18:1,ω7	0.80	9.0×10^{-5}	PC 38:4 18:1/20:3,ω6	0.82	2.9×10^{-5}
Positive	18:1,ω7	0.80	6.4×10^{-5}	18:1,ω9	0.79	1.1×10^{-4}	Lyso PE 22:4,ω6	0.80	5.3×10^{-5}
Positive	Lyso PC 20:3,ω6	0.74	5.3×10^{-4}	Lyso PC 20:3,ω6	0.74	6.7×10^{-4}	PG 38:4 18:1/20:3,ω6	0.80	5.6×10^{-5}
Positive	Lyso PE 20:3,ω6	0.73	6.7×10^{-4}	16:0	0.73	8.1×10^{-4}	PG 38:5 18:1/20:4,ω6	0.79	7.0×10^{-5}
Positive	PC 38:4 18:1/20:3,ω6	0.72	1.1×10^{-3}	Lyso PE 20:3, ω6	0.72	9.7×10^{-4}	PG 38:1 20:0/18:1	0.79	7.0×10^{-5}
Positive	Lyso PC 18:1,ω9	0.71	1.2×10^{-3}	PC 38:4 18:1/20:3,ω6	0.71	1.3×10^{-3}	PG 40:6 18:1/22:5,ω6	0.78	1.1×10^{-4}
Positive	SM d35:1 d14:0/21:1	0.71	1.2×10^{-3}	PC 21:3e 18:3e/3:0	0.71	1.3×10^{-3}	PG 38:2 18:1/20:1	0.78	1.1×10^{-4}
Positive	SM d36:2 d14:0/22:2	0.70	1.4×10^{-3}	Lyso PC 18:1,ω9	0.71	1.3×10^{-3}	PG 40:5 18:1/22:4,ω6	0.78	1.1×10^{-4}
Positive	PA 36:2 18:1/18:1	0.70	1.4×10^{-3}	SM d36:2 d14:0/22:2	0.69	2.2×10^{-3}	PG 36:2 18:1/18:1	0.77	1.5×10^{-4}
Negative	PA 34:3 16:1,ω7/18:2,ω6	-0.77	1.9×10^{-4}	PA 34:3 16:1,ω7/18:2,ω6	-0.75	4.8×10^{-4}	Lyso PE 18:2,ω6	-0.57	1.3×10^{-2}
Negative	PE 34:2 16:0/18:2,ω6	-0.75	3.7×10^{-4}	PE 34:2 16:0/18:2,ω6	0.73	7.1×10^{-4}	8,9-DiHETE	-0.56	1.5×10^{-2}
Negative	PI 36:3 16:0/20:3,ω6	-0.73	7.2×10^{-4}	PI 36:3 16:0/20:3,ω6	-0.71	1.2×10^{-3}	11,12-DiHETE	-0.56	1.5×10^{-2}
Negative	PI 36:2 18:1/18:1	-0.72	8.7×10^{-4}	PI 36:2 18:1/18:1	-0.71	1.3×10^{-3}	8,9-EpETE	-0.56	1.5×10^{-2}
Negative	PC 35:2 13:1/22:1	-0.71	1.1×10^{-3}	PI 36:4 16:0/20:4,ω6	-0.69	1.9×10^{-3}	14,15-EpETE	-0.56	1.7×10^{-2}
Negative	PI 36:4 16:0/20:4,ω6	-0.71	1.1×10^{-3}	PC 35:2 13:1/22:1	-0.69	2.0×10^{-3}	17,18-DiHETE	-0.54	2.0×10^{-2}
Negative	PE 36:2 18:1/18:1	-0.70	1.5×10^{-3}	PE 36:2 18:1/18:1	-0.69	2.2×10^{-3}	20:5,ω3	-0.54	2.2×10^{-2}
Negative	PE 36:2 18:0/18:2,ω6	-0.68	2.4×10^{-3}	PE 36:2 18:0/18:2,ω6	-0.66	3.7×10^{-3}	PI 36:4 16:0/20:4,ω6	-0.53	2.3×10^{-2}
Negative	PA 34:2 16:0/18:2,ω6	-0.66	3.5×10^{-3}	10,11-DiHDPE	-0.65	4.3×10^{-3}	PS 40:6 18:0/22:6,ω3	-0.53	2.3×10^{-2}
Negative	7,8-DiHDPE	-0.66	3.8×10^{-3}	PE 34:3e 16:1,ω7e/18:2,ω6	-0.65	4.4×10^{-3}	10,11-EpDPE	-0.52	2.6×10^{-2}

[1] Associations between NASH inflammation markers and lipids were determined using the statistical package "Pattern Hunter in Metabolanalyst [66]. [2] CC, correlation coefficient; [3] q-value, see Statistical Analysis, Materials and methods.

3. Discussion

The aim of this study was to use a lipidomic approach to identify potential lipid mediators of inflammation and fibrosis associated with WD-induced NASH and DHA-mediated NASH remission. Accordingly, we identified and quantified hepatic membrane lipids and non-esterified oxylipins in a preclinical mouse model of NASH. Feeding mice the WD significantly increased the saturation index of many, but not all membrane lipids (Figure 2). The WD increased SFA and MUFA in several membrane lipids, i.e., PA, PG, lyso PC, lyso PE, lyso PI, lyso PS, ePC, and SM. Surprisingly, addition of DHA to the WD had little effect on the membrane saturation index, despite the fact that DHA and its metabolites were assimilated into all lipid classes, except SM (Table S1). We suspect the assimilation of DHA and its metabolites into membranes has local effects on membrane fluidity, lipid raft composition, and membrane cholesterol content that potentially affects receptor-mediated mechanisms emanating from membranes [58,59].

On a more granular level, we identified strong associations between diet-induced changes in hepatic membrane lipid composition, membrane derived signaling molecules, and the expression of genes linked to WD-induced hepatic inflammation and fibrosis (Tables 1 and 2). We identified two membrane derived lipid classes that are known to play a role in cell signaling, i.e., lysophospholipids (Lyso PL) and oxylipins. Lyso PLs form in the process in *de novo* membrane lipid synthesis (Kennedy Pathway) and membrane lipid remodeling (Lands Pathway). Our untargeted lipidomic analysis cannot distinguish between these pathways, nor can it distinguish between acyl chains in the sn1 or sn2 positions of the lyso PLs. Dietary fat content clearly affected the acyl chain composition of these lyso PLs (Figure 4). Oxylipin precursors, i.e., non-esterified fatty acids (NEFA), are generated as a result of membrane remodeling and involves phospholipase activation. NEFA excised from membranes are substrates for several enzymatic pathways that are active in the liver, including cyclooxygenases (Cox (-1 and -2), arachidonate lipoxygenases (Alox (-5, -12/15, -15)), cytochrome P450 class 2 ((Cyp2 (C and J)), and epoxide hydrolases (Ephx 1 and 2) (Figure 8).

Lyso PLs and oxylipins functioning as ligands have the potential to regulated cell function through multiple receptor-mediated mechanisms. Both bioactive lipids regulate cell function through G-protein receptors (GPR) and nuclear receptors. Lyso PLs signal through GPR23, GPR34, GPR44, GPR92, GPR93, and GPR174, while oxylipins signal through GPR for eicosanoids (prostaglandins (PGE2), thromboxanes (TBXA2), and prostacyclins (PGI2)). Lyso PLs and oxylipins also signal through nuclear receptors, e.g., PPARα, β/δ, γ1, γ2) [68–75]. Our studies clearly establish that both the WD and DHA have major effects on membrane lipid composition and the type and abundance of hepatic lyso PLs and oxylipins derived from PUFA (Figures 4–8).

We took advantage of our transcriptomic data [52] to identify associations between membrane lipids, oxylipins, and markers of inflammation and fibrosis, key markers of NASH (Tables 1 and 2). Hepatic levels of lyso PC and lyso PE containing C_{20-22} ω6 PUFA were positively associated with the expression of inflammation (Opn, CD68) and fibrosis (Col1A2, Timp1, LOX) markers (Tables 1 and 2). As such, changes in the hepatic abundance of lyso PL enriched in C_{20-22} ω6 PUFA, acting through membrane GPR and/or nuclear receptors, may contribute to hepatic pathology. Key enzymes involved in lyso PL metabolism include phospholipases (PLA, multiple subtypes) and lysophosphatidyl choline acyl transferases (LpCAT; 4 subtypes). We previously established that hepatic phospholipase (PLA2g6) and LpCAT1 and LpCAT2 were induced by the WD, while DHA, but not EPA, suppressed LpCAT 1 and 2 expression [50]. Thus, DHA has the potential to regulate cellular levels of LpCAT-derived ligands controlling specific G-protein (GPRs) and nuclear receptors.

Oxylipins represent the second group of regulatory lipids examined in this study (Figures 5–8). Prostaglandins and leukotrienes are well-studied oxidation products of PUFA that are generated by cyclooxygenases (Cox) and lipoxygenases (Alox), respectively. The products of these enzymes are short-lived oxidized lipids that bind to and activated G-protein receptors (GPRs) that induce changes in intracellular second messengers, i.e., cAMP and calcium, affecting multiple signaling pathways [76]. These active products are rapidly degraded to relatively inactive compounds. Because of the short-lived nature of these active products, the inactive compounds are quantified as surrogates for in vivo synthesis of the bioactive Cox/Alox products [76]. Two 20:4, ω6-derived oxylipins identified in our analysis include 6-keto-PGF1α and TXB2; these are degradation products of PGI2 and TXA2, respectively. PGI2 and TXA2 are involved in platelet aggregation, vasodilation, and inflammation, while PGD2 and PGE2 are involved in inflammation and vasodilation [61]. Increased hepatic levels of these products are associated with the induction of expression of Cox1 and Cox2 mRNAs in response to the WD (Figure 7). Dietary DHA, however, lowers hepatic TBX2, 6-keto-PGF1α, and PGE2. This response parallels DHA-mediated suppression of hepatic ARA levels, as opposed to DHA-mediated suppression of Cox1 and Cox2 expression (Figures 5 and 7). Alox products (5 HETE, 12-HETE and 15-HETE) are also lower in livers of WDD-fed mice. Like the Cox products, hepatic levels of Alox products paralleled changes in hepatic ARA.

Other ω6 PUFA derived oxylipins include 9(S)-HODE and 13(S)-HODE, both of which are derived from linoleic acid by enzymatic (Alox) and non-enzymatic (oxidative stress) pathways. These products affect ER-stress, apoptosis, inflammation, cellular adhesions, and PPARγ function [77]. Since there was little effect of diet on hepatic Alox5, Alox12/15, or Alox15 expression, hepatic oxidative stress likely accounts for the increased hepatic levels of 9(S)-HODE and 13(S)-HODE in response to the WD [50]. The decline in these oxylipins parallel the WD-mediated suppression of hepatic LA content (Figure 5A). Feldstein et al. recently reported increased levels of these oxylipins in NASH patients, when compared to patients with benign steatosis [78]. This finding contrast with our findings and may reflect differences in hepatic oxidative stress management in human versus mouse livers. This group also reported no significant change in 5-HETE, 12-HETE, or 15-HETE in normal, steatotic, or NASH livers of patients. These results are similar to our findings (Figure 5F).

The other class of oxylipins examined included products generated by epoxygenases (Cyp2C, Cyp2J) and a soluble epoxide hydrolase (Ephx2). Like the Cox products, the epoxide products of Cyp2C and CYP2J are bioactive compounds. Moreover, Cyp2C and Cyp2J products are rapidly degraded to dihydroxy fatty acids with low bioactivity [79]. The WD has little effect on the formation of the ARA-derived products, but DHA lowered hepatic levels of the epoxy (11,12-EpETrE; 14,15-EpETrE) and dihydroxy (14,15-DiHETrE) products derived from ARA. Since there was little effect of diet on the expression of the Cyp2C, Cyp2J, and Ephx2 (Figure 7), we attribute the declined in Cyp2C, Cyp2J, and Ephx2 products to DHA-mediated suppression of hepatic ARA content (Figure 5). However, we cannot exclude post-translational mechanisms controlling the activity of these enzymes.

ARA-derived epoxygenase products are anti-inflammatory, pro-resolving bioactive mediators [79]. A decline in the hepatic abundance of these metabolites suggest an increase in hepatic inflammation. However, we previously reported that the WD increased hepatic markers of inflammation while the WD supplemented with DHA suppressed hepatic inflammation [52]. To explain this outcome, our analysis revealed a massive suppression (> 70%) of C_{20-22} ω3 PUFA-derived oxylipins (Figures 7 and 8B) in livers of WDO30 fed mice. In WDD30 fed mice, however, the Cyp2C and Cyp2F-derived ω3-PUFA oxylipins were restored to levels at or above levels seen in mice fed the RD. Changes in C_{20-22} ω3 PUFA-derived oxylipins are inversely associated with transcriptomic markers of hepatic inflammation and fibrosis ($q \leq 0.026$; Tables 1 and 2). The concept of an inverse association between tissue levels of C_{20-22} ω3 PUFA and inflammation is not new [80]. In fact, other investigators using the choline-methionine-deficient rat [81] and mouse [82] models of NAFLD reported a similar inverse association between tissue levels of DHA and liver injury. Our studies extend these observations by showing how specific classes of bioactive lipids are responsive to diet and associated with NASH markers (Figures 4–8; Tables 1 and 2).

The outcome of our lipidomic analysis supports the notion that dietary supplementation with DHA mitigates WD-induced NASH progression, at least in part, by lowering hepatic pro-inflammatory oxylipins derived from C_{20-22} ω6 PUFA and increasing hepatic reparative/anti-inflammatory oxylipins derived from C_{20-22} ω3 PUFA. While there is limited information on the differential bioactivity of ω3 PUFA versus ω6 PUFA-derived Cyp2C and Cyp2J, Lopez-Vicario et al. reported that, when compared to ω6 PUFA-derived epoxides, ω3 PUFA-derived epoxides were more effective inhibitors of inflammation and autophagy in insulin sensitive tissues, like liver [83]. As such, tissue levels of ω3 PUFA-derived epoxides may be a good predictor of liver health status in the context of WD-induced NASH. Key next steps will be to identify mechanisms linking specific ω3 PUFA- and ω6 PUFA-derived oxylipins to the expression of specific genes involved in hepatic inflammation and fibrosis.

4. Materials and Methods

4.1. Study Design for DHA-Mediated NASH Remission in Male Ldlr $^{-/-}$ Mice

This study was carried out in strict accordance with the recommendations in the Guide for the Care and Use of Laboratory Animals of the National Institutes of Health. All procedures for the use and care of animals for laboratory research were approved by the Institutional Animal Care and Use Committee at Oregon State University (Permit Number: A3229-01). Liver samples used in this lipidomic analysis were obtained from our previously published study assessing the capacity to DHA to promote NASH remission [52]. Briefly, male mice (B6;129S7-Ldlr$^{tm1Her/J}$, stock# 002207 purchased from Jackson Labs) were group housed (4 mice/cage) and maintained on a 12 h light/dark cycle. Mice were acclimatized to the Oregon State University (OSU) animal facilities for 2 weeks before proceeding with experiments.

At 10 wks of age, mice were fed a chow (Purina Pico Lab diet 5053) and served as a reference diet (RD) group. The RD group was maintained of the RD for the duration of the study, i.e., 30 wks (RD30, $n = 5$) (Figure 1). Ldlr $^{-/-}$ mice were also fed the western diet (Research Diets, D12079B). The WD consists of 41% energy as fat, 43% energy as carbohydrate, 17% energy as protein, and 0.15% w/w cholesterol [52]. After 22 wks on the WD, a group of WD-fed mice was euthanized for recovery of blood and liver. This group (WD22, $n = 5$) served as a baseline for disease progression. The remainder of the WD-fed mice were switched to a diet supplemented with olive oil or DHASCO. DHASCO is a dietary supplement provided by DSM Nutritional Products; it contains DHA in a triglyceride form. DHA represents ~40% of total acyl chains in DHASCO and DHASCO contains no EPA, DPA (22:5, ω3), ARA, or LA [50]. DHA is present in the diet at 2% total calories (WDD30, $n = 7$). In order to have isocaloric diets, olive oil was added to the WD diet, i.e., WDO30. The WDO30 and WDD30 groups were maintained on their respective diets for 8 wks. Mice were then fasted overnight and euthanized for the collection of liver and blood. All samples were stored at −80 °C until used for extraction. The design of this study allowed for the assessment of disease progression from 22 to 30 weeks and the capacity of DHA to affect disease progression (Figure 1).

4.2. RNA Extraction and qRTPCR

Liver RNA was extracted using Trizol (Ambion by Life Technologies, Carlsbad, CA, USA), quantified, and used for qRTPCR as described previously [52]. Primers use for qRTPCR are described in our previous study [60]. Relative quantitation was determined using the delta C_T methods using cyclophilin as the reference gene. The delta C_T value was used for all statistical analyses.

4.3. Sample Preparation for Lipidomic Analysis

Liver lipids were extracted using a biphasic solvent system of cold methanol, methyl tert-butyl ether (MTBE), and water with some modifications [84]. Liver (~20–25 mg) was transferred to 2 mL pre-weighted polypropylene tubes containing ceramic beads and of LC–MS-grade cold methanol (240 μL). Deuterated lipid recovery standards (5 μL of Splash$^®$ Lipidomix$^®$ Mass Spec Standards (Avanti Polar Lipids, Alabaster, AL, USA) were added to each sample. Samples were homogenized in a Precellys$^®$ 24 bead-based homogenizer for 2 min at 1350 rpm. Cold MTBE (750 μL) was added to the samples, followed by vortexing (10 s) and shaking (6 min) at 4 °C. Phase separation was induced by adding LC–MS-grade water (188 μL) followed vortexing and centrifugation (14,000 rpm, 2 min). The upper organic phase (300 μL) was recovered and evaporated using a Labconco centrivap vacuum concentrator (Kansas City, MO, USA). Dried lipid extracts were resuspended in a methanol/toluene (9:1, v/v, 100 μL) mixture containing CUDA (1-cyclohexyl ureido, 3-dodecanoic acid, 50 ng/mL; Cayman Chemical, Ann Arbor, MI, USA) as an additional internal standard. Samples were vortexed (10 s) and centrifuged (14,000 rpm, 2 min) prior to LC–MS/MS analysis.

4.4. Sample Preparation for Oxylipins Analysis

Oxylipins were extracted from liver using the approach described by Pedersen et al. [85], with minor modifications. Liver (~20–25 mg) was transferred 2 mL pre-weighted polypropylene tubes containing ceramic beads. Cold LC–MS-grade methanol (35 μL) and an anti-oxidant solution [0.2 mg mL^{-1} solution BHT (butylated hydroxytoluene) in 1:1 methanol:water] (5 μL) was added to each sample. Each sample also received 10 μL of a deuterated oxylipin recovery standard solution; the standards included 20 deuterated oxylipins (Table S1) in methanol at a concentration of 5 ng/μL each. Ten mM ammonium formate +1% formic acid in isopropanol (550 μL) and water (100 μL) was added and the tubes were placed in a Precellys® 24 bead-based homogenizer for 2 min at 1350 rpm. Samples were centrifuged (9000 rpm for 5 min) at room temperature. Supernatants were transferred to a 96-well Ostro Pass Through Sample Preparation Plate (Waters Corp, Milford, MA, USA) and eluted into glass inserts containing 10 μL 20% glycerol in methanol by applying a vacuum (15 mm Hg) for 10 min. Eluents were dried by vacuum centrifugation in a Labconco centrivap vacuum concentrator for 2 h at room temperature. Once dry, samples were reconstituted with 100 μL of methanol: acetonitrile (50:50), containing the internal standard (CUDA at 50 ng/mL). Samples were transferred to a spin filter (0.22 μm PVDF membrane, Millipore-Sigma, Burlington, MA, USA) and centrifuged (3 min at 6 °C at 9000 rpm) before transferred to 2 mL amber LC–MS vials. Extracts were stored at −20 °C until analysis by ultra-performance liquid chromatography tandem mass spectrometry (UPLC–MS/MS). The internal oxylipin standards added to the samples (Table S3) were used to correct the recovery of the quantified oxylipins [86].

4.5. Chromatographic and Mass Spectrometry Conditions for Lipids and Oxylipins Analysis

4.5.1. Untargeted Lipidomics

UHPLC was performed using a Shimadzu Nexera system (Shimadzu, Columbia, MD, USA) coupled to a triple time-of-flight (TOF)™ 5600 mass spectrometer (AB SCIEX, Framingham, MA, USA). Compounds were separated using a Waters Acquity UPLC CSH C18 column (100 mm length × 2.1 mm id; 1.7 μm particle size) with an additional Waters Acquity VanGuard CSH C18 pre-column (5 mm × 2.1 mm id; 1.7 μm particle size) held constant at 65 °C while utilizing a flow rate of 0.6 mL min^{-1}. Resuspended samples were injected at 2 μL and 3 μL for electrospray ionization (ESI) positive and negative modes, respectively. To improve lipid coverage, different mobile phase modifiers were used for positive and negative mode analysis [87]. For positive mode, 10 mM ammonium formate + 0.1% formic acid was used, while 10 mM ammonium acetate (Sigma–Aldrich, St. Louis, MO, USA) was used for negative mode. Both positive and negative modes used the same mobile phase composition of (A) 60:40 v/v acetonitrile: water (LC–MS grade) and (B) 90:10 v/v isopropanol:acetonitrile. To enhance solubilization of ammonium formate and ammonium acetate after its addition in the mobile phase, the salts were dissolved first in small volume of water before their addition in the mobile phases (0.631 g ammonium formate or 0.771 g ammonium acetate/1 mL water/1 L mobile phase). Each mobile phase with modifiers was mixed, sonicated for 15 min to achieve complete dissolving of modifiers, mixed again, and then sonicated for another 15 min [88]. The separation was conducted under the following gradient: 0 min 15% (B), 0–2 min 30% (B), 2–2.5 min 48% (B), 2.5–11 min 82% (B), 11–11.5 min 99% (B), 11.5–12 min 99% (B), 12–12.1 min 15% (B), and 12.1–15 min 15% (B), at a flow rate of 0.6 mL min^{-1}. All samples were kept at 4 °C throughout the analysis.

All analyses were performed at the high-resolution mode in MS^1 (~35,000 full width at half maximum (FWHM)) and at the high sensitivity mode (~15,000 FWHM) in MS^2. Sequential window acquisition of all theoretical fragment-ion spectra (SWATH) in positive/negative ion mode was used as the data independent acquisition (DIA) system for all samples. Data dependent acquisition (DDA) on a separate quality control (QC) pool sample was used in order to verify the annotations from SWATH acquisition for the most abundant lipid species. Detailed information of SWATH conditions included in Supplemental Information entitled SWATH parameters for untargeted analysis.

The mass calibration was automatically performed every 6 injections using an APCI positive/negative calibration solution (AB SCIEX) via a calibration delivery system (CDS). Quality control was assured by (i) randomization of the sequence, (ii) injection of QC pool samples at the beginning and the end of the sequence and between each 10 actual samples, (iii) procedure blank analysis, and (iv) checking the peak shape and the intensity of spiked internal standards and the internal standard added prior to injection.

4.5.2. Targeted Oxylipidomics

High Performance Liquid Chromatography (HPLC) was performed using a Shimadzu system (Shimadzu, Columbia, MD, USA) coupled to a QTRAP 4000 (AB SCIEX, Framingham, MA, USA). Employing dynamic multi-reaction monitoring (dMRM) we evaluated 39 oxylipins, 17 deuterated oxylipins, CUDA, and the deuterated surrogates eicosapentaenoic acid-d5 (EPA-d5), docosahexaenoic acid-d5 (DHA-d5), and arachidonic acid-d8 (ARA-d8) in a 22 min LC-run in a targeted approach (Figure S1). For each compound, optimal transitions were determined by flow injection of pure standards using the optimizer application, and transitions were compared to literature values when available for certain compounds. The detailed list of MRM transitions is in Table S4. In the dMRM acquisition mode the triple quadrupole MS system focuses directly on the expected analyte retention time (RT) with a defined detection window instead of user-defined time segments to capture groups of closely eluting compounds. Establishing a constant cycle time for each transition improves peak symmetry and allows for a more accurate quantification of narrow chromatographic peaks. For co-eluting metabolites, compound specific precursor ions and their corresponding fragment ions were used for selective detection and quantification of those compounds. For instance, for 11,12-EpETE (m/z 317→195) and 12-HETE (m/z 319→135), both elute at RT 16.14 min.

Compounds were separated using a Waters Acquity UPLC CSH C18 column (100 mm length × 2.1 mm id; 1.7 μm particle size) with an additional Waters Acquity VanGuard CSH C18 pre-column (5 mm × 2.1 mm id; 1.7 μm particle size) held constant at 60 °C. The mobile phase and gradient elution conditions were adopted from Pedersen and Newman [85]. In summary, the mobile phase consisted of (A) water (0.1% acetic acid) and (B) acetonitrile/isopropanol (ACN/IPA) (90/10, v/v) (0.1% acetic acid). Gradient elution conditions were carried out for 22 min at a flow rate of 0.15 mL min^{-1}. Gradient conditions were: 0–1.0 min, 0.1–25% B; 1.0–2.5 min, 25–40% B; 2.5–4.5 min, 40–42% B; 4.5–10.5 min, 42–50% B; 10.5–12.5 min, 50–65% B; 12.5–14 min, 65–75% B; 14–14.5 min, 75–85% B; 14.5–20 min, 85–95% B; 20–20.5 min, 95–95% B; 20.5–22 min, 95–25% B. A 5 μL aliquot of each sample was injected onto the column. Limits of detection (LOD) and quantification (LOQ) (Table S3) were calculated based on one concentration point (0.1 ng μL^{-1}) for each oxylipin and deuterated surrogate.

4.6. Data Processing

4.6.1. Untargeted Lipidomics

MS-DIAL (v. 2.80) was the software program used for data processing [89]. This open-source software permits processing of LC–MS data acquired either in MS^1 only or with accompanying MS/MS information collected in data-dependent or data-independent mode from different MS platforms. We used LipidBlast [90] for lipid identification. Chromatographic peaks were annotated based on different levels of identification [91]. Peak intensities were normalized using the internal standard CUDA and the QC pool sample to correct for differences in injection volume and platform stability throughout the fully randomized batch of samples. The SPLASH Lipidomics Mix was used for the precise identification of major lipid classes and to perform relative quantitation.

4.6.2. Targeted Analysis of Oxylipins

Oxylipin data obtained by HPLC-dMRM-based analyses was processed using our in-house library on MultiQuant™ software.

4.6.3. Statistical Analyses

Annotated metabolites were used for multivariate statistical analysis. Pathway analysis, principal component analysis (PCA) and heat map plots were generated with MetaboAnalyst 4.0 [66]. The significance of individual metabolites between the treatment groups was assessed with a one-way ANOVA followed by Fisher's post hoc analysis and Holm FDR-correction, with a q-value of <0.05 indicating significance. If needed, data was logarithmically transformed to correct for unequal variance or non-normal distribution. No outliers were excluded from the statistical analyses. Differences in oxylipins among treatments were analyzed in GraphPad Prism 7.03 (La Jolla, CA, USA). Discovery was determined using the two-stage linear step-up procedure of Benjamini et al., [92], with q-value = 5% (cutoff for FDR = 0.05). Each compound was analyzed individually, without assuming a consistent standard deviation. Figures were generated with GraphPad Prism 7.03 (La Jolla, CA), PowerPoint 2018 (Microsoft, Redmond, WA, USA), and MetaboAnalyst 4.0 [66].

Supplementary Materials: Figure S1. LC-MS/MS chromatogram of 60 transitions in a 22 min LC-run allowing monitoring 39 oxylipins, 17 deuterated oxylipins, CUDA, and the deuterated surrogates eicosapentaenoic acid-d5 (EPA-d5), docosahexaenoic acid-d5 (DHA-d5), and arachidonic acid-d8 (ARA-d8). Analysis were performed on a SCIEX linear ion trap (LIT) QTRAP 4000 using the dMRM method implemented from Pedersen et al., [80]. The use of a quadrupole mass spectrometer with a linear ion trap significantly enhances platform performance by increasing ion capacity, improving injection and trapping efficiencies, and increasing duty cycle, Table S1. Diet effects on all lipids, Table S2. Lipids significantly affected by diet, Table S3. Detailed list of multi-reaction monitoring (MRM) transitions for the deuterated-oxylipins (surrogates) and CUDA (12-[[(cyclohexylamino) carbonyl] amino]-dodecanoic acid) used as internal standards for our analysis. Compounds are ordered based on retention time (RT), Table S4. Detailed list of multi-reaction monitoring (MRM) transitions for the oxylipins contained in our in-house library. Compounds are ordered based on retention time (RT).

Author Contributions: Conceptualization: K.A.L. and D.B.J.; Data curation: M.G.-J., K.A.L., M.H.S. and D.B.J.; Formal analysis: M.G.-J., K.A.L., M.H.S. and D.B.J.; Funding acquisition: D.B.J.; Investigation: M.G.-J., K.A.L., M.H.S. and D.B.J.; Methodology: M.G.-J., K.A.L., M.H.S. and D.B.J.; Project administration: D.B.J.; Resources: D.B.J.; Supervision: D.B.J.; Validation: M.G.-J., K.A.L., M.H.S. and D.B.J.; Visualization: M.G.-J. and D.B.J.; Writing-original draft: M.G.-J. and D.B.J.; Writing-review and editing: M.G.-J., K.A.L., M.H.S. and D.B.J.

References

1.   Bellentani, S.; Scaglioni, F.; Marino, M.; Bedogni, G. Epidemiology of non-alcoholic fatty liver disease. *Dig. Dis.* **2010**, *28*, 155–161. [CrossRef] [PubMed]

2.   Younossi, Z.; Anstee, Q.M.; Marietti, M.; Hardy, T.; Henry, L.; Eslam, M.; George, J.; Bugianesi, E. Global burden of NAFLD and NASH: Trends, predictions, risk factors and prevention. *Nat. Rev. Gastroenterol. Hepatol.* **2018**, *15*, 11–20. [CrossRef] [PubMed]

3.   Younossi, Z.M.; Golabi, P.; de Avila, L.; Paik, J.M.; Srishord, M.; Fukui, N.; Qiu, Y.; Burns, L.; Afendy, A.; Nader, F. The global epidemiology of NAFLD and NASH in patients with type 2 diabetes: A systematic review and meta-analysis. *J. Hepatol.* **2019**, *4*, 793–801. [CrossRef] [PubMed]

4.   Angulo, P.; Lindor, K.D. Non-alcoholic fatty liver disease. *J. Gastroenterol. Hepatol.* **2002**, *17*, S186–S190. [CrossRef] [PubMed]

5.   Neuschwander-Tetri, B.A.; Caldwell, S.H. Nonalcoholic steatohepatitis: Summary of an AASLD Single Topic Conference. *Hepatology* **2003**, *37*, 1202–1219. [CrossRef]

6.   Farrell, G.C.; Larter, C.Z. Nonalcoholic fatty liver disease: From steatosis to cirrhosis. *Hepatology* **2006**, *43*, S99–S112. [CrossRef]

7. Cohen, J.C.; Horton, J.D.; Hobbs, H.H. Human fatty liver disease: Old questions and new insights. *Science* **2011**, *332*, 1519–1523. [CrossRef]

8. Lauby-Secretan, B.; Scoccianti, C.; Loomis, D.; Grosse, Y.; Bianchini, F.; Straif, K. Body fatness and cancer-viewpoint of the IARC working group. *N. Engl. J. Med.* **2016**, *375*, 794–798. [CrossRef]

9. Amarapurkar, D.; Kamani, P.; Patel, N.; Gupte, P.; Kumar, P.; Agal, S.; Baijal, R.; Lala, S.; Chaudhary, D.; Deshpande, A. Prevalence of non-alcoholic fatty liver disease: Population based study. *Ann. Hepatol.* **2007**, *6*, 161–163. [CrossRef]

10. Center for Disease Control and Prevention. Adult Obesity Facts. 2015. Available online: http://www.cdc. gov/obesity/data/adult.html (accessed on 21 September 2019).

11. Center for Disease Control and Prevention. Childhood Obesity Facts. 2015. Available online: http: //www.cdc.gov/obesity/data/childhood.html (accessed on 21 September 2019).

12. Spooner, M.H.; Jump, D.B. *Omega-3 Fatty Acids and Nonalcoholic Fatty Liver Disease in Adults and Children: Where Do We stand? Current Opinion in Clinical Nutrition and Metabolic Care*; Wolters Kluwer: Alphen aan den Rijn, The Netherlands, 2019.

13. Cussons, A.J.; Watts, G.F.; Mori, T.A.; Stuckey, B.G. Omega-3 fatty acid supplementaion decreases liver fat content in polycystic ovary syndrome: A randomized controlled trial employing proton magnetic resonance spectroscopy. *J. Clin. Endocrinol. Metabol.* **2009**, *94*, 3842–3848. [CrossRef]

14. Soderberg, C.; Stal, P.; Askling, J.; Glaumann, H.; Lindberg, G.; Marmur, J.; Hultcrantz, R. Decreased survival of subjects with elevated liver function tests during a 28-year follow-up. *Hepatology* **2010**, *51*, 595–602. [CrossRef] [PubMed]

15. Ekstedt, M.; Franzen, L.E.; Mathiesen, U.L.; Thorelius, L.; Holmqvist, M.; Bodemar, G.; Kechagias, S. Long-term follow-up of patients with NAFLD and elevated liver enzymes. *Hepatology* **2006**, *44*, 865–873. [CrossRef] [PubMed]

16. Adams, L.A.; Lymp, J.F.; St Sauver, J.; Sanderson, S.O.; Lindor, K.D.; Feldstein, A.; Angulo, P. The natural history of nonalcoholic fatty liver disease: A population-based cohort study. *Gastroenterology* **2005**, *129*, 113–121. [CrossRef] [PubMed]

17. Chalasani, N.; Younossi, Z.; Lavine, J.E.; Diehl, A.M.; Brunt, E.M.; Cusi, K.; Charlton, M.; Sanyal, A.J. The diagnosis and management of non-alcoholic fatty liver disease: Practice guideline by the American Association for the Study of Liver Diseases, American College of Gastroenterology, and the American Gastroenterological Association. *Am. J. Gastroenterol.* **2012**, *107*, 811–826. [CrossRef]

18. Alberti, K.G.; Zimmet, P.; Shaw, J. The metabolic syndrome—A new worldwide definition. *Lancet* **2005**, *366*, 1059–1062. [CrossRef]

19. Day, C.P.; James, O.F. Steatohepatitis: A tale of two "hits"? *Gastroenterology* **1998**, *114*, 842–845. [CrossRef]

20. LaBrecque, D.; Abbas, Z.; Anania, F.; Ferenci, P.; Gahafoor Kahn, A.; Goh, K.-L.; Hamid, S.S.; Isakov, V.; Lizarzabal, M.; Mojica Pernaranda, M.; et al. *Nonalcoholic Fatty Liver Disease and Nonalcoholic Steatohepatitis*; World Gastroentrology Organization Global Guidelines: Milwaukee, WI, USA, 2012; pp. 1–29.

21. Tilg, H.; Moschen, A.R. Evolution of inflammation in nonalcoholic fatty liver disease: The multiple parallel hits hypothesis. *Hepatology* **2010**, *52*, 1836–1846. [CrossRef]

22. Schuppan, D.; Kim, Y.O. Evolving therapies for liver fibrosis. *J. Clin. Invest.* **2013**, *123*, 1887–1901. [CrossRef]

23. Buzzetti, E.; Pinzani, M.; Tsochatzis, E.A. The multiple-hit pathogenesis of non-alcoholic fatty liver disease (NAFLD). *Metabolism* **2016**, *65*, 1038–1048. [CrossRef]

24. Angulo, P. Nonalcoholic fatty liver disease. *N. Engl. J. Med.* **2002**, *346*, 1221–1231. [CrossRef]

25. Friedman, S.L. Mechanisms of hepatic fibrogenesis. *Gastroenterology* **2008**, *134*, 1655–1669. [CrossRef] [PubMed]

26. Koyama, Y.; Brenner, D.A. New therapies for hepatic fibrosis. *Clin. Res. Hepatol. Gastroenterol.* **2015**, *39*, S75–S79. [CrossRef] [PubMed]

27. Rosenbloom, J.; Mendoza, F.A.; Jimenez, S.A. Strategies for anti-fibrotic therapies. *Biochim. Biophys. Acta* **2013**, *1832*, 1088–1103. [CrossRef] [PubMed]

28. Vilar-Gomez, E.; Martenez-Perez, Y.; Calzadilla-Bertot, L.; Torres-Gonzalez, A.; Gra-Oramas, B.; Gonzalez-Fabian, L.; Friedman, S.L.; Diago, M.; Romero-Gomez, M. Weight loss through lifestyle modification significantly reduces features of nonalcoholic steatohepatitis. *Gastroenterology* **2015**, *149*, 367–378. [CrossRef] [PubMed]

29. Chan, H.L.; de Silva, H.J.; Leung, N.W.; Lim, S.G.; Farrell, G.C. How should we manage patients with non-alcoholic fatty liver disease in 2007. *J. Gastroenterol. Hepatol.* **2007**, *22*, 801–808. [CrossRef] [PubMed]
30. Leslie, M. The liver's weight problem. *Science* **2015**, *6243*, 18–20.
31. Chalasani, N.; Younossi, Z.; Lavine, J.E.; Diehl, A.M.; Brunt, E.M.; Cusi, K.; Charlton, M.; Sanyal, A.J. The diagnosis and management of non-alcoholic fatty liver disease: Practice guideline by the American Gastroenterological Association, American Association for the Study of Liver Diseases, and American College of Gastroenterology. *Gastroenterology* **2012**, *142*, 1592–1609. [CrossRef]
32. Lee, Y.A.; Wallace, M.C.; Friedman, S.L. Pathology of liver fibrosis: A translational success story. *Gut* **2015**, *64*, 830–841. [CrossRef]
33. Kappler, R. From crawl to sprint: The race to treat NASH. *Life Sci. VC* **2015**. Available online: https://lifescivc.com/2015/05/from-crawl-to-sprint-the-race-to-treat-nash/ (accessed on 21 September 2019).
34. Musso, G.; Cassader, M.; Rosina, F.; Gambino, R. Impact of current treatments on liver disease, glucose metabolism and cardiovascular risk in non-alcoholic fatty liver disease (NAFLD): A systematic review and meta-analysis of randomised trials. *Diabetologia* **2012**, *55*, 885–904. [CrossRef]
35. Petit, J.M.; Guiu, B.; Duvillard, L.; Jooste, V.; Brindisi, M.C.; Athias, A.; Bouillet, B.; Habchi, M.; Cottet, V.; Gambert, P.; et al. Increased erythrocytes n-3 and n-6 polyunsaturated fatty acids is significantly associated with a lower prevalence of steatosis in patients with type 2 diabetes. *Clin. Nutr.* **2012**, *31*, 520–525. [CrossRef] [PubMed]
36. Zheng, J.S.; Xu, A.; Huang, T.; Yu, X.; Li, D. Low docosahexaenoic acid content in plasma phospholipids is associated with increased non-alcoholic fatty liver disease in China. *Lipids* **2012**, *47*, 549–556. [CrossRef] [PubMed]
37. Parker, H.M.; Johnson, N.A.; Burdon, C.A.; Cohn, J.S.; O'Connor, H.T.; George, J. Omega-3 supplementation and non-alcoholic fatty liver disease: A systematic review and meta-analysis. *J. Hepatol.* **2012**, *56*, 944–951. [CrossRef] [PubMed]
38. Di Minno, M.N.; Russolillo, A.; Lupoli, R.; Ambrosino, P.; Di Minno, A.; Tarantino, G. Omega-3 fatty acids for the treatment of non-alcoholic fatty liver disease. *World J. Gastroenterol.* **2012**, *18*, 5839–5847. [CrossRef]
39. Nobili, V.; Bedogni, G.; Alisi, A.; Pietrobattista, A.; Rise, P.; Galli, C.; Agostoni, C. Docosahexaenoic acid supplementation decreases liver fat content in children with non-alcoholic fatty liver disease: Double-blind randomised controlled clinical trial. *Arch. Dis. Child.* **2011**, *96*, 350–353. [CrossRef]
40. Shapiro, H.; Tehilla, M.; Attal-Singer, J.; Bruck, R.; Luzzatti, R.; Singer, P. The therapeutic potential of long-chain omega-3 fatty acids in nonalcoholic fatty liver disease. *Clin. Nutr.* **2011**, *30*, 6–19. [CrossRef]
41. Glass, L.M.; Dickson, R.C.; Anderson, J.C.; Sufiawinata, A.A.; Putra, J.; Berk, B.S.; Toor, A. Total body weight loss of ≥10% is associated with improved hepatic fibrosis in patients with nonalcoholic steatohepatitis. *Dig. Dis. Sci.* **2015**, *60*, 1024–1030. [CrossRef]
42. Sofi, F.; Casini, A. Mediterranean diet and non-alcoholic fatty liver disease. *World J. Gastroenterol.* **2014**, *20*, 7339–7346. [CrossRef]
43. Marchesini, G.; Mazzotti, A. NAFLD incidence and remission: Only a matter of weight gain and weight loss. *J. Hepatol.* **2015**, *62*, 15–17. [CrossRef]
44. Panera, N.; Barbaro, B.; Della Corte, C.; Mosca, A.; Nobili, V.; Alisi, A. A review of the pathogenic and therapeutic role of nutrition in pediatric nonalcoholic fatty liver disease. *Nutr. Res.* **2018**, *58*, 1–16. [CrossRef]
45. Sumida, Y.; Yoneda, M. Current and future pharmacological therapies for NAFLD/NASH. *J. Gastroenterol.* **2018**, *53*, 362–376. [CrossRef] [PubMed]
46. Albhaisi, S.; Sanyal, A. Recent advances in understanding and managing non-alcoholic fatty liver disease. *F1000Research* **2018**, *7*, 1–11. [CrossRef] [PubMed]
47. Jump, D.B.; Lytle, K.A.; Depner, C.M.; Tripathy, S. Omega-3 polyunsaturated fatty acids as a treatment strategy for nonalcoholic fatty liver disease. *Pharmacol. Ther.* **2018**, *181*, 108–125. [CrossRef] [PubMed]
48. Banini, B.A.; Sanyal, A.J. Current and future pharmacologic treatment of nonalcoholic steatohepatitis. *Curr. Opin. Gastroenterol.* **2017**, *33*, 134–141. [CrossRef] [PubMed]
49. McCollough, A.J. Epidemiology of the metabolic syndrome in the USA. *J. Dig. Dis.* **2011**, *12*, 333–340. [CrossRef] [PubMed]
50. Depner, C.M.; Philbrick, K.A.; Jump, D.B. Docosahexaenoic acid attenuates hepatic inflammation, oxidative

stress, and fibrosis without decreasing hepatosteatosis in a Ldlr(-/-) mouse model of western diet-induced nonalcoholic steatohepatitis. *J. Nutr.* **2013**, *143*, 315–323. [CrossRef]

51. Lytle, K.A.; Jump, D.B. Is western diet-induced nonalcoholic steatohepatitis in Ldlr-/- mice reversible. *PLoS ONE* **2016**, *11*, e0146942. [CrossRef]

52. Lytle, K.A.; Wong, C.P.; Jump, D.B. Docosahexaenoic acid blocks progression of western diet-induced nonalcoholic steatohepatitis in obese Ldlr-/- mice. *PLoS ONE* **2017**, *12*, e0173376. [CrossRef]

53. Simopoulos, A.P. n-3 fatty acid-enriched eggs, lipids, and Western diet: Time for change. *Nutrition* **1993**, *9*, 561–562.

54. Cordain, L.; Eaton, S.B.; Sebastian, A.; Mann, N.; Lindeberg, S.; Watkins, B.A.; O'Keefe, J.H.; Brand-Miller, J. Orgins and evolution of the western diet: Health implications for the 21st century. *Am. J. Clin. Nutr.* **2005**, *81*, 341–354. [CrossRef]

55. Allard, J.B.; Aghdassi, E.; Mohammed, S.; Raman, M.; Avand, G.; Arendt, B.M.; Jalali, P.; Kandasamy, T.; Prayitno, N.; Sherman, M.; et al. Nutrition assessment and hepatic fatty acid composition in non-alcoholic fatty liver disease (NAFLD): A cross-sectional study. *J. Hepatol.* **2007**, *48*, 300–307. [CrossRef] [PubMed]

56. Arendt, B.M.; Comelli, E.M.; Ma, D.W.; Lou, W.; Teterina, A.; Kim, T.; Fung, D.K.H.; McGilvray, I.; Fischer, S.E.; Allard, J.P. Altered hepatic gene expression in non-alcoholic fatty liver disease is associated with lower n-3 and n-6 polyunsaturated fatty acids. *Hepatology* **2015**, *61*, 1565–1578. [CrossRef] [PubMed]

57. Spahis, S.; Alverez, F.; Dubois, J.; Ahmed, N.; Peretti, N.; Levy, E. Plasma fatty acid composition in French-Canadian children with non-alsocholic fatty liver disease: Effect of n-3 PUFA supplementation. *Prostaglandins Leukot. Essent. Fat. Acids* **2015**, *99*, 25–34. [CrossRef] [PubMed]

58. Jump, D.B. The biochemistry of n-3 polyunsaturated fatty acids. *J. Biol. Chem.* **2002**, *277*, 8755–8758. [CrossRef] [PubMed]

59. Jump, D.B.; Tripathy, S.; Depner, C.M. Fatty Acid-regulated transcription factors in the liver. *Ann. Rev. Nutr.* **2013**, *33*, 249–269. [CrossRef] [PubMed]

60. Garcia-Jaramillo, M.; Spooner, M.H.; Loehr, C.V.; Wong, C.P.; Zhang, W.; Jump, D.B. Lipidomic and transcriptomic analysis of western diet-induced nonalcoholic steatohepatitis (NASH) in female Ldlr-/- mice. *PLoS ONE* **2019**, *14*, E0214387. [CrossRef]

61. Gabbs, M.; Leng, S.; Devassy, J.G.; Monirujjaman, M.; Aukema, H.M. Advances in our understanding of oxylipins derived from dietary PUFAs. *Adv. Nutr.* **2015**, *6*, 513–540. [CrossRef]

62. Jump, D.B.; Depner, C.M.; Tripathy, S. Omega-3 fatty acid supplementation and cardiovascular disease. *J. Lipid Res.* **2012**, *53*, 2525–2545. [CrossRef]

63. Scorletti, E.; Bhatia, L.; McCormick, K.G.; Clough, G.F.; Nash, K.; Hodson, L.; Moyses, H.E.; Calder, P.C.; Byrne, C.D.; The Welcome Study Investigators. Effects of purified eicosapentaenoic and docosahexaenoic acids in non-alcoholic fatty liver disease: Results from the *WELCOME study. *Hepatology* **2014**, *60*, 1211–1221. [CrossRef]

64. Sanyal, A.J.; Abdelmalek, M.F.; Suzuki, A.; Cummings, O.W.; Chojkier, M. No significant effects of ethyl-eicosapentaenoic acid on histologic features of nonalcoholic steatohepatitis in a Phase 2 trial. *Gastroenterology* **2014**, *147*, 377–384. [CrossRef]

65. Barter, P.; Ginsberg, H.N. Effectiveness of combined statin plus omega-3 fatty acid therapy for mixed dyslipidemia. *Am. J. Cardiol.* **2008**, *102*, 1040–1045. [CrossRef] [PubMed]

66. Chong, J.; Soufan, O.; Li, C.; Caraus, I.; Li, S.; Bourque, G.; Wishart, D.S.; Xia, J. MetaboAnalyst 4.0: Towards more transparent and integrative metabolomics analysis. *Nucleic Acids Res.* **2018**, *46*, W486–W494. [CrossRef] [PubMed]

67. Mater, M.K.; Thelen, A.P.; Jump, D.B. Arachidonic acid and PGE2 regulation of hepatic lipogenic gene expression. *J. Lipid Res.* **1999**, *40*, 1045–1052.

68. Lopane, C.; Agosti, P.; Gigante, I.; Sabba, C.; Mazzocca, A. Implications of the lysophosphatidic acid signaling axis in liver cancer. *Biochim. Biophys. Acta* **2017**, *1868*, 277–282. [CrossRef]

69. Ishii, I.; Fukushima, N.; Ye, X.; Chun, J. Lysophospholipid receptors: Signaling and biology. *Ann. Rev. Biochem.* **2004**, *73*, 321–354. [CrossRef]

70. Gardell, S.E.; Dubin, A.E.; Chun, J. Emerging medicinal roles for lysophospholipid signaling. *Trends Mol. Med.* **2006**, *12*, 65–75. [CrossRef]

71. Frasch, S.C.; Bratton, D.L. Emerging roles for lysophosphatidylserine in resolution of inflammation. *Prog. Lipid Res.* **2012**, *51*, 199–207. [CrossRef]

72. Tsukahara, T.; Matsuda, Y.; Haniu, H. Lysophospholipid-Related Diseases and PPARgamma Signaling Pathway. *Int. J. Mol. Sci.* **2017**, *18*, 2730. [CrossRef]

73. D'Souza, K.; Paramel, G.V.; Kienesberger, P.C. Lysophosphatidic Acid Signaling in Obesity and Insulin Resistance. *Nutrients* **2018**, *10*, 399. [CrossRef]

74. Brown, A.J.; Jupe, S.; Briscoe, C.P. A family of fatty acid binding receptors. *DNA Cell Biol.* **2005**, *24*, 54–61. [CrossRef] [PubMed]

75. Funk, C.D. Prostaglandins and leukotrienes: Advances in eicosanoid biology. *Science* **2001**, *294*, 1871–1875. [CrossRef] [PubMed]

76. Kostenis, E. A glance at G-protein-coupled receptors for lipid mediators: A growing receptor family with remarkably diverse ligands. *Pharmacol. Ther.* **2004**, *102*, 243–257. [CrossRef] [PubMed]

77. Graves, J.P.; Gruzdev, A.; Bradbury, J.A.; DeGraff, L.M.; Li, H.; House, J.S.; Hoopes, S.L.; Edin, M.L.; Zeldin, D.C. Quantitative Polymerase Chain Reaction Analysis of the Mouse Cyp2j Subfamily: Tissue Distribution and Regulation. *Drug Metab. Dispos.* **2015**, *43*, 1169–1180. [CrossRef] [PubMed]

78. Feldstein, A.E.; Lopez, R.; Tamimi, T.A.; Yerian, L.; Chung, Y.M.; Berk, M.; Zhang, R.; McIntyre, T.M.; Hazen, S.L. Mass spectrometric profiling of oxidized lipid products in human nonalcoholic fatty liver disease and nonalcoholic steatohepatitis. *J. Lipid Res.* **2010**, *51*, 3046–3054. [CrossRef] [PubMed]

79. Hasegawa, E.; Inafuku, S.; Mulki, L.; Okunuki, Y.; Yanai, R.; Smith, K.E.; Kim, C.B.; Klokman, G.; Bielenberg, D.R.; Puli, N.; et al. Cytochrome P450 monooxygenase lipid metabolites are significant second messengers in the resolution of choroidal neovascularization. *Proc. Natl. Acad. Sci. USA* **2017**, *114*, E7545–E7553. [CrossRef] [PubMed]

80. Calder, P.C. Marine omega-3 fatty acids and inflammatory processes: Effects, mechanisms and clinical relevance. *Biochim. Biophys. Acta* **2015**, *1851*, 469–484. [CrossRef] [PubMed]

81. Palladini, G.; Di Pasqua, L.G.; Berardo, C.; Siciliano, V.; Richelmi, P.; Mannucci, B.; Croce, A.C.; Rizzo, V.; Perlini, S.; Vairetti, M.; et al. Fatty Acid Desaturase Involvement in Non-Alcoholic Fatty Liver Disease Rat Models: Oxidative Stress Versus Metalloproteinases. *Nutrients* **2019**, *11*, 799. [CrossRef]

82. Stankovic, M.N.; Mladenovic, D.; Ninkovic, M.; Ethuricic, I.; Sobajic, S.; Jorgacevic, B.; de Luka, S.; Vukicevic, R.J.; Radosavljević, T.S. The effects of alpha-lipoic acid on liver oxidative stress and free fatty acid composition in methionine-choline deficient diet-induced NAFLD. *J. Med. Food.* **2014**, *17*, 254–261. [CrossRef]

83. Lopez-Vicario, C.; Alcaraz-Quiles, J.; Garcia-Alonso, V.; Rius, B.; Hwang, S.H.; Titos, E.; Clària, J. Inhibition of soluble epoxide hydrolase modulates inflammation and autophagy in obese adipose tissue and liver: Role for omega-3 epoxides. *Proc. Natl. Acad. Sci. USA* **2015**, *112*, 536–541. [CrossRef]

84. Matyash, V.; Liebisch, G.; Kurzchalia, T.V.; Shevchenko, A.; Schwudke, D. Lipid extraction by methyl-tert-butyl ether for high-throughput lipidomics. *J. Lipid Res.* **2008**, *49*, 1137–1146. [CrossRef]

85. Pedersen, T.L.; Newman, J.W. Establishing and performing targeted multi-residue analysis for lipid mediators and fatty acids in small clinical plasma samples. *Methods Mol. Biol.* **2018**, *1730*, 175–212. [PubMed]

86. La Franko, M.R.; Hernandez-Carretero, A.; Weber, N.; Borkowski, K.; Pedersen, T.L.; Osborn, O.; Newman, J.W. Diet-induced obesity and weight loss alter bile acid concentrations and bile acid-sensitive gene expression in insulin target tissues of C57BL/6J mice. *Nutr. Res.* **2017**, *46*, 11–21. [CrossRef] [PubMed]

87. Cajka, T.; Fiehn, O. Increasing lipidomic coverage by selecting optimal mobile-phase modifiers in LC-MS of blood plasma. *Metabolomics* **2016**, *12*, 1–11. [CrossRef]

88. Cajka, T.; Davis, R.; Austin, K.J.; Newman, J.W.; German, J.B.; Feihn, O.; Smilowitz, J.T. Using a lipidomics approach for nutritional phenotyping in resposne to a test meal containing gamma-linolenic acid. *Metabolomics* **2016**, *12*, 1–22. [CrossRef]

89. Tsugawa, H.; Cajka, T.; Kind, T.; Ma, Y.; Higgins, B.; Ikeda, K.; Kanazawa, M.; VanderGheynst, J.; Fiehn, O.; Arita, M. MS-DIAL: Data-independent MS/MS deconvolution for comprehensive metabolome analysis. *Nat. Methods.* **2015**, *12*, 523–526. [CrossRef] [PubMed]

90. Kind, T.; Liu, K.H.; Lee, D.Y.; DeFelice, B.; Meissen, J.K.; Fiehn, O. LipidBlast in silico tandem mass spectrometry database for lipid identification. *Nat. Methods* **2013**, *10*, 755–758. [CrossRef]

91. Sumner, L.W.; Amberg, A.; Barrett, D.; Beale, M.H.; Beger, R.; Daykin, C.A.; Fan, T.W.; Fiehn, O.; Goodacre, R.; Griffin, J.L.; et al. Proposed minimum reporting standards for chemical analysis Chemical Analysis Working Group (CAWG) Metabolomics Standards Initiative (MSI). *Metabolomics* **2007**, *3*, 211–221. [CrossRef]

92. Benjamini, Y.; Krieger, A.M.; Yekutieli, D. Adaptive linear step-up procedures that control the false discovery rate. *Biometrika* **2006**, *93*, 491–507. [CrossRef]

8

Exposure of HepaRG Cells to Sodium Saccharin Underpins the Importance of Including Non-Hepatotoxic Compounds when Investigating Toxicological Modes of Action using Metabolomics

Matthias Cuykx [1,2,*], **Charlie Beirnaert** [3,4], **Robim Marcelino Rodrigues** [2], **Kris Laukens** [3,4], **Tamara Vanhaecke** [2,†] and **Adrian Covaci** [1,*,†]

[1] Toxicological Centre, University of Antwerp, Universiteitsplein 1, 2610 Wilrijk, Belgium
[2] Research Group In Vitro Toxicology and Dermato-Cosmetology (IVTD), Vrije Universiteit Brussel, Laarbeeklaan 103, 1090 Jette, Belgium; Robim.marcelino.rodrigues@vub.be (R.M.R.); Tamara.vanhaecke@vub.be (T.V.)
[3] Department of Mathematics & Computer Science, University of Antwerp, Middelheimlaan 1, 2020 Antwerp, Belgium; Charlie.beirnaert@uza.be (C.B.); Kris.laukens@uantwerpen.be (K.L.)
[4] Biomedical Informatics Network Antwerpen (Biomina), University of Antwerp, Middelheimlaan 1, 2020 Antwerp, Belgium
[*] Correspondence: matthiascuykx@gmail.com (M.C.); Adrian.Covaci@uantwerpen.be (A.C.)
[†] These authors contributed equally to this work.

Abstract: Metabolites represent the most downstream information of the cellular organisation. Hence, metabolomics experiments are extremely valuable to unravel the endogenous pathways involved in a toxicological mode of action. However, every external stimulus can introduce alterations in the cell homeostasis, thereby obscuring the involved endogenous pathways, biasing the interpretation of the results. Here we report on sodium saccharin, which is considered to be not hepatotoxic and therefore can serve as a reference compound to detect metabolic alterations that are not related to liver toxicity. Exposure of HepaRG cells to high levels of sodium saccharin (>10 mM) induced cell death, probably due to an increase in the osmotic pressure. Yet, a low number ($n = 15$) of significantly altered metabolites were also observed in the lipidome, including a slight decrease in phospholipids and an increase in triacylglycerols, upon daily exposure to 5 mM sodium saccharin for 72 h. The observation that a non-hepatotoxic compound can affect the metabolome underpins the importance of correct experimental design and data interpretation when investigating toxicological modes of action via metabolomics.

Keywords: in vitro; HepaRG; sodium saccharin; reference toxicants

1. Introduction

Since the introduction of metabolomics as a new "-omics" domain in 1999, the field of research has proved to be a valuable source of information for the actual phenotype or state of organisms [1]. Metabolomics is defined as the study of the biochemical profile of small molecules in an organism [1]. Because the metabolome is the most downstream level in the biomolecular organisation of a system, metabolomics fingerprints are very dynamic and alterations may be induced even by small external triggers [2,3]. Many of these stimuli, such as gender, age (young vs. old), dietary status (e.g., fasting vs. fed) and activity (rested vs. active) potentially form biases that obscure the metabolic signature related to exposure. These biases are important, but can be anticipated through strict subject selection criteria and proper randomisation [4].

An effect often not considered is the exposure itself. Although this placebo effect is well-known in medicine, precautions are often not taken during metabolomics studies. The "exposure bias" is relevant when combining metabolomics with in vitro experiments, since it is one of the main potential sources of bias. Although the biological variation and bias is reduced in cell culture experiments, confounding factors still pose a risk during metabolomics investigations. Indeed, the mere presence of a xenobiotic may theoretically cause a metabolic shift, even though this compound is not considered harmful. This confounding factor of "exposure" can generate results falsely interpreted to be related to toxicity [5].

Sodium saccharin is an artificial sweetener that has been used for over a century. Except for a case study describing an idiosyncratic reaction after exposure to different pharmaceutical products containing the sweetener, no evidence of human hepatotoxicity has been reported so far [6,7]. The safe characteristics of sodium saccharin make it a good candidate to investigate potential metabolic alterations triggered in vitro upon exposure to a non-hepatotoxic molecule.

2. Materials and Methods

2.1. Materials and Methods

Materials, exposure and acquisition methods have been performed as described previously [8]. A brief description highlighting the principles is mentioned in-text and full details concerning the experimental protocols are provided in the Supplementary Materials SM-1 to SM-5.

2.2. Determination of Testing Concentrations

Seven days after initial cell seeding, the wells were divided into two negative control groups and eight groups that were exposed to sodium saccharin at different concentrations ranging from 0.40 to 40 mM for a period of 72 h in a repeated dose exposure, in which the medium was refreshed every 24 h. Viability was assessed using the neutral red uptake (NRU) assay [9,10]. Full details are available in the Supplementary Materials SM-2.

2.3. Metabolomics Experiments

2.3.1. Seeding of the HepaRG® Cells and Exposure to Sodium Saccharin

Cryopreserved differentiated HepaRG® cells were thawed and seeded in collagen-coated two-well Lab-Tek chamber slides at a density of 1.03×10^6 cells/well. Two additional blank chamber slides were treated identically to serve as blanks during further analysis. After seven days of cultivation, the cell cultures were visually checked for hepatocyte/biliary cell ratio and block randomised in three groups: a negative control group in comparison to a dose of sodium saccharin at a concentration of 5.5 mM (high dose) and a 1/10 dilution of the high dose, i.e., 0.5 mM (low dose). Higher concentrations of sodium saccharin were not applied because of hyperosmotic toxic effects (additional osmotic pressure >20 mOsm/L). Each group contained six replicates, which is often considered an adequate sample size for in vitro metabolomics experiments [5,11]. The cell cultures were exposed for 72 h with a medium refreshment every 24 h. The exposure experiment has been performed twice to reduce false positive results [8].

2.3.2. Sample Preparation

The cell cultures were harvested according to previously described protocols, full details are available in SM-3 [12,13]. Briefly, cells were prepared for extraction with a wash in phosphate buffered saline (37 °C) followed by freezing on liquid nitrogen. Cells were scraped from the surface three times with 200 μL of a cooled (−80 °C) 80% (v/v) methanol (MeOH)/milliQ water solution. Liquid/liquid extraction was performed using ultrapure water, methanol, and chloroform. Quality control (QC) pools were generated through the collection of aliquots of all samples for the polar and non-polar phases [14]. Both fractions were evaporated to dryness and reconstituted in LC-MS-compatible solvents.

2.3.3. LC-MS Analysis

LC-MS analysis was performed using separation mechanisms described in SM-4 [8,15]. The non-polar fraction was analysed using reversed phase chromatography on a Kinetex XB-C18 (150 × 2.1 mm; 1.7 μm particle size, Phenomenex, Utrecht, the Netherlands). Mobile phase compositions were mixtures of methanol, isopropanol (IPA) and water with ammonium acetate (pH 6.7) and of acetonitrile (ACN), IPA and water with an acetate buffer (pH 4.2) for negative and positive ionisation modes, respectively.

The polar fractions were analysed using HILIC systems using an iHILIC column (100 × 2.1 mm; 1.8 μm particle size, HILICON, Umea, Sweden) with ACN, MeOH and water with an ammonium formate buffer (pH 3.15) for the positive ionisation mode, and a polymeric iHILIC Fusion Column (100 × 2.1 mm, 5 μm particle size, HILICON) in combination with ACN, MeOH and water with an ammonium carbonate ($(NH_4)_2CO_3$) buffer (pH 9.0) for the negative ionisation mode. LC-separation was performed on an Agilent Infinity 1290 UPLC (Agilent Technologies, Santa Clara, CA, USA), connected to an Agilent 6530 QTOF with Agilent Jet Stream nebuliser (Agilent Technologies). The LC-MS system was equilibrated using 15 QC-injections at the start of the data acquisition. The injection order of the samples was block-randomised to prevent bias related to instrumental drift. One QC injection was performed after every four sample injections to monitor instrumental drifts.

2.3.4. Data Analysis

Data Quality Control

Internal standards were used to evaluate the precision of the retention time and m/z-accuracy within and between experimental batches. The raw data were searched for the internal standards using the Find by Formula algorithm (Agilent Technologies) with the following parameters: formula matching ± 10 ppm, expected variation 2 mDa ± 8 ppm. Samples were only considered when internal standards were detected and the number of molecular features was comparable to those of the other samples. The absence of internal standards and/or molecular features in an acquired LC-MS run may indicate analytical issues during the run and, therefore, the removal of the failed runs was considered to improve the quality of the final dataset. The results of internal standard quality control were used to set the parameters for further data processing.

Data Pretreatment

Acquired data were imported on the MassHunter Qualitative software (Agilent Technologies, v 2.06.00) and converted to centroid m/z data. The generic datafiles were processed using the XCMS package in the R workspace [16,17]. Features representing the ions of the extracted metabolites were searched using the centWave algorithm. Features were aligned with the Obiwarp algorithm and grouped by density [18]. Missing peaks were re-extracted using the fillPeaks algorithm [17].

The dataset was cleaned by removing isotopes and features present in blank samples. Other applied filters were based on a high number of missing values and within-group variability. All preprocessing functions were executed using the MetaboMeeseeks package [19]. A principal component analysis (PCA) was performed and outliers were removed for further analysis ($n = 4$) (Figure S6). After outlier removal, the filter process was re-iterated and samples were normalised using BatchCorr normalisation [20]. Missing values imputation was considered but not applied, since it had no positive impact on the within-group variance. The final dataset was once more evaluated using a PCA to assess important trends and their potential impact on the subsequent multivariate analysis. All parameters of feature extraction and data clean-up are mentioned in SM-5.

Statistical Analysis

Univariate statistical analysis was performed through the non-parametric Mann–Whitney U test with a Benjamini–Hochberg correction for multiple testing using the multtest package in R [21]. In addition, a partial least squares discriminant analysis (PLS-DA) and a random forest classification were performed as multivariate analyses [19,22]. Performances were checked using leave-one-out cross-validation. Metabolic alterations were defined based on significance in the univariate tests (q-value <0.05) and on importance in the multivariate models (based on the covariance of the latent values of the first component of the PLS-DA and the bimodal distribution of the variable importance measure (VIM) of the random forest classifier model). The raw signals of the selected signals were manually checked to confirm the result.

Metabolite Annotation

The details of metabolite annotation are mentioned in SM-6. Briefly, annotation was performed in Mass Hunter using the molecular feature extractor algorithm: the signals corresponding to the altered metabolite were selected, the complete result set was extracted and the Molecular Formula Generator (MFG) generated a list of possible chemical formulas. The identification was based on the m/z-value, the isotope pattern, the measured retention time and the fragmentation spectra acquired during the equilibration runs. Results were reported according to the standards of the CAWG and MSI [23,24]. Level 2 and level 3 identifications were considered of sufficient quality to infer a biological interpretation to the outcome of the experiments. All metabolites, including molecular features with lower levels of confidence in annotation (levels 4–5), are reported in Table S4.

3. Results

3.1. Experimental Observations

The dose–response curves of the viability assay in Figure 1 showed a clear decrease in viability from 10 mM sodium saccharin onwards. Indeed, concentrations of 10 mM increased the osmotic pressure over 20 mOsm/L to supra-physiological ranges [25]. Hyperosmolarity is a form of toxicity not related to physiological hepatotoxicity, and such high exposures are therefore not considered as a good reference for investigating the chemical hazard of the product. A high-dose exposure of 5 mM induced an osmotic pressure of ±10 mOsm/L, yet no cytotoxic effects were observed.

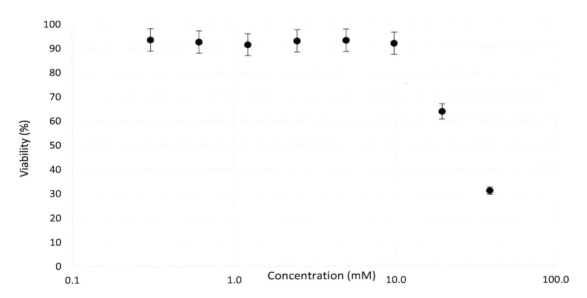

Figure 1. Averaged viability curve for the neutral red uptake (NRU)-assay upon daily exposure to sodium saccharin for a period of 72 h. Cytotoxicity is observed from 10 mM onwards, which is equal to an osmotic pressure of ±20 mOsm/L.

3.2. Data Quality

The injections that were not considered during statistical analysis are reported in Table S2. For the non-polar fraction, injections QC-1 and QC-2 were excluded from the analysis because of failed injections, reflected by the absence of internal standards in the chromatogram and the absence of the typical chromatogram.

As shown in Table S3, standard deviations were higher during the first experimental batch due to autosampler thermostatic issues. The high mRSDs for QCs in comparison to all other experiments using lipidomics approaches can be explained by the shift in retention times between the two experimental batches. To correctly match corresponding peaks, the parameters for alignment and grouping were less strict, which introduced extra noise in the data.

3.3. Selection of Potential Endogenous Markers of Exposure

As shown in the PCA plots in Figure 2 and Figures S7–S10, no clear distinction between all exposure groups was observed. The overlap between the different exposure groups indicated that the source of variation in the dataset was probably not related to the exposure. This was also reflected by the poor performance of both multivariate and univariate tests: all AUCs for the random forest classifiers reported in Table 1 were below 0.7, except for the high-dose exposure conditions. According to the R^2 and Q^2 values in Table 2, the PLS-models overfit, with Q^2 values < 0.2. The R^2 of the non-polar fraction in positive mode was good (>0.8), but the cross-validation showed this was an overfit value, and the Q^2 was reduced to 0.40.

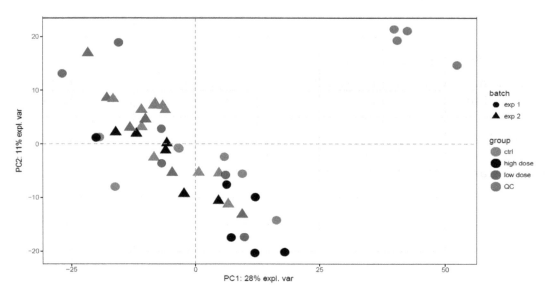

Figure 2. PCA plots of the non-polar fraction in positive mode during the 72-h exposure showing PC1 vs. PC2. There is strong overlapping of the different exposure groups in all principal components, indicating the variance is not related to exposure. Only a slight trend is visible between the negative control group and the group exposed to the higher dose.

Univariate tests did not reveal major differences between the exposure groups and the negative control group. Only 15 features were observed to be significantly different between the negative control group and the high-dose exposure group, and only for the non-polar fraction in positive mode.

The identified features given in Table S4 represent a decreased presence of six phosphatidylethanolamines, two phosphatidylinositols and one sphingomyelin. Further differences included the increase of two low-saturated triacylglycerols. Their respective boxplots are represented in Figure S10.

Table 1. AUCs of the random forest classifiers comparing the negative control group against the different exposures.

Exposure	Non-Polar Positive	Non-Polar Negative	Polar Positive	Polar Negative
Low Dose	0.51	0.55	0.59	0.17
High Dose	0.95	0.40	0.69	0.21

Table 2. R^2 and Q^2 values for the PLS-DA discrimination between the exposure groups and the negative control group.

Exposure	Non-Polar Positive		Non-Polar Negative		Polar Positive		Polar Negative	
	R^2	Q^2	R^2	Q^2	R^2	Q^2	R^2	Q^2
Low Dose	0.01	0.01	0.1	0.06	0.22	0.14	0.21	0.05
High Dose	0.84	0.4	0.42	0.10	0.08	0.03	0.33	0.04

4. Discussion

The metabolome is a dynamic level of the cellular organisation. External stimuli theoretically invoke a response of the cell, resulting in a change of the metabolome. Sodium saccharin is considered to be a non-hepatotoxic chemical, which makes it an ideal compound to select markers of exposure not necessarily related to hepatotoxicity [8,9].

The acquisition of the metabolome of cells exposed to a hepatotoxicant in comparison to vehicle only would reveal alterations that would all be addressed to a toxic mode of action. The main consequence of this assumption is the questionable predictive value of the observed metabolic alterations, especially in small-scale experiments (one dose, one time point exposure of a single chemical exposure). This consideration stresses the importance of an exposure to a non-toxic negative control during the experiment.

Few features of the lipidome were changed significantly ($n = 15$) and included the presence of triacylglycerols and a lower presence of phospholipids. The absence of significant changes in the polar fraction suggested that the cell culture did not implement major adaptations in metabolism as a response to the external stimuli.

Effects related to hyperosmolarity have also been described in human cell cultures, which showed the increased presence of monosaccharides and amino acids to retain the osmotic balance [26]. However, it is possible that these effects were not observed in this current experiment due to the deliberate choice to avoid these hyperosmolar (non-physiological) concentrations. The choice of a supra-physiological dose would imply a bias to select metabolic alterations related to modes of action not relevant in physiological conditions. This bias is especially relevant in in vitro techniques, as exposure concentrations can be increased to unrealistic, non-physiological levels. A potential prevention is the use of toxicokinetic data to confirm the plausibility of the exposure conditions.

García-Cañaveras et al. [27] and Ramirez et al. [28] classified different toxicants according to the mode of action, observing specific fingerprints for different end-points of toxicity. Ramirez et al. described the downregulation of carnitine, creatine, phosphocreatine, and pantothenic acid during exposure to peroxisome proliferating agents, the decrease of oleic acid, galactose and acetyl aspartate in combination with an increase of tryptophan and alanine during exposure to enzyme-inducing xenobiotics [28]. Garcia et al. compared the fingerprint of xenobiotics inducing oxidative stress, steatosis and phospholipidosis, in which they observed alterations in glutamate levels, oxido-reductive status, lysophospholipid/phospholipid ratio and lipid accumulation [27]. The inclusion of non-hepatotoxic compounds in their experimental design, such as citrate and ketotifen, states the importance of reference compounds for non-hepatotoxicity as metabolic changes were observed, albeit with a different fingerprint.

A qualitative comparison of the metabolic alterations for steatosis and cholestasis obtained in previous experiments are presented in Table 3 [8,29]. The clear alterations of the metabolome during hepatotoxic modes of action can be discriminated from the exposure to a non-hepatotoxic toxicant. Next to significant differences in the polar metabolome, the lipidome of a cell culture exposed to hepatotoxic compounds showed clear and strong alterations, with multiple lipid species of several classes involved in the downstream effect, whereas the effects during exposure to sodium saccharin were not substantial.

Table 3. Heat map for the endogenous markers of toxicity for hepatotoxicants inducing steatosis (sodium valproate) [8] and cholestasis (bosentan) [29] showing their up- (red) or down-regulation (green) in comparison to a negative control group (sodium saccharin). Common alterations indicate the importance of the use of non-hepatotoxic reference compounds as a negative control to prevent an exposure bias, especially in the lipidomics group.

Time Frame	Bosentan				Sodium Valproate				Sodium Saccharin
	24 h		72 h		24 h		72 h		72 h
Concentration (µg/mL)	23	230	9.5	95	230	2300	66.5	665	1000
Acetylcholine									
Acetylspermidine									
Aminergic Oligopeptides									
Carnitine									
citric-acid N-sugar									
Choline									
Cholesterol Sulfate									
Creatine									
diacetylspermidine									
GTP									
Isoputreanine									
Methylbutyryl Carnitine									
Methylhydroxylysine									
Nucleotides									
Ornithine									
Pantothenic Acid									
Phosphocholine									
Phosphorylated Metabolites									
Phosphorylethanolamine									
Putrescine									
SAM									
Spermidine									
Taurine									
Trimethylammonium Butanoic Acid									
UDP Glucuronic Acid									
Bile Acids									
Ceramide									
Ceramide, Derivative									
Diacylglycerol									
Glycosfingolipid									
LPE 18:1									
PC									
PE (non PUFA)									
PE (PUFA)									
PE (P)									
PS									
Sfingomyelin									
Triacylglycerol (O)									
Triacylglycerol (>50, PUFA)									
Triacylglycerol (>50, non PUFA)									
Triacylglycerol (<50)									

(A)

Abbreviations: GTP, guanosyl triphosphate; LPE, lysophosphatidylethanolamine; PC, phosphatidylcholine; PE, phosphatidylethanolamine; PI, phosphaditylinositol; PS, phosphatidylserine; SAM, S-adenosyl methionine; TG, triacylglycerol.

Colour						
Number of Lipid Species	>3	1–3	0	1–3	4–10	>10
Signal Abundance	Lower	Lower	N/A	Higher	Higher	Higher

(B)

A mechanistic interpretation based on the observed metabolic alterations provides an additional value to the localisation of the specific molecular initiating event and the potential adverse outcome, as this observation is an additional argument for a toxic cascade. Although metabolic alterations were observed upon exposure to sodium saccharin, no specific affected pathway could be identified. Based on all observations, the use of a non-hepatotoxic compound instead of a vehicle-only negative control group may help reducing false positive results without jeopardising the sensitivity of toxic insults.

5. Conclusions

The exposure of HepaRG cells to high levels of sodium saccharin induced cell death, possibly due to osmotic pressure. The exposure concentration should not solely be determined from viability curves, but should also be checked for physiological relevance to prevent unrealistic exposure scenarios. Although sodium saccharin is not considered to be a hepatotoxicant, minor changes were observed in the lipidome, including a slight decrease in phospholipids and an increase in saturated triacylglycerols. The metabolome was altered upon exposure to non-hepatotoxic compounds, indicating the importance of reference compounds when investigating toxicological insults. The metabolic changes were less pronounced than those of reference hepatotoxicants and can therefore be used as a background response to prevent false positive results related to the exposure bias.

Supplementary Materials: Figure S1: Viability curves for the NRU-assay 72 h of exposure., Figure S2: Extracted ion chromatogram for all samples in experiment 1 for m/z 162.1139 at a retention time of 8.7. Figure S3: Boxplots for m/z 162 at rt 8.7 min. Figure S4: Annotation of the molecular formula using the Agilent Molecular Formula Generator reveals a match for the proton, sodium and potassium adduct of a molecule with formula $C_7H_{15}NO_3$, Figure S5: MS/MS spectrum of the molecular feature (up), which matches with the MS/MS spectrum of L-carnitine in the METLIN database (down), Figure S6: PCA reflecting the outlier position of QC-1 and IC10-6 for the dataset of the non-polar fraction in negative ionisation mode, Figure S7: PCA plots of the non-polar fraction in negative mode during the 72 h exposure showing PC1 vs. PC2 (upper) and PC3 vs. PC4 (lower), Figure S8: PCA plots of the non-polar fraction in positive mode during the 72 h exposure showing PC1 vs. PC2 (upper) and PC3 vs. PC4 (lower), Figure S9: PCA plots of the polar fraction in negative mode during the 72 h exposure PC1 vs. PC2 (upper) and PC3 vs. PC4 (lower), Figure S10: PCA plots of the polar fraction in positive mode during the 72 h exposure showing PC1 vs. PC2 (upper) and PC3 vs. PC4 (lower), Table S1: Concentration range (in µg/mL) for the NRU-assay of sodium saccharin on HepaRG cells for a period of 72 h, Table S2: Samples which did not meet QC criteria., Table S3: Median relative standard deviations (mRSDs) for all subgroups in the experiments, Table S4: AUCs of the random forest classifiers comparing the negative control group against the different exposures, Table S5: R^2 and Q^2 values for the PLS-DA discrimination between the exposure groups and the negative control group, Table S6: Metabolites identified as potential metabolites of interest for all exposure models.

Author Contributions: Conceptualization, R.M.R. and T.V.; Data curation, C.B. and K.L.; Investigation, M.C., T.V. and A.C.; Methodology, M.C., C.B. and R.M.R.; Software, C.B.; Supervision, R.M.R., K.L., T.V. and A.C.; Writing—original draft, M.C.; Writing—review & editing, K.L., T.V. and A.C.

References

1.   Nicholson, J.K.; Lindon, J.C.; Holmes, E. "Metabonomics": Understanding the metabolic responses of living systems to pathophysiological stimuli via multivariate statistical analysis of biological NMR spectroscopic data. *Xenobiotica* **1999**, *29*, 1181–1189. [CrossRef]

2.   Balcke, G.U.; Kolle, S.N.; Kamp, H.; Bethan, B.; Looser, R.; Wagner, S.; Landsiedel, R.; van Ravenzwaay, B. Linking energy metabolism to dysfunctions in mitochondrial respiration—A metabolomics in vitro approach. *Toxicol. Lett.* **2011**, *203*, 200–209. [CrossRef]

3.   Ramirez, T.; Daneshian, M.; Kamp, H.; Bois, F.Y.; Clench, M.R.; Coen, M.; Donley, B.; Fischer, S.M.; Ekman, D.R.; Fabian, E.; et al. Metabolomics in toxicology and preclinical research. *ALTEX* **2013**, *30*, 209–225. [CrossRef]

4.   Broadhurst, D.I.; Kell, D.B. Statistical strategies for avoiding false discoveries in metabolomics and related experiments. *Metabolomics* **2006**, *2*, 171–196. [CrossRef]

5.   Cuykx, M.; Rodrigues, R.M.; Laukens, K.; Vanhaecke, T.; Covaci, A. In vitro assessment of hepatotoxicity by metabolomics: A review. *Arch. Toxicol.* **2018**, *92*, 3007–3029. [CrossRef] [PubMed]

6.   Negro, F.; Mondardine, A.; Palmas, F. Hepatotoxicity of saccharin. *N. Engl. J. Med.* **1994**, *330*, 134–135. [CrossRef] [PubMed]

7.   US National Library of Medicine Toxnet: Hazardous Substance Database—Saccharin. Available online: http://toxnet.nlm.nih.gov (accessed on 1 October 2018).

8.   Cuykx, M.; Claes, L.; Rodrigues, R.M.; Vanhaecke, T.; Covaci, A. Metabolomics profiling of steatosis progression in HepaRG® cells using sodium valproate. *Toxicol. Lett.* **2018**, *286*, 22–30. [CrossRef] [PubMed]
9.   Zhang, S.-Z.; Lipsky, M.M.; Trump, B.F.; Hsu, I.-C. Neutral red (NR) assay for cell viability and xenobiotic-induced cytotoxicity in primary cultures of human and rat hepatocytes. *Cell Biol. Toxicol.* **1990**, *6*, 219–234. [CrossRef]
10. Ates, G.; Vanhaecke, T.; Rogiers, V.; Rodrigues, R.M. Assaying cellular viability using the Neutral Red Uptake assay. Cell Viability Assays. In *Methods in Molecular Biology*; Humana Press: New York, NY, USA, 2017; pp. 19–26.
11. 1Hayton, S.; Maker, G.L.; Mullaney, I.; Trengove, R.D. Experimental design and reporting standards for metabolomics studies of mammalian cell lines. *Cell. Mol. Life Sci.* **2017**, *74*, 4421–4441. [CrossRef]
12. Wu, H.; Southam, A.D.; Hines, A.; Viant, M.R. High-throughput tissue extraction protocol for NMR- and MS-based metabolomics. *Anal. Biochem.* **2008**, *372*, 204–212. [CrossRef]
13. Cuykx, M.; Mortelé, O.; Rodrigues, R.M.; Vanhaecke, T.; Covaci, A. Optimisation of in vitro sample preparation for LC-MS metabolomics applications on HepaRG cell cultures. *Anal. Methods* **2017**, *9*, 3704–3712. [CrossRef]
14. Dunn, W.B.; Wilson, I.D.; Nicholls, A.W.; Broadhurst, D. The importance of experimental design and QC samples in large-scale and MS-driven untargeted metabolomic studies of humans. *Bioanalysis* **2012**, *4*, 2249–2264. [CrossRef] [PubMed]
15. Cuykx, M.; Negreira, N.; Beirnaert, C.; Van den Eede, N.; Rodrigues, R.; Vanhaecke, T.; Laukens, K.; Covaci, A. Tailored LC-MS analysis improves the coverage of the intracellular metabolome of HepaRG cells. *J. Chromatogr.* **2017**, *1487*, 168–178. [CrossRef] [PubMed]
16. R Core Team. *R: A Language and Environment for Statistical Computing*; R Foundation for Statistical Computing: Vienna, Austria, 2014.
17. Smith, C.A.; Want, E.J.; Maille, G.O.; Abagyan, R.; Siuzdak, G. XCMS: Processing mass spectrometry data for metabolite profiling using nonlinear peak alignment, matching, and identification. *ACS Publ.* **2006**, *78*, 779–787. [CrossRef]
18. Prince, J.T.; Marcotte, E.M. Chromatographic alignment of ESI-LC-MS proteomics data sets by ordered bijective interpolated warping. *Anal. Chem.* **2006**, *78*, 6140–6152. [CrossRef]
19. Beirnaert, C.; Cuykx, M.; Bijtebier, S. MetaboMeeseeks: Helper functions for metabolomics analysis. *R Package*. 2019. version 0.1.10044. Available online: https://github.com/Beirnaert/MetaboMeeseeks (accessed on 25 September 2019).
20. Wehrens, R.; Hageman, J.A.; van Eeuwijk, F.; Kooke, R.; Flood, P.J.; Wijnker, E.; Keurentjes, J.J.; Lommen, A.; van Eekelen, H.D.; Hall, R.D.; et al. Improved batch correction in untargeted MS-based metabolomics. *Metabolomics* **2016**, *12*, 88. [CrossRef]
21. Pollard, K.S.; Dudoit, S.; Van der Laan, M.J. Multiple Testing Procedures: The multtest Package and Applications to Genomics. In *Bioinformatics and Computational Biology Solutions Using R and Bioconductor*; Springer: New York, NY, USA, 2005; pp. 249–271.
22. Rohart, F.; Gautier, B.; Singh, A.; le Cao, K.-A. Le mixOmics: An R package for 'omics feature selection and multiple data integration. *PLoS Comput. Biol.* **2017**, *13*, e1005752. [CrossRef]
23. Schymanski, E.L.; Jeon, J.; Gulde, R.; Fenner, K.; Ruff, M.; Singer, H.P.; Hollender, J. Identifying small molecules via high resolution mass spectrometry: Communicating confidence. *Environ. Sci. Technol.* **2014**, *48*, 2097–2098. [CrossRef]
24. Sumner, L.W.; Amberg, A.; Barrett, D.; Beale, M.H.; Beger, R.; Daykin, C.A.; Fan, T.W.M.; Fiehn, O.; Goodacre, R.; Griffin, J.L.; et al. Proposed minimum reporting standards for chemical analysis: Chemical Analysis Working Group (CAWG) Metabolomics Standards Initiative (MSI). *Metabolomics* **2007**, *3*, 211–221. [CrossRef]
25. Burtis, C.; Ashwood, E.; Bruns, D. *Tietz Textbook of Clinical Chemistry and Molecular Diagnostics*; Elsevier: St. Louis, MO, USA, 2006; ISBN 13 978-0-7216-0189-2.
26. Sévin, D.C.; Stählin, J.N.; Pollak, G.R.; Kuehne, A.; Sauer, U. Global metabolic responses to salt stress in fifteen species. *PLoS ONE* **2016**, *11*, e0148888. [CrossRef]
27. García-Cañaveras, J.C.; Castell, J.V.; Donato, M.T.; Lahoz, A. A metabolomics cell-based approach for anticipating and investigating drug-induced liver injury. *Sci. Rep.* **2016**, *6*, 27239. [CrossRef] [PubMed]

28. Ramirez, T.; Strigun, A.; Verlohner, A.; Huener, H.A.; Peter, E.; Herold, M.; Bordag, N.; Mellert, W.; Walk, T.; Spitzer, M.; et al. Prediction of liver toxicity and mode of action using metabolomics in vitro in HepG2 cells. *Arch. Toxicol.* **2017**, *92*, 839–906. [CrossRef] [PubMed]
29. Cuykx, M.; Beirnaert, C.; Rodrigues, R.M.; Laukens, K.; Vanhaecke, T.; Covaci, A. Untargeted liquid chromatography-mass spectrometry metabolomics to assess drug-induced cholestatic features in HepaRG® cells. *Toxicol. Appl. Pharmacol.* **2019**, *379*, 114666. [CrossRef] [PubMed]

9

Nicotinamide and NAFLD: Is there Nothing New Under the Sun?

Maria Guarino [1,2] **and Jean-François Dufour** [1,3,*]

[1] Hepatology, Department for BioMedical Research, University of Bern, 3008 Bern, Switzerland
[2] Gastroenterology, Department of Clinical Medicine and Surgery, University of Naples Federico II, 80131 Naples, Italy
[3] University Clinic of Visceral Surgery and Medicine, Inselspital Bern, 3008 Bern, Switzerland
* Correspondence: jean-francois.dufour@dbmr.unibe.ch

Abstract: Nicotinamide adenine dinucleotide (NAD) has a critical role in cellular metabolism and energy homeostasis. Its importance has been established early with the discovery of NAD's therapeutic role for pellagra. This review addresses some of the recent findings on NAD physiopathology and their effects on nonalcoholic fatty liver disease (NAFLD) pathogenesis, which need to be considered in the search for a better therapeutic approach. Reduced NAD concentrations contribute to the dysmetabolic imbalance and consequently to the pathogenesis of NAFLD. In this perspective, the dietary supplementation or the pharmacological modulation of NAD levels appear to be an attractive strategy. These reviewed studies open the doors to growing interest in NAD metabolism for NAFLD diagnosis, prevention, and treatment. Future rigorous clinical studies in humans will be necessary to validate these preliminary but promising results.

Keywords: nicotinamide; NAFLD; steatosis

1. Introduction

The global diabesity (diabetes and obesity) [1] epidemic has dramatically increased the prevalence of nonalcoholic fatty liver disease (NAFLD), such that it is the most frequent cause of chronic liver disease. NAFLD is considered to be the liver manifestation of the metabolic syndrome, because of its frequent association with dyslipidemia, cardiovascular disease, obstructive sleep apnea, vitamin D deficiency, and other components of the metabolic syndrome, and insulin resistance is central to its pathogenesis [2,3].

Liver steatosis is the hallmark histologic feature of NAFLD, and it is the result of triglyceride accumulation in the hepatocytes cytoplasm. Liver lipid accumulation arises from an imbalance between lipid accumulation and removal, which is linked to increased liver lipogenesis, increased lipid uptake, and/or reduced triglyceride export or β-oxidation [4,5]. Liver secretion of triglycerides as very low-density lipoprotein (VLDL) particles for delivery to peripheral tissues is a crucial pathway for the mobilization of hepatic fat. Defects in VLDL processing are directly linked to hepatic steatosis. Jiang et al. showed that non-alcoholic steatohepatitis (NASH) was related to an increment in VLDL particle size, while hepatic fibrosis was related to a reduction in the concentration of small VLDL particles [6]. Moreover, there is a relationship between choline deficiency and accumulation of liver lipid, which is why choline-deficient diets are often used to induce NAFLD in animal models. Within hepatocytes, choline may be oxidized for phosphatidylcholine synthesis. Liver phosphatidylcholine is used to build the monolayers of VLDL, and its deficiency increases de novo hepatic lipogenesis [7].

The present model for NAFLD pathophysiology, called "the multiple-hit hypothesis", defines NAFLD as the manifestation of environmental and genetic factors, including the dysfunction of different organs and organelles, together with the intricate interaction between hepatocytes and other cells (such as stellate cells and Kupffer) in the liver [8]. Additionally, the liver is a hub for several metabolic pathways defining NAFLD as a multistep, progressive systemic disease.

2. NAD: Behind Its Metabolism

Nicotinamide adenine dinucleotide (NAD) is a hydride acceptor producing the reduced NADH, as well as the derivate phosphorylated dinucleotide pair NADP/NADPH, which is required for many cellular biosynthetic pathways and for protecting cells from reactive oxygen species (ROS). The keystone function of NAD is to facilitate hydrogen transfer in metabolic pathways as enzyme cofactors dealing with hydrogen transfer in reductive or oxidative metabolic reaction. So, it plays a central role in basic energy metabolism such as assisting with mitochondrial electron transport, glycolysis, the oxidation of fatty acids and amino acids in mitochondria, and the citric acid cycle. NAD is also a substrate for signaling enzymes such as poly (ADP ribose) polymerase (PARP), sirtuins (SIRTs), and ADP ribosyl transferases, called "NAD consumers" [9] (Figure 1). For example, it is involved in repairing and maintaining genomic integrity, thanks to PARP, which transfers ADP-ribose from NAD to itself, histones, and other proteins at sites of DNA damage.

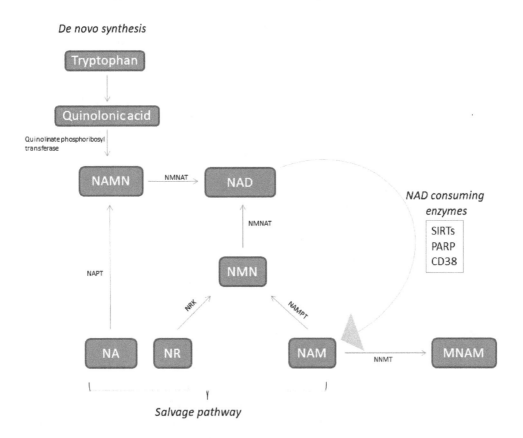

Figure 1. NAD synthesis pathways. NA, nicotinic acid; NAD, nicotinamide adenine dinucleotide; NAM, nicotinamide; NAMN, nicotinic acid mononucleotide; NAPT, nicotinic acid phosphoribosyltransferase; NMN, nicotinamide mononucleotide; NMNAT, nicotinamide nucleotide adenylyltransferase; NR, nicotinamide riboside; NRK, NR kinase; NNMT, nicotinamide-N-methyltransferase; PARP, poly (ADP ribose) polymerase; NNMT, nicotinamide N-methyltransferase; NAMPT, nicotinamide phosphoribosyltransferase; SIRT, sirtuin.

The cellular NAD pool is created by a balance between the activity of NAD-consuming and synthesizing enzymes [10–12]. NAD concentrations display the cell energy state and are modulated by physiological processes. In fact, during fasting, caloric restriction, and exercise, NAD levels increase. Conversely, caloric excess and aging diminish NAD levels [13].

NAD is synthesized from four distinct biosynthetic precursors in two different pathways (Figure 1). De novo synthesis (the deamidated pathway) uses as precursor the dietary amino acid tryptophan, which is metabolized to create biosynthetic intermediates. In particular, the creation of unstable α-amino-β-carboxymuconate-ε-semialdehyde (ACMS) forms a branching point of the deaminated pathway. The ACMS is subjected to both non-enzymatic cyclization or complete enzymatic oxidation to quinolinic acid, and this is the first limiting step [14]. The second limiting mechanism involves the catalytic conversion of quinolinic acid to nicotinic acid mononucleotide (NAMN) by quinolinate phosphoribosyl transferase. Next, NAMN is transformed into NAD by the nicotinamide mononucleotide adenylyltransferase (NMNAT) enzyme. This pathway is recognized as the minor contributor to the total NAD pool [14].

Dietary vitamin B3 compounds, including nicotinic acid (NA), also known as niacin, NAM, and nicotinamide riboside (NR), supply as NAD biosynthetic precursors and are rescued from the diet (the amidated pathway) for generating cellular NAD. This salvage pathway is the most relevant for NAD homeostasis [15]. NA is converted to NAMN by nicotinic acid phosphoribosyltransferase (NAPT), which is afterward converted to NAD by NMNAT. The NAM and NR are transformed into NMN by nicotinamide phosphoribosyltransferase (NAMPT) and NR kinase (NRK) enzymes, respectively. Finally, NMN is enzymatically transformed into NAD by NMNAT [15].

NAMPT, also known with the name visfatin, is a highly conserved protein with cytokine functions, which is expressed in almost all tissues and cells (Figure 1) [16]. In particular, it is an essential regulator of the intracellular NAD pool by catalyzing the formation of nicotinamide mononucleotide (NMN) from nicotinamide and 5′-phosphoribosyl-1-pyrophosphate, which is the limiting step in the NAD salvage pathway [17]. NAMPT has both intracellular and extracellular forms in mammals. The extracellular NAMPT (eNAMPT) is secreted from adipocytes [18], hepatocytes [19], and leucocytes [20] and circulates in the blood where, additionally to its enzymatic function, it has also cytokine-like actions [16,21,22]. In virtue of its NAD biosynthetic activity, intracellular NAMPT (iNAMPT) controls the activity of NAD-dependent and consuming enzymes, such as SIRTs [23], the NADase CD38 (a cyclic ADP-ribose synthesis) [24], and PARPs [25], by which it controls mitochondrial biogenesis, cellular metabolism [26], and adaptive responses to oxidative, inflammatory, genotoxic, and proteotoxic stress [27]. Genotoxic stress and nutrient deprivation activate NAMPT, which protects cells from these stresses through the maintenance of the mitochondrial NAD level [23].

The NAD levels are also regulated by the cytosolic enzyme nicotinamide-N-methyltransferase (NNMT), which methylates nicotinamide to produce N1-methyl nicotinamide (MNAM) toward the universal methyl donor S-adenosylmethionine as a methyl donor (Figure 1). NNMT is mainly expressed in the liver, but also in other organs such as muscle, adipose tissue, and heart. An increase of NNMT expression has been observed in obesity and diabetes [28–30].

SIRTs are NAD-dependent deacylases [31]. SIRTs have key roles in response to environmental and nutritional perturbations, such as DNA damage, oxidative stress, and fasting. For this reason, SIRTs have to be considered as nutritional sensors that operate in regulating glucose and lipid homeostasis, inflammatory responses, and cell death [23,32–34]. Additionally, SIRTs influence cells' metabolism through the regulation of the circadian clock machinery with the deacetylation of central clock components in the liver [35,36]. Accordingly, NAD synthesis is controlled by the circadian machinery to furnish a crucial link from the clock oscillator to metabolic pathways [37]. NAD is synthesized with circadian oscillations, leading to a circadian schedule of SIRT activation and mitochondrial metabolism, such as the oxidation of fatty acids [38]. SIRTs' activity is dependent on its cofactor NAD and it is sensitive to the cellular NAD levels [39], designating NAD as a rate-limiting substrate for their reactions [32,40,41]. As NAM is the product of SIRT-catalyzed deacetylation reactions, high levels of NAM have been used as a SIRTs inhibitor [42]. This drives speculation that enzymes involved in NAD synthesis could control SIRTs' activity. For example, an increment in NAD was proposed by Lin et al. to mediate the health span and extension of life by dietary restriction [43], and recently, studies demonstrated that the activity of SIRTs declines with aging by a systemic reduction in NAD levels [44,45].

3. NAD Involvement in NAFLD Pathogenesis

In the last years, an emerging role of NAD metabolism in protection against NAFLD stimulated a growing interest. Von Shönfels et al. performed a small-molecule metabolite screen of human hepatic tissue to find metabolic markers related to NASH histology. According to its concentration in liver tissue, they suggested a protective effect of NA, which was subsequently verified in a nutritional animal model of NAFLD showing a marked effect on steatosis and transaminases levels with NA supplementation [46]. NAD deficiency decreases the oxidation of fatty acids, promoting steatosis [47]. Usually, the triglycerides are broken down into glycerol and fatty acids, so they can enter into the mitochondria and proceed on with fatty acid oxidation. Fatty acids shift in this pathway as Coenzyme A (CoA) derivatives utilizing NAD. The acetyl groups created by the β-oxidation of the fatty acid take part in the activity of the Krebs cycle, causing the formation of NADH. The reduced coenzyme (NADH) is oxidized by leaving the protons and electrons to oxygen in the mitochondria to synthesize ATP in the electron transport system [48]. So, NAD deficiency causes a reduction of β-oxidation, and consequently the accumulation of triglycerides in the hepatocytes (steatosis).

The control of rate-limiting enzymes of NAD biosynthesis avoids the negative effects of high-fat diet (HFD) and keeps up insulin sensitivity and glucose homeostasis. Penke et al. [49] reported increased hepatic NAD levels in mice under HFD thanks to increased NAMPT expression. So, it seems that NAD deficiency is a crucial risk factor for NAFLD resulting from having compromised the NAMPT-controlled NAD salvage pathway in liver [50]. Plasma levels of eNAMPT may be closely linked to NAFLD, obesity, diabetes, and atherosclerosis [51–54]. Moreover, decreased NAMPT expression in NAMPT +/− mice, which reduced circulating NMN levels and decreased NAD levels in brown adipose tissue, impaired glucose-stimulated insulin secretion [22]. This event can be rescued by NMN supplementation, suggesting that the maintenance of NAD concentrations is critical for pancreatic function [22].

The mechanisms of NAMPT protecting the liver from HFD are depicted in Figure 2. NAMPT induces the production of NAD by activating the NAD salvage pathway, and consecutively, the augmented NAD (as a substrate) activates the SIRT 1 and 3 signaling pathways, alleviating HFD-induced hepatic steatosis. De novo lipogenesis (DNL) is known to be high in individuals with NAFLD, and provides about 26% of hepatic lipids [55,56]. The NAMPT is critical for the formation of acetyl-CoA and for the increase of fatty acid oxidation by providing NAD for SIRT3 with the activation of acetyl-CoA synthetase (ACS) [57]. At the same time, the activation of SIRT1 by NAMPT promotes the deacetylation of sterol regulatory element-binding protein 1 (SREBP1), which inhibits SREBP1 activity, resulting in the lower expression of lipogenesis genes, including fatty acid synthase (FAS) and acetyl-CoA carboxylase (ACC). Additionally, SIRT 1 directly activates AMP-activated protein kinase (AMPK), which further inhibits SREBP1 activity. All together, these results show that NAMPT modulates processes involved in NAFLD pathogenesis (such as de novo lipogenesis and fatty acid oxidation). Accordingly, Zhou et al. showed that dominant negative-NAMPT transgenic mice, under normal chow, display systemic NAD decrease and had a moderate NASH phenotype, with enhanced oxidative stress, lipid accumulation, impaired insulin sensitivity, and triggered inflammation in liver. These features deteriorate further under HFD [50].

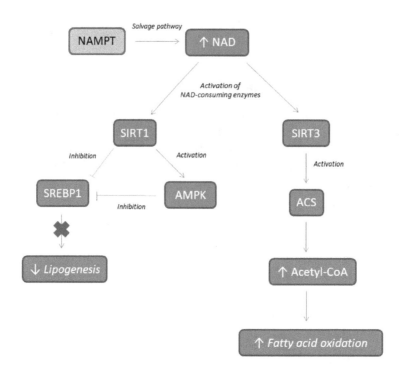

Figure 2. NAMPT involvement in lipids metabolism. NAMPT, nicotinamide phosphoribosyltransferase; NAD, nicotinamide adenine dinucleotide; ACS, acetyl-CoA synthetase; AMPK, AMP-activated protein kinase; SIRT, sirtuin; SREBP1, sterol regulatory element-binding protein 1.

NNMT has also been associated to the development of diabetes, obesity, and metabolic syndrome [28–30]. An increase of NNMT expression has been observed in obesity and diabetes [28–30], probably because NNMT controls lipid, cholesterol, and glucose metabolism by stabilizing SIRTs [58]. In humans, adipose tissue NNMT expression and its product MNAM correlate positively with insulin resistance. Kannt et al. [29] showed an increased expression of NNMT in the adipose tissue of diabetic patients according to the insulin resistance severity, suggesting that NNMT could be a "bad actor" limiting fuel oxidation and promoting fat storage. NNMT protein levels are upregulated in the liver and adipose tissue of mouse models of insulin resistance and obesity, and NNMT knockdown has a protective effect against the metabolic consequences of HFD [28], suggesting that NNMT may have a critical role in NAFLD pathogenesis. The dietary regulation of liver NNMT expression, the site of its major expression, shows some interesting patterns. The ketogenic diet suppresses liver NNMT expression, contributing to the increased liver and serum cholesterol levels in this model [59]. Conversely, caloric restriction increased NNMT liver expression, promoting SIRT1 protein stability, which mediates several metabolic effects of caloric restriction [60]. Liver NNMT expression inversely correlates with serum triglycerides (TGs), cholesterol, and free fatty acid levels, suggesting that increased liver NNMT expression is associated with a better metabolic profile, contrary to its expression in adipose tissue [28,29]. Furthermore, a genome-wide association study showed significant associations between the risk of developing NASH and a specific single-nucleotide polymorphisms (SNPs) in the NNMT gene (rs694539) [61]: in this case, subjects with the AA genotype showed a statistically significant increased NASH risk, while the GG genotype seemed to be protective. Similarly, Hasan et al. showed that the AA genotype correlates with the degree of steatosis as detected by the controlled attenuation parameter, even if it does not correlate with the degree of fibrosis detected by FibroScan [62].

4. NAD as Biomarker for NAFLD Diagnosis

The identification of non-invasive biomarkers has become a major focus of interest in NAFLD. Since the diagnosis of NASH is still a histological one, the dramatic increase in the prevalence of

NAFLD and its severity spectrum mean that liver biopsy is not feasible for all patients. Current plasma biomarkers include predictive models for diagnosing or grading steatosis (such as the fatty liver index) or staging fibrosis (such as the NAFLD fibrosis score), and other ones specific to NAFLD (such as the BARD and NAFLD fibrosis scores), even if some have been initially developed in a hepatitis C setting (AST/ALT ratio, APRI, FIB-4) [63].

Several studies evaluated the relationship between NAD metabolism and NAFLD [29,64–68] (Table 1). Human studies investigated how plasma and liver NAMPT protein levels are affected in subjects with steatosis and NAFLD [64–68]. Gaddipati et al. [64] showed that a significant reduction in the NAMPT levels of the visceral adipose tissue is associated to degree of steatosis in NAFLD patients. Similarly, Amirkalali et al. [68] showed that higher serum NAMPT is associated with lower liver DNL in female subjects (probably associated with a higher adipose tissue DNL according to the higher fat mass), while the only significant association in male subjects was between serum NAMPT and liver fat content, probably for the inflammatory role of NAMPT. Thus, the plasma NAMPT levels could have a different meaning for each sex because of the opposing effects of liver and adipose tissue DNL on NAFLD pathogenesis. Conversely, Kannt et al. [29] showed that NNMT mRNA in adipose tissue and 1-methylnicotinamide serum concentrations are higher in patients with insulin resistance and correlate with insulin resistance severity. An additional interesting result is that improvements of insulin sensitivity obtained with exercise and bariatric surgery are associated with a reduction of NNMT expression in adipose tissue and of 1-methylnicotinamide serum levels [29].

5. NAD Supplementation for NAFLD Prevention

The evidence for using dietary supplementation to prevent chronic disease is a longstanding issue of debate. Several evidences are emerging to support the hypothesis that supplementation with NAD precursors could protect against metabolic imbalance and liver steatosis (Table 2) [12,49,69–71]. A supplementation study with NMN showed its property to restore NAD levels either in nuclear and mitochondrial cells compartments and to prevent diet-induced and age-induced diabetes in C57BL/6 mice [12]. Tao et al. showed that NAMPT gives resistance to hepatic steatosis through NAD synthesis [69], and NR supplementation gives protection against steatosis in mice under high-fat/high-sucrose diet [70,71]. NAM supplementation protects hepatocytes from palmitate-induced cell death, and autophagy induction contributes to the anti-lipotoxic property of NAM through SIRT1 activation in hepatocytes. Additionally, NAM prevents hepatic alterations in glucose-6-phosphate dehydrogenase and the redox state, and attenuates increased serum FFA, oxidative stress, inflammation, and hepatic damage in high fructose or high glucose consumption-induced liver steatosis in rats [72]. Lastly, Komatsu et al. showed that NNMT and NAM supplementation causes liver steatosis and fibrosis, although increased lipid metabolism and decreased adiposity. NNMT overexpression induces genes for liver steatosis and fibrosis by decreasing tissue NAD content and methylation pool, suggesting that NNMT connects NAD and methionine metabolism and causes NAFLD progression [73]. Thus, NAD supplementation may represent a preventive treatment for metabolic dysfunctions such as diabetes, and NAFLD spectrum disease, from steatosis to NASH.

6. NAD Supplementation for NAFLD Treatment

The relevance of dietary NAD precursors in health is well known, thanks to the historical use of NA and NAM in the treatment of dietary tryptophan deficits (pellagra) and hyperlipidemia, although high-dose NA use is limited by painful flushing, while high-dose NAM is hepatotoxic [74,75]. In fact, the use of NA is associated with a flush of face and chest and a sensation of warmth or burning. NA causes flushing principally by releasing prostaglandins D2 and E2 from skin cells, which afterwards dilates skin arterioles [76,77]. The precursors NA, NMN, and NR, but also PARP or CD38 inhibitors, rise NAD levels in different mice cells and tissues [12,13,70]. Boosting NAD concentrations can be therapeutic in metabolic diseases such as diabetes [12,53] and NAFLD [70], and potentially protects against obesity [51] and age-related disorders (Table 3).

Due to its ability to increase NAD synthesis without inducing side effects [44,70], NR has been used in mice to increase NAD metabolism and improve health in models of metabolic stress, showing that NR abolishes DNA damage in HFD-fed mice [70,78]. Canto et al. [70] treated mice with NR (400 mg/kg animal weight per day), demonstrating an increase of NAD levels in muscle and liver. Mice under HFD were protected from body weight increase and showed an improvement of mitochondrial function and fatty acids oxidation as a fuel source. In accordance with increases in tissue NAD levels, SIRT1 and SIRT3 were upregulated [70]. NR also ameliorated insulin sensitivity in weight-matched mice [70]. Similarly, Zhou et al. [50] demonstrated that the oral administration of NR corrects NAFLD phenotypes induced by NAD deficiency alone or combined with HFD. Trammell et al. [79] performed a clinical study enrolling 12 healthy subjects receiving three single doses of NR, demonstrating that NR supplementation safely induces NAD metabolism at all doses. They also demonstrated that NR is more orally bioavailable than NAM, which is more orally bioavailable than NA. The capability of NR to increase ADPR is threefold higher than NAM. This validates NR as the preferred NAD precursor vitamin for boosting NAD and NAD-consuming activities in liver. No dose-dependent side effects of NR have been reported, contrary to high-dose NAM, which may lead to liver damage [15]. Shi et al. [80] carried out a dose–response dietary intervention mice study using a wide range of NR (from 5 to 900 mg NR per kg of an obesogenic diet), concluding that 30 mg/kg diet constitutes the best concentration to reinforce metabolic health. These studies showed the powerful biological effects of NR in mitigating the negative consequences of HFDs [70,71,81,82], suggesting that NAD substrates supplementation may be a promising therapeutic strategy for preventing and treating NAFLD/NASH.

Another possibility to modulate NAD levels consists of using NMN. Supplementation with NMN, an enzymatic product of NAMPT, improves diabetes [12,13] and other damages such as vascular dysfunction, oxidative stress [83], and cognitive impairment [84]. Yoshino et al. demonstrated that increasing NAD biosynthesis by the intraperitoneal injection of NMN improves glucose homeostasis in obese mice, and that NAMPT activity is altered by HFD and can cause diabetes [12]. Similarly, supplementation with MNAM significantly reduces hepatic cholesterol and triglycerides concentrations, by suppressing fatty acid and cholesterol synthesis and the expression of lipogenic and cholesterol synthesis genes [58]. MNAM supplementation produces a selective reduction in larger lipoprotein particles but not high-density lipoprotein, suggesting that MNAM or its derivatives could be used to reduce low-density lipoprotein levels [58].

Another attractive angle to modulate NAD levels consists in targeting the activity of NAD-consuming enzymes, such as CD38 [10] and PARPs [11]. Several studies showed that CD38 knockout (KO) mice have higher NAD levels than Wild-type (WT) animals, and are protected against obesity and metabolic syndrome [10,85]. The treatment of obese mice with CD38 inhibitors augments intracellular NAD concentrations and improves glucose and lipid homeostasis [86]. Increased PARP activity causes an elevated consumption of cellular NAD, which is associated to increased ATP consumption, compromising energy balance and facilitating cell death [87]. Upon persistent PARP activation, decreased mitochondrial ATP production inhibits NAD re-synthesis, creating a feed-forward loop in ATP-consuming processes, and resulting in metabolic catastrophe and cell death. PARP inhibition causes an increase in NAD levels. Rucaparib (a PARP inhibitor) significantly increases hepatic NAD levels, as previously described with NAM treatment [88], while in PARP1 KO liver, NAD levels were similar to those in treated PARP1 WT liver. So, CD38 and PARP inhibition combined with NAD precursors may be an intriguing therapeutic perspective for NAFLD [13].

Finally, Katsiuba et al. presented an additional mechanism for increasing NAD levels toward the inhibition of the ACMS decarboxylase with a selective inhibitor recently developed, TES-991. ACMS decarboxylase inhibition in a mouse model of diet-induced NAFLD increased levels of NAD and the activation of SIRT1 with improvement of the NAFLD phenotype, without systemic side effects [14].

Table 1. NAD as biomarker for NAFLD diagnosis.

Biomarker	Study Design	Analyzed Tissue	Results	Ref.
NAMPT	77 NAFLD patients vs. 38 control patients (all undergoing diagnostic laparoscopy)	Visceral adipose tissue (VAT)	Reduction of NAMPT levels in VAT according to the degree of steatosis	Gaddipati et al. [64]
NAMPT	69 obese women with NAFLD vs. 19 obese women vs. 38 healthy women	Liver tissue and serum	Serum NAMPT and its liver expression are higher in obese women with NAFLD, irrespective of the presence of diabetes	Auguet et al. [65]
NAMPT	58 NAFLD patients vs. 27 healthy controls	Liver tissue and serum	NAFLD patients had decreased NAMPT expression both in serum and in liver tissue, with no difference between simple steatosis and NASH	Dahl et al. [52]
NAMPT	40 severely obese patients with NAFLD	Liver tissue	Positive association between NAMPT expression and the fibrosis stage in NAFLD	Kukla et al. [67]
NAMPT	62 NAFLD patients (32 males, 30 females)	Serum	Higher serum NAMPT in women was associated with a lower hepatic DNL index, while in men, it was associated with higher hepatic fat, and had no association with the DNL index	Amirkalali et al. [68]
NNMT and 1-Methylnicotinamide	199 patients undergoing abdominal surgery (111 diabetic and 88 non-diabetic); 60 individuals on a 12-week exercise program (20 diabetic, 20 insulin-resistant, and 20 with normal glucose tolerance)	Serum and white adipose tissue (WAT)	Patients with diabetes have a twofold higher NNMT expression. There is an inverse correlation between insulin sensitivity and plasma 1-methylnicotinamide and WAT NNMT expression.	Kannt et al. [29]

NAMPT, nicotinamide phosphoribosyltransferase; NNMT, nicotinamide-N-methyltransferase.

Table 2. NAD supplementation for NAFLD prevention.

Preventive Supplementation	Study Design	Results	Ref.
NMN	C57BL/6, HFD vs. control diet	NMN ameliorates glucose intolerance by restoring NAD levels, enhances hepatic insulin sensitivity, and restores gene expression related to oxidative stress, inflammatory response, and circadian rhythm, partly through SIRT1 activation.	Yoshino et al. [12]
Nicotinamide	HepG2 cells and alpha mouse liver (AML)-12 hepatocyte transfected with human SIRT1 siRNA under palmitate-elicited hepatotoxicity	Nicotinamide supplementation protects hepatocytes against palmitate-induced cell death. SIRT1 inhibition abrogates the nicotinamide anti-lipotoxic effect.	Shen et al. [42]
NR	C57Bl/6J, HFD vs. control diet; murine C2C12 myoblasts, murine Hepa1.6, and human HEK293T cells, with or without deletion of the SIRT3 gene	NR prevents diet-induced obesity by enhancing energy expenditure, reducing cholesterol levels, and increasing intracellular and mitochondrial NAD content both in cell and in vivo experiments. NR enhances SIRT1 and SIRT3 activity and energy expenditure, and ameliorates the oxidative performance of skeletal muscle and brown adipose tissue.	Canto et al. [70]
NR	C57BL/6J mice, high-fat and high-sucrose diet vs. control diet; primary hepatocytes from SIRT1 floxed or SIRT3 floxed mice	NR prevents NAFLD by inducing a sirtuin-dependent mitochondrial unfolded protein response, triggering an adaptive mitohormetic pathway to increase hepatic β-oxidation and mitochondrial complex content and activity.	Gariani et al. [71]
NAM	Male Sprague–Dawley rats were randomly distributed into six groups according to the following treatments: (1) Control; (2) Glucose; (3) Glucose+NAM 0.06%; (4) Glucose+NAM 0.12%; (5) Fructose; and (6) Fructose+NAM 0.12%.	NAM attenuates increases in levels of FFA, thiobarbituric acid reactive substances, and markers of hepatic damage induced by high glucose or fructose. NAM decreases hepatic steatosis. NAM only partially prevented changes in the glutathione/glutathione disulfide levels and redox potential, as well as pro-inflammatory conditions. NAM mitigates increases in hepatic glucose-6-phosphate dehydrogenase mRNA, protein levels, and specific activity induced by glucose or fructose.	Mejia et al. [72]
NAM	C57Bl/6J transgenic mice overexpressing NNMT vs. wild type, HFD + water containing 1% NAM	NNMT overactivation decreases the NAD content in the liver and decreases gene activity related to fatty acid oxidation by inhibiting SIRT3 and fibrosis by reducing the tissue NAD content and methylation pool.	Komatsu et al. [73]

NR, nicotinamide riboside; NMN, nicotinamide mononucleotide; HFD, high-fat diet.

Table 3. NAD supplementation for NAFLD treatment.

Treatment	Study design	Results	ref
NR	C57Bl/6J, HFD vs. control diet.	Long-term NR administration in vivo lowers HFD-induced body weight gain by enhancing energy expenditure, and ameliorates insulin-sensitivity and cholesterol profiles.	Canto et al. [70]
NR	Dominant negative (DN)-NAMPT transgenic C57EL/6J, HFD vs. control diet.	DN-NAMPT mice under control diet displays systemic NAD reduction and had moderate NAFLD phenotypes, including lipid accumulation, enhanced oxidative stress, triggered inflammation, and impaired insulin sensitivity in liver. All these NAFLD phenotypes deteriorate further under HFD challenge. Oral administration of NR completely corrects these NAFLD phenotypes induced by NAD deficiency alone or with HFD.	Zhou et al. [50]
NR	C57BL/6JRcc mice. semi-synthetic obesogenic diet containing 0.14% L-tryptophan and either 5, 15, 30, 180, or 900 mg NR per kg diet	There is a dose–response effect to NR; in particular, mice fed a 30 mg NR/kg diet are more metabolically flexible than the wide range of other NR concentrations. Moreover, in epididymal white adipose tissue, the gene expression of Peroxisome-proliferator-activated receptor-γ (Ppar-γ), Superoxide dismutase-2 (SOD2) and Peroxiredoxin 3 (Prdx3) - are significantly upregulated in mice fed 30 mg NR/kg.	Shi et al. [80]
NR	Obese-diabetic KK/HIJ mice, control or NR group	Total cholesterol concentration in the liver, glucose control, and levels of serum insulin and adiponectin are improved by NR. At liver histology, NR rescues the disrupted cellular integrity of the mitochondria and nucleus of obese–diabetic KK mice. In addition, NR treatment significantly improves hepatic pro-inflammatory markers, including tumor necrosis factor-alpha, Interleukin (IL) 6, and IL-1. These results demonstrate that NR attenuates hepatic metaflammation by modulating the NLRP3 inflammasome.	Lee et al. [81]
NR	C57BL/6J, HFD vs. control diet	NR improves glucose tolerance, and reduces weight gain, liver damage, and hepatic steatosis.	Trammell et al. [82]
MNAM	C57BL/6J, HFD vs. control diet	MNAM significantly lowers liver and serum cholesterol and TG levels, while also suppressing fatty acid and cholesterol synthesis and the expression of lipogenic and cholesterol synthesis genes. MNAM-supplemented mice have higher liver SIRT1 protein expression. Consistent with higher SIRT1 protein expression, liver FoxO1 acetylation is significantly lower. MNAM-fed mice had significantly lower liver expression of the pro-inflammatory cytokines.	Hong et al. [58]

Table 3. *Cont.*

Treatment	Study design	Results	ref
Flavonoid Apigenin (CD38 inhibitor)	C57BL/6, HFD vs. control diet	Apigenin inhibits CD38 and is associated with increased NAD and decreased protein acetylation, likely through the activation of SIRT1. Apigenin improves glucose homeostasis in vivo and promotes fatty acid oxidation in the liver.	Escande et al. [86]
PARP-1 inhibitors	HeLa cells exposed to the PARP-1-activating agent N-methyl-N′-nitro-N-nitrosoguanidine (MNNG) or to PARP-1 inhibitors after MNNG exposure.	PARP-1 hyperactivity in the nucleus rapidly impairs ATP production in mitochondria, whereas the release of the pro-apoptotic factors AIF/Cyt-c from mitochondria only occurs several hours after PARP-1 hyperactivation. PARP-1 inhibitors are able to prevent MNNG-induced nucleotide depletion, apoptosis-inducing factor (AIF) release, and cell death.	Cipriani et al. [87]
Rucaparib (PARP1 inhibitor)	PARP1 wild-type (WT) and PARP1 knock-out (KO) mice	In PARP1 WT livers, the NAD concentration in the rucaparib-treated group was significantly higher when compared with the concentration in untreated mice, and similar to the concentration in KO mice.	Almeida et al. [88]
TES-991 (ACMS decarboxylase inhibitor)	C57BL/6J under methionine-choline deficient (MCD) diet	Supplementing the MCD diet with TES-991 increases hepatic NAD, attenuates hepatic steatosis and plasma transaminases levels, protects against hepatic lipid accumulation, attenuates inflammation, recovers hepatic SOD2 activity and ATP content, and reverses NAFLD changes in the transcription of genes involved in ROS defense, β-oxidation, inflammation, and mitochondrial function.	Katsyuba et al. [14]

NR, nicotinamide riboside; MNAM, N1-methyl nicotinamide; PARP1, poly (ADP ribose) polymerase 1; HFD, high fat diet.

7. Conclusions

Until now, there is still no approved drug for the treatment of NAFLD, and although lifestyle modification appears beneficial in patients with NAFLD, no single approach is likely to be suitable for all patients. NAD reduction might be caused by the imbalance in NAD biosynthesis and depletion, both of which occur in NAFLD. NAD reduction may induce NAFLD through decreased SIRT activities in the nucleus and mitochondria. The supplementation of key NAD intermediates, such as NMN and NR, can ameliorate NAFLD.

Author Contributions: Conceptualization, J.-F.D. and M.G.; Literature Analysis, M.G.; Writing—Original Draft Preparation, M.G. and J.-F.D.; Writing—Review and Editing, M.G. and J.-F.D.

Abbreviations

ACC, acetyl-CoA carboxylase; ACMS, amino-β-carboxymuconate-ε-semialdehyde; ACS, acetyl-CoA synthetase; ADPR, ADP ribose; AMPK, AMP-activated protein kinase; DNL, de novo lipogenesis; eNAMPT, extracellular NAMPT; FAS, fatty acid synthase; FFA, free fatty acid; HCC, hepatocellular carcinoma; HFD, high fat diet; iNAMPT, intracellular NAMPT; KO, knock-out; MNAM, N1-methyl nicotinamide; NA, nicotinic acid; NAD, nicotinamide adenine dinucleotide; NADP, phosphorylated nicotinamide adenine dinucleotide; NAFLD, nonalcoholic fatty liver disease; NAM, nicotinamide; NAMN, NA mononucleotide; NAMPT, nicotinamide phosphoribosyltransferase; NAPRT1, nicotinate phosphoribosyltransferase domain containing 1; NASH, non-alcoholic steatohepatitis; NMN, nicotinamide mononucleotide; NMNAT, nicotinamide nucleotide adenylyltransferase 3; NNMT, nicotinamide-N-methyltransferase; NR, nicotinamide riboside; NRK, NR kinase; PARP, poly (ADP ribose) polymerase; ROS, reactive oxygen species; SIRT, sirtuin; SREBP1, sterol regulatory element-binding protein 1; TNF-α, tumor necrosis factor-α; WT, wild-type.

References

1. Kalra, S. Diabesity. *J. Pak. Med. Assoc.* **2013**, *63*, 532–534.
2. Musso, G.; Gambino, R.; De Michieli, F.; Cassader, M.; Rizzetto, M.; Durazzo, M.; Fagà, E.; Silli, B.; Pagano, G. Dietary habits and their relations to insulin resistance and postprandial lipemia in nonalcoholic steatohepatitis. *Hepatology* **2003**, *37*, 909–916. [CrossRef]
3. Sookoian, S.; Burgueno, A.L.; Castano, G.; Pirola, C.J. Should nonalcoholic fatty liver disease be included in the definition of metabolic syndrome? A cross-sectional comparison with adult treatment panel III criteria in nonobese nondiabetic subjects: Response to Musso. *Diabetes Care* **2008**, *31*, e42. [CrossRef]
4. Kawano, Y.; Cohen, D.E. Mechanisms of hepatic triglyceride accumulation in non-alcoholic fatty liver disease. *J. Gastroenterol.* **2013**, *48*, 434–441. [CrossRef]
5. Koo, S.H. Nonalcoholic fatty liver disease: Molecular mechanisms for the hepatic steatosis. *Clin. Mol. Hepatol.* **2013**, *19*, 210–215. [CrossRef]
6. Jiang, Z.G.; Tapper, E.B.; Connelly, M.A.; Pimentel, C.F.; Feldbrügge, L.; Kim, M.; Krawczyk, S.; Afdhal, N.; Robson, S.C.; Herman, M.A.; et al. Steatohepatitis and liver fibrosis are predicted by the characteristics of very low density lipoprotein in nonalcoholic fatty liver disease. *Liver Int.* **2016**, *36*, 1213–1220. [CrossRef]
7. Sherriff, J.L.; O'Sullivan, T.A.; Properzi, C.; Oddo, J.L.; Adams, L.A. Choline, its potential role in nonalcoholic fatty liver disease, and the case for human and bacterial genes. *Adv. Nutr.* **2016**, *7*, 5–13. [CrossRef]
8. Buzzetti, E.; Pinzani, M.; Tsochatzis, E.A. The multiple-hit pathogenesis of non-alcoholic fatty liver disease (NAFLD). *Metabolism* **2016**, *65*, 1038–1048. [CrossRef]
9. Canto, C.; Auwerx, J. NAD$^+$ as a signaling molecule modulating metabolism. *Cold Spring Harb. Symp. Quant. Biol.* **2011**, *76*, 291–298. [CrossRef]
10. Barbosa, M.T.; Soares, S.M.; Novak, C.M.; Sinclair, D.; Levine, J.A.; Aksoy, P.; Chini, E.N. The enzyme CD38 (a NAD glycohydrolase, EC 3.2.2.5) is necessary for the development of diet-induced obesity. *FASEB J.* **2007**, *21*, 3629–3639. [CrossRef]
11. Bai, P.; Cantó, C.; Oudart, H.; Brunyánszki, A.; Cen, Y.; Thomas, C.; Yamamoto, H.; Huber, A.; Kiss, B.; Houtkooper, R.H.; et al. PARP-1 inhibition increases mitochondrial metabolism through SIRT1 activation. *Cell Metab.* **2011**, *13*, 461–468. [CrossRef]
12. Yoshino, J.; Mills, K.F.; Yoon, M.J.; Imai, S.I. Nicotinamide mononucleotide, ia key NAD(+) intermediate, treats the pathophysiology of diet- and age-induced diabetes in mice. *Cell Metab.* **2011**, *14*, 528–536. [CrossRef]

13. Mouchiroud, L.; Houtkooper, R.H.; Auwerx, J. NAD$^+$ metabolism: A therapeutic target for age-related metabolic disease. *Crit. Rev. Biochem. Mol. Biol.* **2013**, *48*, 397–408. [CrossRef]

14. Katsyuba, E.; Mottis, A.; Zietak, M.; De Franco, F.; van der Velpen, V.; Gariani, K.; Ryu, D.; Cialabrini, L.; Matilainen, O.; Liscio, P.; et al. De novo NAD$^+$ synthesis enhances mitochondrial function and improves health. *Nature* **2018**, *563*, 354–359. [CrossRef]

15. Bogan, K.L.; Brenner, C. Nicotinic acid, nicotinamide, and nicotinamide riboside: A molecular evaluation of NAD$^+$ precursor vitamins in human nutrition. *Annu. Rev. Nutr.* **2008**, *28*, 115–130. [CrossRef]

16. Samal, B.; Sun, Y.; Stearns, G.; Xie, C.; Suggs, S.; McNiece, I. Cloning and characterization of the cDNA encoding a novel human pre-B-cell colony enhancing factor. *Mol. Cell Biol.* **1994**, *14*, 1431–1437. [CrossRef]

17. Rongvaux, A.; Shea, R.J.; Mulks, M.H.; Gigot, D.; Urbain, J.; Leo, O.; Andris, F. Pre-B cell colony-enhancing factor, whose expression is up-regulated in activated lymphocytes, is a nicotinamide phosphoribosyltransferase, a cytosolic enzyme involved in NAD biosynthesis. *Eur. J. Immunol.* **2002**, *32*, 3225–3234. [CrossRef]

18. Tanaka, M.; Nozaki, M.; Fukuhara, A.; Segawa, K.; Aoki, N.; Matsuda, M.; Komuro, R.; Shimomura, I. Visfatin is released from 3T3-L1 adipocytes via a non-classical pathway. *Biochem. Biophys. Res. Commun.* **2007**, *359*, 194–201. [CrossRef]

19. Garten, A.; Petzold, S.; Barnikol-Oettler, A.; Körner, A.; Thasler, W.E.; Kratzsch, J.; Kiess, W.; Gebhardt, R. Nicotinamide phosphoribosyltransferase (NAMPT/PBEF/visfatin) is constitutively released from human hepatocytes. *Biochem. Biophys. Res. Commun.* **2010**, *391*, 376–381. [CrossRef]

20. Friebe, D.; Neef, M.; Kratzsch, J.; Erbs, S.; Dittrich, K.; Garten, A.; Petzold-Quinque, S.; Blüher, S.; Reinehr, T.; Stumvoll, M.; et al. Leucocytes are a major source of circulating nicotinamide phosphoribosyl transferase (NAMPT)/pre-B cell colony (PBEF)/visfatin linking obesity and inflammation in humans. *Diabetologia* **2011**, *54*, 1200–1211. [CrossRef]

21. Yang, H.; Lavu, S.; Sinclair, D.A. Nampt/PBEF/Visfatin: A regulator of mammalian health and longevity? *Exp. Gerontol.* **2006**, *41*, 718–726. [CrossRef] [PubMed]

22. Revollo, J.R.; Körner, A.; Mills, K.F.; Satoh, A.; Wang, T.; Garten, A.; Dasgupta, B.; Sasaki, Y.; Wolberger, C.; Townsend, R.R.; et al. Nampt/PBEF/Visfatin regulates insulin secretion in beta cells as a systemic NAD biosynthetic enzyme. *Cell Metab.* **2007**, *6*, 363–375. [CrossRef] [PubMed]

23. Yang, H.; Yang, T.; Baur, J.A.; Perez, E.; Matsui, T.; Carmona, J.J.; Lamming, D.W.; Souza-Pinto, N.C.; Bohr, V.A.; Rosenzweig, A.; et al. Nutrient-sensitive mitochondrial NAD$^+$ levels dictate cell survival. *Cell* **2007**, *130*, 1095–1107. [CrossRef] [PubMed]

24. Bowlby, S.C.; Thomas, M.J.; D'Agostino, R.B., Jr.; Kridel, S.J. Nicotinamide phosphoribosyl transferase (Nampt) is required for de novo lipogenesis in tumor cells. *PLoS ONE* **2012**, *7*, e40195. [CrossRef] [PubMed]

25. Pillai, J.B.; Isbatan, A.; Imai, S.; Gupta, M.P. Poly(ADP-ribose) polymerase 1 dependent cardiac myocyte cell death during heart failure is mediated by NAD$^+$ depletion and reduced Sir2α deacetylase activity. *J. Biol. Chem.* **2005**, *280*, 43121–43130. [CrossRef]

26. Rodgers, J.T.; Lerin, C.; Gerhart-Hines, Z.; Puigserver, P. Metabolic adaptations through the PGC 1 α and SIRT1 pathways. *FEBS Lett.* **2008**, *582*, 46–53. [CrossRef]

27. Luo, X.; Kraus, W.L. On PAR with PARP: Cellular stress signaling through poly (ADP-ribose) and PARP 1. *Genes Dev.* **2012**, *26*, 417–432. [CrossRef]

28. Kraus, D.; Yang, Q.; Kong, D.; Banks, A.S.; Zhang, L.; Rodgers, J.T.; Pirinen, E.; Pulinilkunnil, T.C.; Gong, F.; Wang, Y.C.; et al. Nicotinamide Nmethyltransferase knockdown protects against diet-induced obesity. *Nature* **2014**, *508*, 258–262. [CrossRef]

29. Kannt, A.; Pfenninger, A.; Teichert, L.; Tönjes, A.; Dietrich, A.; Schön, M.R.; Klöting, N.; Blüher, M. Association of nicotinamide-N-methyltransferase mRNA expression in human adipose tissue and the plasma concentration of its product, 1-methylnicotinamide, with insulin resistance. *Diabetologia* **2015**, *58*, 799–808. [CrossRef]

30. Giuliante, R.; Sartini, D.; Bacchetti, T.; Rocchetti, R.; Klöting, I.; Polidori, C.; Ferretti, G.; Emanuelli, M. Potential involvement of nicotinamide n-methyltransferase in the pathogenesis of metabolic syndrome. *Metab. Syndr. Relat. Disord.* **2015**, *13*, 165–170. [CrossRef]

31. Imai, S.; Armstrong, C.M.; Kaeberlein, M.; Guarente, L. Transcriptional silencing and longevity protein Sir2 is an NAD-dependent histone, deacetylase. *Nature* **2000**, *403*, 795–800. [CrossRef] [PubMed]

32. Pfluger, P.T.; Herranz, D.; Velasco-Miguel, S.; Serrano, M.; Tschöp, M.H. Sirt1 protects against high-fat diet-induced metabolic damage. *Proc. Natl. Acad. Sci. USA* **2008**, *105*, 9793–9798. [CrossRef] [PubMed]

33. Houtkooper, R.H.; Pirinen, E.; Auwerx, J. Sirtuins as regulators of metabolism and healthspan. *Nat. Rev. Mol. Cell Biol.* **2012**, *13*, 225–238. [CrossRef] [PubMed]

34. Caron, A.Z.; He, X.; Mottawea, W.; Seifert, E.L.; Jardine, K.; Dewar-Darch, D.; Cron, G.O.; Harper, M.E.; Stintzi, A.; McBurney, M.W. The SIRT1 deacetylase protects mice against the symptoms of metabolic syndrome. *FASEB J.* **2014**, *28*, 1306–1316. [CrossRef] [PubMed]

35. Asher, G.; Gatfield, D.; Stratmann, M.; Reinke, H.; Dibner, C.; Kreppel, F.; Mostoslavsky, R.; Alt, F.W.; Schibler, U. SIRT1 regulates circadian clock gene expression through PER2 deacetylation. *Cell* **2008**, *134*, 317–328. [CrossRef] [PubMed]

36. Nakahata, Y.; Kaluzova, M.; Grimaldi, B.; Sahar, S.; Hirayama, J.; Chen, D.; Guarente, L.P.; Sassone-Corsi, P. The NAD⁺-dependent deacetylase SIRT1 modulates CLOCK-mediated chromatin remodeling and circadian control. *Cell* **2008**, *134*, 329–340. [CrossRef] [PubMed]

37. Imai, S. "Clocks" in the NAD World: NAD as a metabolic oscillator for the regulation of metabolism and aging. *Biochim. Biophys. Acta* **2010**, *1804*, 1584–1590. [CrossRef] [PubMed]

38. Peek, C.B.; Affinati, A.H.; Ramsey, K.M.; Kuo, H.Y.; Yu, W.; Sena, L.A.; Ilkayeva, O.; Marcheva, B.; Kobayashi, Y.; Omura, C.; et al. Circadian clock NAD⁺ cycle drives mitochondrial oxidative metabolism in mice. *Science* **2013**, *342*, 1243417. [CrossRef]

39. Fulco, M.; Schiltz, R.L.; Iezzi, S.; King, M.T.; Zhao, P.; Kashiwaya, Y.; Hoffman, E.; Veech, R.L.; Sartorelli, V. Sir2 regulates skeletal muscle differentiation as a potential sensor of the redox state. *Mol. Cell* **2003**, *12*, 51–62. [CrossRef]

40. Kendrick, A.A.; Choudhury, M.; Rahman, S.M.; McCurdy, C.E.; Friederich, M.; Van Hove, J.L.; Watson, P.A.; Birdsey, N.; Bao, J.; Gius, D.; et al. Fatty liver is associated with reduced SIRT3 activity and mitochondrial protein hyperacetylation. *Biochem. J.* **2011**, *433*, 505–514. [CrossRef]

41. Ishikawa, S.; Li, G.; Takemitsu, H.; Fujiwara, M.; Mori, N.; Yamamoto, I.; Arai, T. Change in mRNA expression of sirtuin 1 and sirtuin 3 in cats fed on high fat diet. *BMC Vet. Res.* **2013**, *9*, 187. [CrossRef] [PubMed]

42. Shen, C.; Dou, X.; Ma, Y.; Ma, W.; Li, S.; Song, Z. Nicotinamide protects hepatocytes against palmitate-induced lipotoxicity via SIRT1-dependent autophagy induction. *Nutr. Res.* **2017**, *40*, 40–47. [CrossRef] [PubMed]

43. Lin, S.-J.; Ford, E.; Haigis, M.; Liszt, G.; Guarente, L. Calorie restriction extends yeast life span by lowering the level of NADH. *Genes Dev.* **2004**, *18*, 12–16. [CrossRef] [PubMed]

44. Zhang, H.; Ryu, D.; Wu, Y.; Gariani, K.; Wang, X.; Luan, P.; D'Amico, D.; Ropelle, E.R.; Lutolf, M.P.; Aebersold, R.; et al. NAD⁺ repletion improves mitochondrial and stem cell function and enhances life span in mice. *Science* **2016**, *352*, 1436–1443. [CrossRef] [PubMed]

45. Satoh, A.; Stein, L.; Imai, S. The role of mammalian sirtuins in the regulation of metabolism, aging, and longevity. *Handb. Exp. Pharmacol.* **2011**, *206*, 125–162. [CrossRef]

46. Von Schönfels, W.; Patsenker, E.; Fahrner, R.; Itzel, T.; Hinrichsen, H.; Brosch, M.; Erhart, W.; Gruodyte, A.; Vollnberg, B.; Richter, K.; et al. Metabolomic tissue signature in human non-alcoholic fatty liver disease identifies protective candidate metabolites. *Liver Int.* **2015**, *35*, 207–214. [CrossRef] [PubMed]

47. Mukherjee, S.; Chellappa, K.; Moffitt, A.; Ndungu, J.; Dellinger, R.W.; Davis, J.G.; Agarwal, B.; Baur, J.A. Nicotinamide adenine dinucleotide biosynthesis promotes liver regeneration. *Hepatology* **2017**, *65*, 616–630. [CrossRef]

48. Shi, L.; Tu, B.P. Acetyl-CoA and the regulation of metabolism: Mechanisms and consequences. *Curr. Opin. Cell Biol.* **2015**, *33*, 125–131. [CrossRef]

49. Penke, M.; Larsen, P.S.; Schuster, S.; Dall, M.; Jensen, B.A.; Gorski, T.; Meusel, A.; Richter, S.; Vienberg, S.G.; Treebak, J.T.; et al. Hepatic NAD salvage pathway is enhanced in mice on a high-fat diet. *Mol. Cell Endocrinol.* **2015**, *412*, 65–72. [CrossRef]

50. Zhou, C.C.; Yang, X.; Hua, X.; Liu, J.; Fan, M.B.; Li, G.Q.; Song, J.; Xu, T.Y.; Li, Z.Y.; Guan, Y.F.; et al. Hepatic NAD(+) deficiency as a therapeutic target for non-alcoholic fatty liver disease in ageing. *Br. J. Pharmacol.* **2016**, *173*, 2352–2368. [CrossRef]

51. Chang, Y.H.; Chang, D.M.; Lin, K.C.; Shin, S.J.; Lee, Y.J. Visfatin in overweight/obesity, type 2 diabetes mellitus, insulin resistance, metabolic syndrome and cardiovascular diseases: A meta-analysis and systemic review. *Diabetes Metab. Res. Rev.* **2011**, *27*, 515–527. [CrossRef] [PubMed]

52. Dahl, T.B.; Yndestad, A.; Skjelland, M.; Oie, E.; Dahl, A.; Michelsen, A.; Damas, J.K.; Tunheim, S.H.; Ueland, T.; Smith, C.; et al. Increased expression of visfatin in macrophages of human unstable carotid and coronary atherosclerosis: Possible role in inflammation and plaque, destabilization. *Circulation* **2007**, *115*, 972–980. [CrossRef] [PubMed]

53. El-Mesallamy, H.O.; Kassem, D.H.; El-Demerdash, E.; Amin, A.I. Vaspin and visfatin/Nampt are interesting interrelated adipokines playing a role in the pathogenesis of type 2 diabetes mellitus. *Metabolism* **2011**, *60*, 63–70. [CrossRef] [PubMed]

54. Aller, R.; de Luis, D.A.; Izaola, O.; Sagrado, M.G.; Conde, R.; Velasco, M.C.; Alvarez, T.; Pacheco, D.; Gonzalez, J.M. Influence of visfatin on histopathological changes of non-alcoholic fatty liver disease. *Dig. Dis. Sci.* **2009**, *54*, 1772–1777. [CrossRef] [PubMed]

55. Lee, J.J.; Lambert, J.E.; Hovhannisyan, Y.; Ramos-Roman, M.A.; Trombold, J.R.; Wagner, D.A.; Parks, E.J. Palmitoleic acid is elevated in fatty liver disease and reflects hepatic lipogenesis. *Am. J. Clin. Nutr.* **2015**, *101*, 34–43. [CrossRef] [PubMed]

56. Berlanga, A.; Guiu-Jurado, E.; Porras, J.A.; Auguet, T. Molecular pathways in non-alcoholic fatty liver disease. *Clin. Exp. Gastroenterol.* **2014**, *7*, 221–239. [CrossRef]

57. Hallows, W.C.; Lee, S.; Denu, J.M. Sirtuins deacetylate and activate mammalian acetyl-CoA synthetases. *Proc. Natl. Acad. Sci. USA* **2006**, *103*, 10230–10235. [CrossRef]

58. Hong, S.; Moreno-Navarrete, J.M.; Wei, X.; Kikukawa, Y.; Tzameli, I.; Prasad, D.; Lee, Y.; Asara, J.M.; Fernandez-Real, J.M.; Maratos-Flier, E.; et al. Nicotinamide N-methyltransferase regulates hepatic nutrient metabolism through Sirt1 protein stabilization. *Nat. Med.* **2015**, *21*, 887–894. [CrossRef]

59. Kennedy, A.R.; Pissios, P.; Otu, H.; Roberson, R.; Xue, B.; Asakura, K.; Furukawa, N.; Marino, F.E.; Liu, F.F.; Kahn, B.B.; et al. A high-fat, ketogenic diet induces a unique metabolic state in mice. *Am. J. Physiol.* **2007**, *292*, E1724–E1739. [CrossRef]

60. Bordone, L.; Cohen, D.; Robinson, A.; Motta, M.C.; van Veen, E.; Czopik, A.; Steele, A.D.; Crowe, H.; Marmor, S.; Luo, J.; et al. SIRT1 transgenic mice show phenotypes resembling calorie restriction. *Aging Cell* **2007**, *6*, 759–767. [CrossRef]

61. Sazci, A.; Ozel, M.D.; Ergul, E.; Aygun, C. Association of nicotinamide-N-methyltransferase gene rs694539 variant with patients with nonalcoholic steatohepatitis. *Genet. Test. Mol. Biomark.* **2013**, *17*, 849–853. [CrossRef] [PubMed]

62. Hasan, E.M.; Abd Al Aziz, R.A.; Sabry, D.; Darweesh, S.K.; Badary, H.A.; Elsharkawy, A.; Abouelkhair, M.M.; Yosry, A. Genetic Variants in nicotinamide-N-methyltransferase (NNMT) gene are related to the stage of non-alcoholic fatty liver disease diagnosed by controlled attenuation parameter (CAP)-fibroscan. *J. Gastrointest. Liver Dis.* **2018**, *27*, 265–272. [CrossRef]

63. Castera, L.; Friedrich-Rust, M.; Loomba, R. Noninvasive Assessment of Liver Disease in Patients with NAFLD. *Gastroenterology* **2019**, *156*, 1264–1281.e4. [CrossRef] [PubMed]

64. Gaddipati, R.; Sasikala, M.; Padaki, N.; Mukherjee, R.M.; Sekaran, A.; Jayaraj-Mansard, M.; Rabella, P.; Rao-Guduru, V.; Reddy-Duvvuru, N. Visceral adipose tissue visfatin in nonalcoholic fatty liver disease. *Ann. Hepatol.* **2010**, *9*, 266–270. [CrossRef]

65. Auguet, T.; Terra, X.; Porras, J.A.; Orellana-Gavaldà, J.M.; Martinez, S.; Aguilar, C.; Lucas, A.; Pellitero, S.; Hernández, M.; Del Castillo, D.; et al. Plasma visfatin levels and gene expression in morbidly obese women with associated fatty liver disease. *Clin. Biochem.* **2013**, *46*, 202–208. [CrossRef] [PubMed]

66. Dahl, T.B.; Haukeland, J.W.; Yndestad, A.; Ranheim, T.; Gladhaug, I.P.; Damås, J.K.; Haaland, T.; Løberg, E.M.; Arntsen, B.; Birkeland, K.; et al. Intracellular nicotinamide phosphoribosyl transferase protects against hepatocyte apoptosis and is down-regulated in nonalcoholic fatty liver disease. *J. Clin. Endocrinol. Metab.* **2010**, *95*, 3039–3047. [CrossRef] [PubMed]

67. Kukla, M.; Ciupińska-Kajor, M.; Kajor, M.; Wyleżoł, M.; Zwirska-Korczala, K.; Hartleb, M.; Berdowska, A.; Mazur, W. Liver visfatin expression in morbidly obese patients with nonalcoholic fatty liver disease undergoing bariatric surgery. *Pol. J. Pathol.* **2010**, *61*, 147–153. [PubMed]

68. Amirkalali, B.; Sohrabi, M.R.; Esrafily, A.; Jalali, M.; Gholami, A.; Hosseinzadeh, P.; Keyvani, H.; Shidfar, F.; Zamani, F. Association between Nicotinamide Phosphoribosyltransferase and de novo Lipogenesis in Nonalcoholic Fatty Liver Disease. *Med. Princ. Pract.* **2017**, *26*, 251–257. [CrossRef]

69. Tao, R.; Wei, D.; Gao, H.; Liu, Y.; DePinho, R.A.; Dong, X.C. Hepatic FoxOs regulate lipid metabolism via modulation of expression of the nicotinamide phosphoribosyltransferase gene. *J. Biol. Chem.* **2011**, *286*, 14681–14690. [CrossRef]

70. Canto, C.; Houtkooper, R.H.; Pirinen, E.; Youn, D.Y.; Oosterveer, M.H.; Cen, Y.; Fernandez-Marcos, P.J.; Yamamoto, H.; Andreux, P.A.; Cettour-Rose, P.; et al. The NAD(+) precursor nicotinamide riboside enhances oxidative metabolism and protects against high-fat diet-induced obesity. *Cell Metab.* **2012**, *15*, 838–847. [CrossRef]

71. Gariani, K.; Menzies, K.J.; Ryu, D.; Wegner, C.J.; Wang, X.; Ropelle, E.R.; Moullan, N.; Zhang, H.; Perino, A.; Lemos, V.; et al. Eliciting the mitochondrial unfolded protein response by nicotinamide adenine dinucleotide repletion reverses fatty liver disease in mice. *Hepatology* **2016**, *63*, 1190–1204. [CrossRef] [PubMed]

72. Mejía, S.Á.; Gutman, L.A.B.; Camarillo, C.O.; Navarro, R.M.; Becerra, M.C.S.; Santana, L.D.; Cruz, M.; Pérez, E.H.; Flores, M.D. Nicotinamide prevents sweet beverage-induced hepatic steatosis in rats by regulating the G6PD, NADPH/NADP$^+$ and GSH/GSSG ratios and reducing oxidative and inflammatory, stress. *Eur. J. Pharmacol.* **2018**, *818*, 499–507. [CrossRef] [PubMed]

73. Komatsu, M.; Kanda, T.; Urai, H.; Kurokochi, A.; Kitahama, R.; Shigaki, S.; Ono, T.; Yukioka, H.; Hasegawa, K.; Tokuyama, H.; et al. NNMT activation can contribute to the development of fatty liver disease by modulating the NAD$^+$ metabolism. *Sci. Rep.* **2018**, *8*, 8637. [CrossRef] [PubMed]

74. Houtkooper, R.H.; Canto, C.; Wanders, R.J.; Auwerx, J. The secret life of NAD$^+$: An old metabolite controlling new metabolic signaling pathways. *Endocr. Rev.* **2010**, *31*, 194–223. [CrossRef] [PubMed]

75. Knip, M.; Douek, I.F.; Moore, W.P.; Gillmor, H.A.; McLean, A.E.; Bingley, P.J.; Gale, E.A.; European Nicotinamide Diabetes Intervention Trial Group. Safety of high-dose nicotinamide: A review. *Diabetologia* **2000**, *43*, 1337–1345. [CrossRef] [PubMed]

76. Lukasova, M.; Hanson, J.; Tunaru, S.; Offermanns, S. Nicotinic acid (niacin): New lipid independent mechanisms of action and therapeutic potentials. *Trends Pharmacol. Sci.* **2011**, *32*, 700–707. [CrossRef] [PubMed]

77. Yadav, R.; France, M.; Younis, N.; Hama, S.; Ammori, B.J.; Kwok, S.; Soran, H. Extended release niacin with laropiprant: A review on efficacy, clinical effectiveness and safety. *Expert Opin. Pharmacother.* **2012**, *13*, 1345–1362. [CrossRef] [PubMed]

78. Gomes, A.L.; Teijeiro, A.; Burén, S.; Tummala, K.S.; Yilmaz, M.; Waisman, A.; Theurillat, J.P.; Perna, C.; Djouder, N. Metabolic Inflammation-Associated IL-17A Causes Non-alcoholic Steatohepatitis and Hepatocellular Carcinoma. *Cancer Cell* **2016**, *30*, 161–175. [CrossRef]

79. Trammell, S.A.; Schmidt, M.S.; Weidemann, B.J.; Redpath, P.; Jaksch, F.; Dellinger, R.W.; Li, Z.; Abel, E.D.; Migaud, M.E.; Brenner, C. Nicotinamide riboside is uniquely and orally bioavailable in mice and humans. *Nat. Commun.* **2016**, *7*, 12948. [CrossRef] [PubMed]

80. Shi, W.; Hegeman, M.A.; van Dartel, D.A.; Tang, J.; Suarez, M.; Swarts, H.; van der Hee, B.; Arola, L.; Keijer, J. Effects of a wide range of dietary nicotinamide riboside (NR) concentrations on metabolic flexibility and white adipose tissue (WAT) of mice fed a mildly obesogenic diet. *Mol. Nutr. Food Res.* **2017**, *61*. [CrossRef]

81. Lee, H.J.; Hong, Y.S.; Jun, W.; Yang, S.J. Nicotinamide riboside ameliorates hepatic metaflammation by modulating NLRP3 inflammasome in a rodent model of type 2 diabetes. *J. Med. Food* **2015**, *18*, 1207–1213. [CrossRef] [PubMed]

82. Trammell, S.A.; Weidemann, B.J.; Chadda, A.; Yorek, M.S.; Holmes, A.; Coppey, L.J.; Obrosov, A.; Kardon, R.H.; Yorek, M.A.; Brenner, C. Nicotinamide Riboside Opposes Type 2 Diabetes and Neuropathy in Mice. *Sci. Rep.* **2016**, *6*, 26933. [CrossRef] [PubMed]

83. De Picciotto, N.E.; Gano, L.B.; Johnson, L.C.; Martens, C.R.; Sindler, A.L.; Mills, K.F.; Imai, S.; Seals, D.R. Nicotinamide mononucleotide supplementation reverses vascular dysfunction and oxidative stress with aging in mice. *Aging Cell* **2016**, *15*, 522–530. [CrossRef] [PubMed]

84. Wang, X.; Hu, X.; Yang, Y.; Takata, T.; Sakurai, T. Nicotinamide mononucleotide protects against beta-amyloid oligomer-induced cognitive impairment and neuronal death. *Brain Res.* **2016**, *1643*, 1–9. [CrossRef] [PubMed]

85. Aksoy, P.; White, T.A.; Thompson, M.; Chini, E.N. Regulation of intracellular levels of NAD: A novel role for CD38. *Biochem. Biophys. Res. Commun.* **2006**, *345*, 1386–1392. [CrossRef]

86. Escande, C.; Nin, V.; Price, N.L.; Capellini, V.; Gomes, A.P.; Barbosa, M.T.; O'Neil, L.; White, T.A.; Sinclair, D.A.; Chini, E.N. Flavonoid apigenin is an inhibitor of the NAD$^+$ase CD38: Implications for cellular NAD$^+$ metabolism, protein acetylation, and treatment of metabolic syndrome. *Diabetes* **2013**, *62*, 1084–1109. [CrossRef]

87. Cipriani, G.; Rapizzi, E.; Vannacci, A.; Rizzuto, R.; Moroni, F.; Chiarugi, A. Nuclear poly(ADP-ribose) polymerase-1 rapidly triggers mitochondrial dysfunction. *J. Biol. Chem.* **2005**, *280*, 17227–17234. [CrossRef]

88. Almeida, G.S.; Bawn, C.M.; Galler, M.; Wilson, I.; Thomas, H.D.; Kyle, S.; Curtin, N.J.; Newell, D.R.; Maxwell, R.J. PARP inhibitor rucaparib induces changes in NAD levels in cells and liver tissues as assessed by MRS. *NMR Biomed.* **2017**, *30*. [CrossRef]

10

Acupuncture on ST36, CV4 and KI1 Suppresses the Progression of Methionine- and Choline-Deficient Diet-Induced Nonalcoholic Fatty Liver Disease in Mice

Xiangjin Meng [1,2], Xin Guo [1,3,*], Jing Zhang [1], Junji Moriya [2], Junji Kobayashi [2], Reimon Yamaguchi [4] and Sohsuke Yamada [1,3]

[1] Department of Pathology and Laboratory Medicine, Kanazawa Medical University, 1-1 Daigaku, Uchinada, Kahoku, Ishikawa 920-0293, Japan; meng6950@kanazawa-med.ac.jp (X.M.); jing2018@kanazawa-med.ac.jp (J.Z.); sohsuke@kanazawa-med.ac.jp (S.Y.)

[2] Department of General Internal Medicine, Kanazawa Medical University, Ishikawa 920-0293, Japan; moriya@kanazawa-med.ac.jp (J.M.); mary@kanazawa-med.ac.jp (J.K.)

[3] Department of Pathology, Kanazawa Medical University Hospital, Ishikawa 920-0293, Japan

[4] Department of Dermatology, Kanazawa Medical University, Ishikawa 920-0293, Japan; raymon-y@kanazawa-med.ac.jp

* Correspondence: tianqi11211216@yahoo.co.jp

Abstract: Nonalcoholic fatty liver disease (NAFLD) is one of the most common chronic liver diseases worldwide, and its treatment remain a constant challenge. A number of clinical trials have shown that acupuncture treatment has beneficial effects for patients with NAFLD, but the molecular mechanisms underlying its action are still largely unknown. In this study, we established a mouse model of NAFLD by administering a methionine- and choline-deficient (MCD) diet and selected three acupoints (ST36, CV4, and KI1) or nonacupoints (sham) for needling. We then investigated the effects of acupuncture treatment on the progression of NAFLD and the underlying mechanisms. After two weeks of acupuncture treatment, the liver in the needling-nonapcupoint group (NG) mice appeared pale and yellowish in color, while that in the needling-acupoint group (AG) showed a bright red color. Histologically, fewer lipid droplets and inflammatory foci were observed in the AG liver than in the NG liver. Furthermore, the expression of proinflammatory signaling factors was significantly downregulated in the AG liver. A lipid analysis showed that the levels of triglyceride (TG) and free fatty acid (FFA) were lower in the AG liver than in the NG liver, with an altered expression of lipid metabolism-related factors as well. Moreover, the numbers of 8-hydroxy-2'-deoxyguanosine (8-OHdG)-positive hepatocytes and levels of hepatic thiobarbituric acid reactive substances (TBARS) were significantly lower in AG mice than in NG mice. In line with these results, a higher expressions of antioxidant factors was found in the AG liver than in the NG liver. Our results indicate that acupuncture repressed the progression of NAFLD by inhibiting inflammatory reactions, reducing oxidative stress, and promoting lipid metabolism of hepatocytes, suggesting that this approach might be an important complementary treatment for NAFLD.

Keywords: nonalcoholic fatty liver disease; acupuncture; imflammation; lipid metabolism; oxidative stress

1. Introduction

Nonalcoholic fatty liver disease (NAFLD) is one of the most common clinicopathological conditions in chronic liver disease and is characterized by an obvious increase in fat deposition in the hepatocytes of the liver parenchyma [1]. Epidemiologically, NAFLD affects approximately 40% of the population worldwide, and the prevalence is increasing annually all over the world [2]. This disease has been considered to carry a high risk of developing into liver cirrhosis and hepatocellular carcinoma.

However, there are still no effective drugs specifically developed for the treatment of NAFLD, especially in patients with non-alcoholic steatohepatitis (NASH), a severe stage of NAFLD. Although several agents have shown some benefits for patients with NAFLD, even the most promising of such pharmacological agents are associated with significant adverse effects, and none have been approved by the Food and Drug Administration (FDA) for NAFLD therapy [3]. Balancing the benefits and risks in drugs for long-term treatment remains a constant challenge that has hampered the development of therapy strategies for NAFLD [4].

Ectopic fat accumulation in the hepatocytes, a hallmark of NAFLD, is thought to be caused by a complex and multiple mechanism that is still not completely understood but involves several interdependent molecular processes, such as inflammation, lipid metabolism, and oxidative stress [5]. An abnormal lipid metabolism, such as an increased uptake of lipids and the upregulation of de novo lipogenesis in the liver, is the initial trigger of NAFLD. Lipid overload promotes reactive oxygen species (ROS) generation and peroxidation itself, which causes the release of pro-inflammatory cytokines and inflammatory cellular infiltration [6,7]. The activation of the nuclear factor-κB (NF-κB) inflammatory pathway regulating downstream target genes plays very important roles in the progression of NAFLD. These inflammatory cytokines can recruit and activate Kupffer cells/macrophages and further aggravate liver injury and steatohepatitis formation [8].

Oxidative stress caused by the imbalance between oxidants and antioxidants seems to be one of the most important mechanisms leading to NAFLD liver injury, which plays a fundamental role in the progression from simple steatosis to NASH. The enhanced production of ROS can reportedly lead to necroinflammation and fibrosis through lipid peroxidation induced by astrocyte activation [9].

Acupuncture is a treatment method found in traditional Chinese medicine (TCM). Due to its advantages of low cost, few side effects, and simple operation, the role of acupuncture in disease prevention and treatment has recently attracted attention, and a large body of evidence has shown that acupuncture can induce pathophysiological consequences and alleviate the symptoms of diseases in multiple organs [10–12]. A number of clinical trials have also indicated that acupuncture treatment can improve metabolism conditions and exert beneficial effects on patients with NAFLD [13–15], but the mechanisms underlying its action remain unclear.

According to the theory of TCM, fatty liver formation primarily involves metabolic disorders caused by qi and blood stasis, and acupuncture at certain points of related meridians can improve the metabolism by keeping the body in a balanced state between "Yin" and "Yang" [16]. However, from a modern medicine viewpoint, how acupuncture exerts its therapeutic role and what kind of physiological consequences acupuncture causes at different acupoints of meridians are still unclear.

In the present study, we established a mouse model of NAFLD by administering a methionine- and choline-deficient diet (MCD), a classic diet inducing NAFLD [17]. We selected three acupoints of related meridians regulating the metabolism to needle the mice with NAFLD and observed the roles of acupuncture in the progression of NAFLD. Furthermore, we also investigated the pathogenic mechanisms leading to these significant effects through laboratory and molecular biology experiments. Our results suggest that acupuncture might be a useful treatment for NAFLD and provide solid evidence supporting the incorporation of acupuncture into therapy for metabolic syndrome from a modern medicine viewpoint.

2. Results

2.1. Lipid Accumulation was Significantly Reduced in the Livers of AG Mice with NAFLD Induced by an MCD Diet

After two weeks of acupuncture, the livers from the needling-nonapcupoint group (NG) mice were variably pale and yellowish in color. In contrast, the livers from the needling-acupoint group (AG) showed a bright red color (Figure 1A). The mouse body weight and liver weight were significantly lower in AG mice than in those of NG mice ($p < 0.0001$, $n = 17$) (Figure S1). However, the mouse liver/BW ratios were no significant difference between the two groups ($p < 0.0001$, $n = 17$) (Figure 1B).

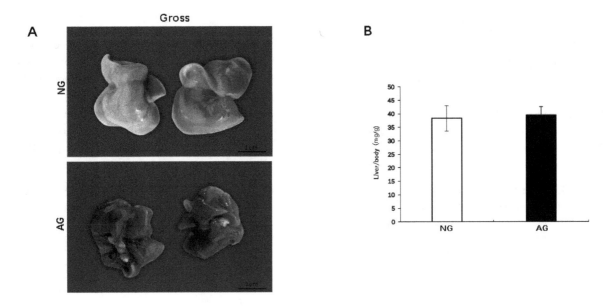

Figure 1. The appearance of the liver and ratio of the liver to the body weight after two weeks of acupuncture. (**A**) The liver tissues of the NG mice were obviously pale and yellowish in color, and while the tissue of the AG liver showed a bright red color. Bar = 1 cm. (**B**) There was no marked difference in the ratio of the liver to the body weight between the two groups. Values are shown as the mean ± SD, * $p < 0.05$, ** $p < 0.001$, *** $p < 0.0001$, $n = 17$. NG: needling-nonacupoint group, AG: needling-acupoint group, MCD diet: methionine- and choline-deficient diet, HF diet: high-fat diet, NAFLD: nonalcoholic fatty liver disease.

Hematoxylin and eosin (H&E) staining showed that the AG liver tended to contain fewer lipid droplets and inflammatory foci than those of NG mice, and there was also a significant histological difference between the two livers. Ballooning of hepatocytes, inflammation, and fibrosis were noted in the livers of NG mice. Furthermore, the NASH score in the AG livers was significantly lower than that in the NG livers after acupuncture ($n = 17$) (Figure 2A and Table 1). Oil red-O staining revealed few lipid droplets in the AG mice, while the numbers of lipid-positive hepatocytes and droplets in each hepatocyte were increased in NG mice ($n = 17$) (Figure 2B). These morphology and histology findings indicate that acupuncture can treat the liver damage caused by a high-fat diet.

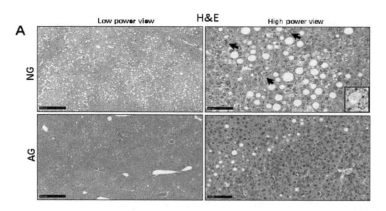
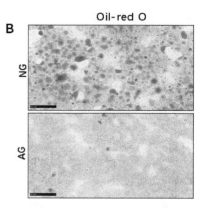

Figure 2. Histological observation of the liver from the two groups of mice. (**A**) Representative photomicrographs of liver (H&E). H&E-stained sections revealed macrovesicular and microvesicular steatosis throughout the entire lobules in the NAFLD livers from NG mice, as well as scattered lobular and perivenular inflammation (arrowhead). (original magnification: ×40 [low]; Bars = 50 μm, ×200 [high]; Bars = 100 μm, n = 17). (**B**) Oil Red-O staining revealed a number of lipid droplets accumulated in NG liver, while fewer lipid droplets were observed in the AG liver (original magnification: ×400, Bars = 50 μm, n = 17). NG: needling-nonacupoint group, AG: needling-acupoint group, H&E: hematoxylin and eosin, NAFLD: nonalcoholic fatty liver disease.

Table 1. Quantitative scoring of the fat accumulation, inflammation and ballooning in the NAFLD livers of model AG and NG mice.

Steatosis Score			
Score	NG	AG	P
0	0	11	<0.001
1	8	6	
2	4	0	
3	5	0	
Inflammation Score			
Score	NG	AG	P
0	0	5	0.003
1	12	12	
2	4	0	
3	1	0	
Ballooning Score			
Score	NG	AG	P
0	5	16	<0.001
1	10	1	
2	2	0	
3	0	0	
NAFLD Score			
Score	NG	AG	P
0–3	7	17	<0.001
4–6	8	0	
7–9	6	0	

Values are shown as the means ± standard deviation, * $p < 0.05$, ** $p < 0.001$, *** $p < 0.0001$, n = 17. NG: needling-nonacupoint group, AG: needling-acupoint group, NAFLD: nonalcoholic fatty liver disease.

2.2. Acupuncture Treatment Inhibits the Inflammation Reaction during the Progression of MCD Diet–Induced NAFLD

IHC for Mac-2 revealed that the AG livers contained a significantly smaller number of infiltrating macrophages (Kupffer cells) than the NG livers (AG 6.7 ± 2.5 vs. NG 12.3 ± 4.7; $p < 0.001$, n = 17)

(Figure 3A). In addition, fibrogenesis and stellate cell activation, as determined by IHC for α-smooth muscle actin (α-SMA), were not apparent in the AG liver, and the specific and linear expression of α-SMA along with the activation of hepatic stellate cells in AG mice was much lower than that in NG mice (AG 18.7 ± 6.1.0 vs. NG 39.4 ± 7.5; $p < 0.0001$, $n = 17$) (Figure 3B).

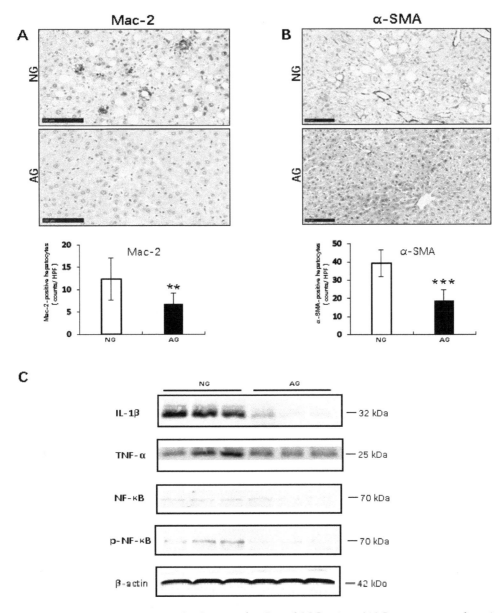

Figure 3. Inflammatory responses in the livers of AG and NG mice. (**A**) Immunocytochemistry (IHC) showed the number of Mac-2-positive infiltrating macrophages in the NAFLD liver. (**B**) α-SMA-positive activated hepatic stellate cells in the NAFLD liver. Values are shown as the means ± SD, Bars = 100 μm * $p < 0.05$, ** $p < 0.001$, *** $p < 0.0001$, $n = 17$. (**C**) The IL-1β, TNFα, NF-κB and p-NF-κB protein expression was determined by Western blotting. Values are normalized β-actin expression (Western blotting) expression and are presented as means ± SD. $n = 7$. NG: needling-nonacupoint group, AG: needling-acupoint group, IHC: immunocytochemistry, α-SMA: α-smooth muscle actin, IL-1β: interleukin 1β, TNFα: tumor necrosis factor-α, NF-κB: nuclear factor-κB, p-NF-κB: phospho-nuclear factor-κB.

A Western blot analysis showed that the expression of proinflammatory signaling factors and inflammatory cytokines or transcriptional factor and their receptors, such as interleukin 1β (IL-1β), tumor necrosis factor-α (TNFα) and the key regulators of inflammation, NF-κB and phospho-nuclear factor-KB (p-NF-κB), was significantly lower in the AG livers than in the NG livers. Therefore, acupuncture can promote liver metabolism by inhibiting inflammatory reaction ($n = 7$) (Figure 3C).

2.3. Acupuncture Treatment Changed the Lipid Profiles and Regulated Lipid Metabolism in the Liver with NAFLD Induced by an MCD Diet

The hepatic triglyceride (TG) and free fatty acid (FFA) levels in liver were significantly lower in AG mice than in NG mice (TG: AG 6.7 ± 3.5 mg/g vs. NG 11.0 ± 5.2 mg/g; $p < 0.05$, $n = 17$; FFA: AG 0.15 ± 0.15 mEq/g vs. NG 0.4 ± 0.2 mEq/g; $p < 0.01$, $n = 17$). However, the liver T-cho levels were not significantly different between AG and NG mice (Figure 4A).

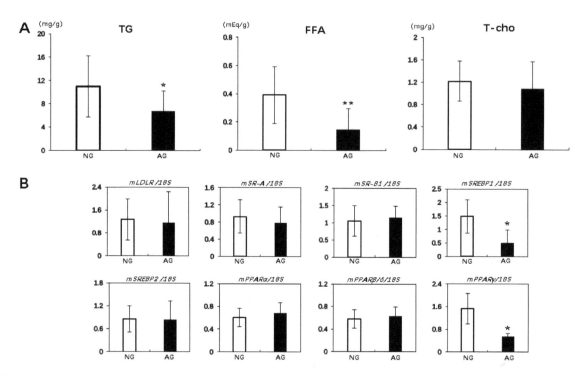

Figure 4. Acupuncture improved the lipid metabolism in the livers of mice with NAFLD. (**A**) A hepatic lipid analysis in NG and AG mice after two weeks of acupuncture. Values are shown as the mean ± SD, * $p < 0.05$, ** $p < 0.001$, *** $p < 0.0001$, $n = 17$. (**B**) Real time PCR revealed that the expression of several proinflammatory signaling factors (SREBP1 and PPARγ) was significantly lower in the livers of AG mice than in those of NG mice. LDLR, SR-A, SR-B1, and SREBP2 showed no significant difference between the groups, nor did PPARα or PPARβ/δ. Values are normalized by the 18S rRNA expression. RT-PCR values are presented as the means ± SD. * $p < 0.05$, ** $p < 0.001$, *** $p < 0.0001$, $n = 7$. NG: needling-nonacupoint group, AG: needling-acupoint group, TG: triglyceride, T-cho: total cholesterol, FFA: free fatty acid, LDLR: low-density lipoprotein receptor, SR-A: scavenger receptor class A, SR-B1: scavenger receptor class B type 1, SREBP: sterol regulatory element-binding protein, PPAR: peroxisome proliferator-activated receptor.

Real Time Reverse Transcription Polymerase Chain Reaction (RT-PCR) showed that no marked differences between the two groups were observed in the expression of some receptors related to the lipid uptake in the liver, including low-density lipoprotein receptor (LDLR), scavenger receptor class A (SR-A) and scavenger receptor class B type 1 (SR-B1) (Figure 4B). However, the expression of transcription factor sterol regulatory element binding protein 1 (SREBP1), an important transcriptional protein that regulates lipid synthesis with a well-studied function in lipid metabolism [18], was significantly lower in the AG livers than in the NG livers ($p < 0.05$, $n = 7$), while that of SREBP2, which primarily regulates cholesterol biosynthesis, showed no significant difference between the two groups (Figure 4B). The expression of SREBP1 target genes, such as fatty acid synthase (FAS) and stearoyl-CoA

9-desaturase 1 (SCD1), was also significantly lower in the AG livers than in the NG livers ($p < 0.05$, $n = 7$) (Figure S2B). Peroxisome proliferator-activated receptors (PPARs) are primary modulators in the metabolism of fatty acids in the liver [19] and include PPARα, PPARβ/δ, and PPARγ. The PPARγ RNA expression was significantly lower in AG livers than NG livers ($p < 0.05$, $n = 7$), as well as the the expression of PPARγ target such as adiponectin receptor 2 (AdipoR2). The expression was significantly lower in AG livers than NG livers ($p < 0.05$, $n = 7$) (Figure S2B), but the PPARα and PPARβ/δ RNA expression did not differ significantly between the groups (Figure 4B). Moreover, the expression of genes involved in hepatic lipid secretion apolipoprotein B (ApoB), apolipoprotein E (ApoE), and microsomal triglyceride transfer protein (MTTP) were significantly higher in the AG livers than in the NG livers ($p < 0.05$, $n = 7$) (Figure S2A).

2.4. Acupuncture Treatment Improved Oxidative Stress Induced by Lipid Accumulation of the NAFLD Liver in Mice

We used IHC to determine the expression of 8-hydroxy-2′-deoxyguanosine (8-OHdG) as a marker for oxidative stress. There were significantly fewer cells positive for 8-OHdG in AG mice than in NG mice after 2 weeks of acupuncture (AG: 104.5 ± 26.4 vs. NG: 221.8 ± 63.9; $p < 0.001$, $n = 17$) (Figure 5A).

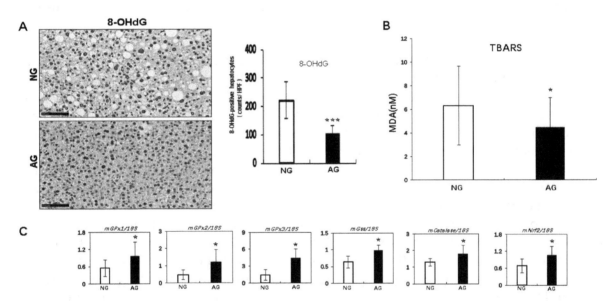

Figure 5. The analysis of hepatic oxidative stress in mice with NAFLD. (**A**) 8-hydroxy-20-deoxyguanosine (8-OHdG) staining revealed significantly fewer accumulated 8-OHdG-positive hepatocytes in the livers of AG mice than in those of NG mice after acupuncture. Values are shown as the mean ± SD, * $p < 0.05$, ** $p < 0.001$, *** $p < 0.0001$, $n = 17$. (**B**) The levels of the oxidative stress marker thiobarbituric acid reactive substances (TBARS) in AG mice were significantly lower than in NG mice after acupuncture. Values are shown as the mean ± SD, * $p < 0.05$, ** $p < 0.001$, *** $p < 0.0001$, $n = 17$. (**C**) Real time PCR showed that the GPx1, GPx2, GPx3, Gss, Catalase, and Nrf2 expression in the liver was significantly higher in AG mice than in NG mice. Values are shown as the means ± SD. * $p < 0.05$, ** $p < 0.001$, *** $p < 0.0001$, $n = 7$. NG: needling-nonacupoint group, AG: needling-acupoint group, GPx: glutathione peroxidase, Gss: glutathionylspermidine synthetase/amidase, Nrf2: nuclear factor erythroid 2-related factor 2.

We next measured the liver levels of another oxidative stress marker, thiobarbituric acid reactive substances (TBARS). The TBARS levels were significantly lower in AG mice than in NG mice after 2 weeks of acupuncture (AG 4.5 ± 2.5 nmol malondialdehyde ([MDA]) protein vs. NG 6.3 ± 3.3 nmol MDA protein, $p < 0.05$, $n = 17$) (Figure 5B).

Real time PCR showed that the hepatic expression of several antioxidant enzymes, including glutathione peroxidase 1, 2, and 3 (GPx1, 2, and 3), glutathionylspermidine synthetase/amidase

(Gss), and catalase and the transcription factor nuclear factor erythroid 2-related factor 2 (Nrf2), were significant higher in AG mice than in NG mice ($p < 0.05$, $n = 7$) (Figure 5C). Therefore, acupuncture may reduce oxidative stress by upregulating the antioxidant expression.

3. Discussion

Acupuncture is a vital component of TCM and has a history of more than 2500 years. Given its safety and few side effects, this major TCM has been widely used to treat various diseases and symptoms, especially chronic metabolic illness [20]. Many modern studies have proven the efficacy of acupuncture against a wide range of diseases [21–23]. However, due to lack of understanding of the mechanisms underlying its action, acupuncture is the subject of severe controversy, with its effects proposed to be placebo effects [24]. To clarify these points and the efficacy of acupuncture on the systemic metabolism, it is necessary to determine the molecular mechanism underlying acupuncture's effects on specific tissues and cell metabolism.

Since it is illegal and unethical to carry out laboratory experiments on the human body without need, animal studies of acupuncture are of great value and show obvious advantages regarding research on the metabolic signal pathways compared to clinical studies [25]. Therefore, in this study, we used a mouse model of MCD + HF diet-induced NAFLD to investigate the mechanisms by which acupuncture treatment improves the conditions of this chronic disease.

According to TCM, the three acupoints of Zusanli (ST36), Yongquan (KI1) and Guanyuan (CV4) were selected for needling model mice in order to harmonize the Yin and Yang and dredge the channel of Qi and Blood. Our pathological and experimental results showed that acupuncture treatment significantly attenuated the progression of NAFLD by inhibiting inflammatory reactions, reducing oxidative stress and promoting lipid metabolism of hepatocytes. These results provide solid evidence from a modern medicine perspective supporting the notion that acupuncturing these three acupoints may be beneficial for patients with NAFLD.

Inflammation plays very important roles in the process of NAFLD progression. Injured liver cells can release damage-associated molecular patterns (DAMPs) to promote the activation of the NF-κB pathway, thus inducing the production of pro-inflammatory cytokines like TNF-α and ILs, which is a key step in the progression from simple steatosis to NASH [26,27]. Many studies have confirmed that acupuncture can downregulate the NF-κB expression [28,29]. Indeed, in the present study, hepatic injury induced by the absence of methionine and choline in the diet clearly upregulated the expression and enhanced the activation of NF-κB, thus increasing the production of downstream factors TNF-α and IL-1β in the livers of NG mice, while acupuncture treatment significantly inhibited the NF-κB inflammatory signals in the AG mice. These cytokines can contribute to the recruitment and activation of macrophages/Kupffer cells (resident hepatic macrophages) to mediate inflammation [30], which is critical in NASH. A significant increase in macrophages has been shown to occur in the liver tissue of patients with NASH compared to those with simple steatosis [31]. In the present study, with the reduction in the TNF-α and IL-1β expression, much fewer Mac-2- and α-SMA-positive cells were observed in the livers of AG mice with simple steatosis than in NG mice showing progression to NASH. These results indicate that acupuncture treatment can improve the pathological progression of NAFLD by inactivating the inflammatory signaling pathways.

The regulatory role of acupuncture in inflammation has also been reported in other studies, but the effects are not the same when needling different acupoints. For example, acupuncture of the Sanyinjiao (SP6) acupoint can increase IL-10 levels [32], while needling Fenglong (ST40) and Neiguan (PC6) acupoints reduced the IL-17 expression [33]. These data imply that although acupuncture treatment at several acupoints can suppresses the inflammation response, different acupoints can achieve the same effect by regulating specific cytokines.

The accumulation of excess lipid in hepatocytes causes organelle failure, such as mitochondrial dysfunction and endoplasmic reticulum stress, and leads to liver injury in patients with NAFLD [34,35]. However, in some NAFLD patients, the accumulation of lipids is not toxic to liver cells, a paradoxical effect that is believed to be related to the type of lipid itself. For example, TG reportedly does not seem toxic, but FFA and cholesterol—including its metabolites—are highly toxic to cells [36,37]. In our MCD-induced NAFLD mouse model, the hepatic total cholesterol levels were not markedly different between NG and AG mice, but the TG and especially the FFA levels were markedly reduced in the livers of AG mice compared to the livers of NG mice. Therefore, a significant decrease in the FFA level in the liver may play a more important role in acupuncture treatment for NAFLD than a reduction in TG. The FFA pool in the circulation is the major source of FFA in the liver [38], but no remarkable difference in the hepatic expression of receptors related to the lipid uptake were noted between NG and AG mice. However, we found that some regulators expressions regarding de novo lipogenesis and lipid storage in the liver were significantly decreased and genes involved in hepatic lipid secretion increased in AG mice compared with NG mice, suggesting that the reduction in hepatic lipid deposition after acupuncture treatment is induced by reducing the synthesis and promoting the metabolism of lipids rather than by inhibiting their uptake in the liver altogether.

Mitochondrial dysfunction and endoplasmic reticulum stress caused by the accumulation of lipids, especially FFA, can also result in the increased production of ROS and lead to oxidative stress that promotes inflammatory reactions, the activation of stellate cells and fibrosis in the liver, which have been recognized as important events in the development of NAFLD [39–41]. In the present study, the number of 8-OHdG-positive cells and the level of MDA in the liver were significantly reduced in AG mice compared to NG mice, showing that acupuncture treatment can also improve the oxidative stress status during NAFLD progression. It seems easy to understand that the lower level of hepatic FFA inhibited organelle failure and repressed the increased production of ROS in AG mice. These results should be rational, however, the consideration is probably oversimplified, as we also found expressions of some protective antioxidants to significantly increase in the livers of AG mice (Figure 5C), which may be the real reason for the inhibition of oxidative stress by the accumulation of lipids. Another interesting finding of the present study was that acupuncture treatment had significant regulatory effects on inflammatory reaction, lipid metabolism and redox homeostasis, which was found to be closely associated with changes in the expression of transcription factors related to these signaling pathways, like NF-κB, PPARs, and Nrf2 (Figure 3C, Figure 4B, and Figure 5C respectively). These results remind us that acupuncture may regulate cell metabolism at the expression level. To confirm this suspicion, more molecular mechanism experiments will be needed in the future.

In summary, from this study, we obtained some novel findings: (1) acupuncture on the three acupoints, ST36, CV4 and KI1, can improve pathological process of NAFLD; (2) acupuncture treatment can inhibit inflammatory reactions, reduce oxidative stress and promote lipid metabolism; (3) acupuncture on different acupoints can inhibit inflammatory reactions by regulating specific cytokines; (4) acupuncture treatment have regulatory effects on the expression of transcription factors. Although some exciting results were found in the present study, there are still some limitations to be noted. First, an MCD + HF diet-induced NAFLD model was used to investigate the roles of acupuncture in inhibiting the progression of NAFLD in this study, but the molecular mechanism underlying special diet-induced NAFLD does not totally reflect the pathogenesis of this disease in human, even though some pathological manifestations are consistent between the two entities. Second, although acupuncture treatment has few side effects, since this was the first instance of observing the effects of needling the three acupoints ST36, KI1, and CV4 in mice with NAFLD, and since this treatment was administered daily for only two weeks, we cannot confirm that no side effects would be noted with this approach over a long period of time. Finally, after two weeks of acupuncture treatment, we also found metabolic changes in other tissues and organs aside from the liver, largely related to gastrointestinal absorption, lipid storage and energy metabolism (data not shown), which have a major influence on metabolic syndrome, such as insulin resistance, obesity and fatty liver. However, in the present study, we ignored these other influences temporarily and instead focused on the metabolic changes in the liver after acupuncture treatment. The influence of other factors should therefore be discussed in future studies.

4. Materials and Methods

4.1. Animals and Experimental Protocol

Experiments were performed using 8-week-old male C57BL/6 mice weighing approximately 20 g that were maintained in a temperature- and light-controlled facility with free access to water. Mice were fed an MCD + HF diet (60% fat; KBT Oriental Corporation, Saga, Japan) for 3 weeks and then given an HF diet for two weeks to maintain their hyperlipidemia. As described previously [17], mice were anesthetized with an injection of ketamine-medetamidine and euthanized by exsanguination. The liver was excised and cut into small pieces, frozen, and fixed in 10% neutral-buffered formalin for the experiments described below.

4.2. Acupuncture Manipulation

The mice were randomly divided into two groups: AG and NG. They were fed an MCD + HF diet for three weeks and then given HF diet for two weeks to maintain their hyperlipidemia. For the needling treatment, three acupoints (AG) or no acupoints (NG) were needled (Figure 6A).

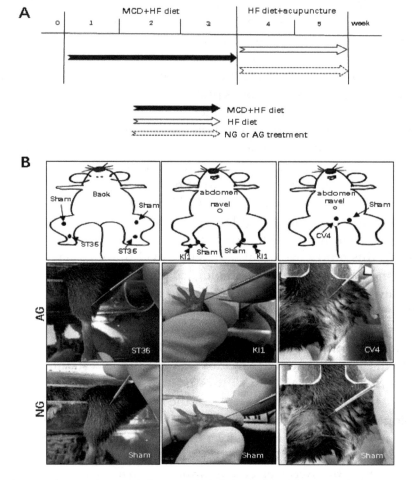

Figure 6. Acupoints and experimental design. (**A**) Schematic diagram of the experimental design. After being fed an MCD + HF diet for three weeks, mice were needled at acupoints or nonacupoints (sham) under a HF diet. (**B**) The acupoints and nonacupoints (sham) are shown in the diagrams (upper pictures). The actual acupoints and nonacupoints (sham) in mice are indicated in the middle and lower pictures. NG: needling-nonacupoint group, AG: needling-acupoint group, ST36: Zusanli, CN4: Guanyuan, KI1: Yongquan, sham: nonacupoints, MCD diet: methionine- and choline-deficient diet, HF diet: High Fat diet.

The ST36 acupoint is located near the knee joint of the hind limb and 1.5 mm from the distal side of the anterior tibial tubercle. The KI1 acupoint is located in the middle of the hind paw. The pubic symphysis was obliquely stabbed at point CV4 at the mouse abdomen median line, 10 mm below the navel [22,42,43] (Figure 6B). AG mice received acupuncture at both sides of ST36 and CV4 with 13-mm needles. Acupuncture was delivered using stainless steel needles (length: 13 mm, diameter: 0.25 mm; Hwatuo, Suzhou Medical Supplies Factory Co., Ltd., Suzhou, China). ST36 and CV4 needling was performed by straightly inserting a stainless steel needle to a depth of 3 mm. KI1 was needled obliquely toward the elbow to a depth of 2 mm. NG mice received nonacupoint needling. All points were rotated slowly at 60 rounds per minute, completed in 2 min, without retaining the needle.

4.3. Ethics

The Ethics Committee of Animal Care and Experimentation, Kanazawa Medical University, Japan, approved the protocols. The project code of the approval, 2019-21, was identified on 3 July 2019. Experiments were performed according to the Institutional Guidelines for Animal Experiments and the Law (no. 105) and Notification (no. 6) of the Japanese government. The number of animals used and their suffering were minimized.

4.4. Histopathology

After fixation in 10% neutral-buffered formalin for 24 h, paraffin-embedded liver specimens were systematically cut into sequential 4-μm-thick sections. For histological analyses of the liver, images of hematoxylin and eosin (H&E), oil red-O, and immunohistochemistry.

IHC sections were captured and quantified using the NanoZoomer Digital Pathology Virtual Slide Viewer software program (Hamamatsu Photonics Corp, Hamamatsu, Japan). To evaluate the degree of lipid accumulation (steatosis score and lipid accumulation score for the liver), we performed oil red-O staining using frozen liver sections and categorized the tissues into 4 grades, as follows: no lipid droplets (score = 0); lipid droplets in <33% of hepatocytes (score = 1); lipid droplets 33%–66% of hepatocytes (score = 2) and lipid droplets in >66% of hepatocytes (score = 3). In addition, the degree of liver cell ballooning injury (ballooning score) was classified into three grades as follows: none (score = 0); few balloon cells (score = 1) or many balloon cells/prominent ballooning (score = 2).

4.5. IHC

To evaluate the severity of NAFLD, we determined the intensity of inflammation (inflammatory score) using an anti-mouse Mac-2 monoclonal antibody (1:1000; Cedarlane Laboratories Ltd., Burlington, Ontario, Canada). As described previously [44], we counted the number of positive macrophages in 10 randomly selected fields per liver section (original magnification: ×200). The NAFLD liver tissues were then classified into four (inflammation score) grades, as follows: no inflammation (score = 0); <10 inflammatory foci, each consisting of > 5 inflammatory cells (score = 1); ≥10 inflammatory foci (score = 2) or uncountable diffuse or fused inflammatory foci (score = 3). We used the HistoMouse™–Plus Kit (Invitrogen Corporation, Camarillo, CA, USA) to block endogenous IgG and then stained tissue with a monoclonal mouse anti-human α-SMA antibody (1:1000; Dako Cytomation, Carpenteria, CA, USA.). The number of activated stellate cells was then counted in 10 randomly selected fields per section (original magnification: ×200), as described previously [44]. To determine the ROS/oxidative stress or expression in hepatocytes after acupuncture, we used an 8-OHdG monoclonal antibody (1:200; Japan Institute for the Control of Aging, Fukuroi, Japan) and quantified the number of hepatocytes positive for either antibodies in 10 randomly selected fields per section (original magnification: ×200), as previously described. For IHC studies, we examined at least 1 section from each of 17 mice per experimental group.

All histological and immunohistochemical slides were evaluated by two independent observers (certified surgical pathologists in our department; X.G. and S.Y.) using a blind protocol design (observers blinded to the mice treatment data). The agreement between the observers was excellent (more than 95%) for all antibodies investigated.

4.6. Western Blotting

Liver protein samples were separated by electrophoresis on 10% sodium dodecyl sulfate-polyacrylamide gel electrophoresis (SDS-PAGE) gels and transferred onto Immun-Blot PVDF membranes (Bio-Rad Laboratories, K.K., Tokyo, Japan). The membranes were then incubated overnight at 4 °C with IL-1β antibody (#12242; Cell Signaling,), TNF-α antibody (#11948; Cell Signaling), NF-κB antibody (#8242; Cell Signaling), phospho-NF-κB antibody (#3033; Cell Signaling) and anti-β-actin monoclonal antibody (Wako Pure Chemical Co., Osaka, Japan) diluted in Can Get Signal solution 1 (Toyobo, Osaka, Japan), after which the membranes were incubated for 1 h at room temperature with a horseradish peroxidase-conjugated goat anti-rabbit antibody (Vector Laboratories, Burlingame, CA, USA).

4.7. Analyses of Lipid Contents from the Liver

To examine the hepatic lipid profiles, each snap-frozen tissue (70 mg) was homogenized and extracted with chloroform-methanol (2/1 v/v), as described previously [45]. The organic phase was dried and resolubilized in 2-propanol. The TG, FFA, and TCHO levels were then determined using commercial assay kits (Wako Pure Chemical Co.)

4.8. Real Time Reverse Transcription Polymerase Chain Reaction (RT-PCR)

Real time PCR was used to analyze the gene expression in the liver. Total RNA was extracted from mouse liver using the extracted by ReliaPrep™ RNA Tissue Miniprep kit (Promega, Leiden, Netherlands). The whole extraction process was performed under RNase-free conditions in order to prevent RNA degradation. Custom primers and TaqMan probe for gene amplification were purchased from Life Technologies. The mRNA expression of SREBP1, LDLR, SR-A, SREBP2, SR-B1, PPARγ, PPARα, PPARβ/δ, GPx1, GPx2, GPx3, Gss, catalase, and Nrf2 was analyzed by real time PCR (TaqMan probes Applied Biosystems, Warrington, UK). The relative expression of each gene was normalized to that of 18S ribosomal RNA using random primers.

4.9. The Measurement of the TBARS Levels

We measured the liver TBARS levels using a TBARS Assay Kit (Cayman Chemical Company, Ann Arbor, MI, USA). Liver tissue specimens were homogenized in 250 RIPA buffer solution. A 100-μL aliquot of the homogenate was added to a reaction mixture containing 200 μL of 8.1% (w/v) SDS, 1.5 mL of 20% (v/v) acetic acid, pH 3.5, 1.5 mL of 0.8% (w/v) thiobarbituric acid, and 700 μL of distilled water. Samples were then boiled for 1 h at 95 °C and centrifuged at 1600× g for 10 min. The absorbance of the supernatant was measure spect rophotometrically at a wavelength of 530–540 nm [46].

4.10. Statistical Analyses

The results are expressed as the means ± standard deviation (SD). Significant differences were analyzed using Student's t-test, Welch's t-test or a one-way analysis of variance (ANOVA), where appropriate. Values of $p < 0.05$ were considered to be statistically significant.

Supplementary Materials: Figure S1: The body weight and liver weight after two weeks of acupuncture. (**A**) The body weight was significantly lower in AG mice than in those of NG mice. Values are shown as the mean ± SD, * $p < 0.05$, ** $p < 0.001$, *** $p < 0.0001$, n = 17. (**B**) The liver weight was significantly lower in AG mice than in those of NG mice. Values are shown as the mean ± SD, * $p < 0.05$, ** $p < 0.001$, *** $p < 0.0001$, n = 17. NG: needling-nonacupoint group, AG: needling-acupoint group, MCD diet: methionine- and choline-deficient diet, HF diet: high-fat diet, NAFLD: nonalcoholic fatty liver disease.; Figure S2: Acupuncture improved the lipid metabolism in the livers of mice with NAFLD. (**A**) Real time PCR revealed that the expression of ApoB, ApoE and MTTP were significantly higher in the livers of AG mice than in those of NG mice. ApoC-III showed no significant difference between the groups. (**B**)The expression of Fas, SCD1 and

AdipoR2 were significantly lower in the livers of AG mice than in those of NG mice. Values are normalized by the 18S rRNA expression. RT-PCR values are presented as the means± SD. * $p < 0.05$, ** $p < 0.001$. *** $p < 0.0001$, n = 7. NG: needling-nonacupoint group, AG: needling-acupoint group, ApoB: apolipoproteinsB, ApoE: apolipoproteinsE, MTTP: microsomal triglyceride transfer protein, ApoC-III: apolipoproteins C-III, Fas: fat acid syntheas, SCD1: stearoyl-CoA 9-desaturase 1, AdipoR2: adiponectin receptor 2.

Author Contributions: X.M., X.G., and S.Y. conceptualized and designed the experiments; X.M., J.Z., R.Y., and X.G. carried out the experiments; X.M., X.G., J.Z., J.M., and J.K. analyzed the data; X.M. and X.G. wrote the manuscript; X.G., S.Y., and X.M. edited the manuscript.

Acknowledgments: We would like to thank Yuka Hiramatsu and Manabu Yamashita for their expert technical assistance.

References

1. Marjot, T.; Moolla, A.; Cobbold, J.F.; Hodson, L.; Tomlinson, J.W. Non-alcoholic fatty liver disease in adults: Current concepts in etiology, outcomes and management. *Endocr. Rev.* **2019**, bnz009. [CrossRef]

2. Bugianesi, E.; Gentilcore, E.; Manini, R.; Natale, S.; Vanni, E.; Villanova, N.; David, E.; Rizzetto, M.; Marchesini, G. A randomized controlled trial of metformin versus vitamin E or prescriptive diet in nonalcoholic fatty liver disease. *Am. J. Gastroenterol.* **2005**, *100*, 1082–1090. [CrossRef]

3. Neuschwander-Tetri, B.A.; Brunt, E.M.; Wehmeier, K.R.; Oliver, D.; Bacon, B.R. Improved nonalcoholic steatohepatitis after 48 weeks of treatment with the PPAR-gamma ligand rosiglitazone. *Hepatology* **2003**, *38*, 1008–1017. [CrossRef]

4. Abd El-Kader, S.M.; El-Den Ashmawy, E.M. Non-alcoholic fatty liver disease: The diagnosis and management. *World J. Hepatol.* **2015**, *7*, 846–858. [CrossRef]

5. Zhang, Y.; Cui, Y.; Wang, X.L.; Shang, X.; Qi, Z.G.; Xue, J.; Zhao, X.; Deng, M.; Xie, M.L. PPARalpha/gamma agonists and antagonists differently affect hepatic lipid metabolism, oxidative stress and inflammatory cytokine production in steatohepatitic rats. *Cytokine* **2015**, *75*, 127–135. [CrossRef]

6. Pham, D.D.; Bruelle, C.; Thi Do, H.; Pajanoja, C.; Jin, C.; Srinivasan, V.; Olkkonen, V.M.; Eriksson, O.; Jauhiainen, M.; Lalowski, M.; et al. Caspase-2 and p75 neurotrophin receptor (p75NTR) are involved in the regulation of SREBP and lipid genes in hepatocyte cells. *Cell Death Dis.* **2019**, *10*, 537. [CrossRef]

7. Liu, Q.; Pan, R.; Ding, L.; Zhang, F.; Hu, L.; Ding, B.; Zhu, L.; Xia, Y.; Dou, X. Rutin exhibits hepatoprotective effects in a mouse model of non-alcoholic fatty liver disease by reducing hepatic lipid levels and mitigating lipid-induced oxidative injuries. *Int. Immunopharmacol.* **2017**, *49*, 132–141. [CrossRef]

8. Zhang, B.; Li, M.; Zou, Y.; Guo, H.; Zhang, B.; Xia, C.; Zhang, H.; Yang, W.; Xu, C. NFkappaB/Orai1 Facilitates Endoplasmic Reticulum Stress by Oxidative Stress in the Pathogenesis of Non-alcoholic Fatty Liver Disease. *Front. Cell Dev. Biol.* **2019**, *7*, 202. [CrossRef]

9. Murray, P.J.; Allen, J.E.; Biswas, S.K.; Fisher, E.A.; Gilroy, D.W.; Goerdt, S.; Gordon, S.; Hamilton, J.A.; Ivashkiv, L.B.; Lawrence, T.; et al. Macrophage activation and polarization: nomenclature and experimental guidelines. *Immunity* **2014**, *41*, 14–20. [CrossRef]

10. Dong, W.; Yang, W.; Li, F.; Guo, W.; Qian, C.; Wang, F.; Li, C.; Lin, L.; Lin, R. Electroacupuncture Improves Synaptic Function in SAMP8 Mice Probably via Inhibition of the AMPK/eEF2K/eEF2 Signaling Pathway. *Evid. Based Complement. Altern. Med.* **2019**, 8260815. [CrossRef]

11. Zhang, Y.Y.; Li, X.H.; Wu, M.X. Effect of electroacupuncture at Wnt/beta-catenin signaling pathway on inhibiting cartilage degeneration in rats with knee osteoarthritis. *Zhongguo Zhen Jiu* **2019**, *39*, 1081–1086. [PubMed]

12. Guo, Z.Q.; Huang, Y.; Jiang, H.; Wang, W.B. Randomized clinical trials of early acupuncture treatment of limb paralysis in traumatic brain injury patients and its mechanism. *Zhen Ci Yan Jiu* **2019**, *44*, 589–593. [PubMed]

13. Gao, Y.; Chen, R.; Liang, F. Mechanisms of acupuncture for non-alcoholic fatty liver disease: Researches progress and prospects. *Zhongguo Zhen Jiu* **2018**, *38*, 109–113. [PubMed]

14. Liang, F.; Koya, D. Acupuncture: Is it effective for treatment of insulin resistance? *Diabetes Obes. Metab.* **2010**, *12*, 555–569. [CrossRef] [PubMed]

15. Wang, H.Y.; Liang, C.M.; Cui, J.W.; Pan, L.; Hu, H.; Fang, H.J. Acupuncture improves hepatic lipid metabolism by suppressing oxidative stress in obese nonalcoholic fatty liver disease rats. *Zhen Ci Yan Jiu* **2019**, *44*, 189–194. [PubMed]

16. Dela Peña, A.; Leclercq, I.; Field, J.; George, J.; Jones, B.; Farrell, G. NF-kappaB activation, rather than TNF, mediates hepatic inflammation in a murine dietary model of steatohepatitis. *Gastroenterology* **2005**, *129*, 1663–1674. [CrossRef]

17. Nawata, A.; Noguchi, H.; Mazaki, Y.; Kurahashi, T.; Izumi, H.; Wang, K.Y.; Guo, X.; Uramoto, H.; Kohno, K.; Taniguchi, H.; et al. Overexpression of Peroxiredoxin 4 Affects Intestinal Function in a Dietary Mouse Model of Nonalcoholic Fatty Liver Disease. *PLoS ONE* **2016**, *11*, e0152549. [CrossRef]

18. Li, W.; Tai, Y.; Zhou, J.; Gu, W.; Bai, Z.; Zhou, T.; Zhong, Z.; McCue, P.A.; Sang, N.; Ji, J.Y.; et al. Repression of endometrial tumor growth by targeting SREBP1 and lipogenesis. *Cell Cycle* **2012**, *11*, 2348–2358. [CrossRef]

19. Korbecki, J.; Bobinski, R.; Dutka, M. Self-regulation of the inflammatory response by peroxisome proliferator-activated receptors. *Inflamm. Res.* **2019**, *68*, 443–458. [CrossRef]

20. Yang, J.W.; Li, Q.Q.; Li, F.; Fu, Q.N.; Zeng, X.H.; Liu, C.Z. The holistic effects of acupuncture treatment. *Evid. Based Complement. Alternat. Med.* **2014**, *2014*, 739708. [CrossRef]

21. Yan, Z.K.; Yang, Z.J.; Chen, F. Effect of electroacupuncture stimulation of "Housanli" (ST 36) and "Zhongwan" (CV 12) on serum leptin and hepatocellular JAK 2-STAT 3 signaling in obese rats. *Acupunct. Res.* **2015**, *40*, 1–5.

22. Kim, S.; Zhang, X.; O'Buckley, S.C.; Cooter, M.; Park, J.J.; Nackley, A.G. Acupuncture Resolves Persistent Pain and Neuroinflammation in a Mouse Model of Chronic Overlapping Pain Conditions. *J. Pain* **2018**, *19*, 1384 e1–1384 e14. [CrossRef]

23. Li, Z.X.; Zhang, H.H.; Lan, D.C.; Chen, X.Z.; Sun, J. Progress of researches on mechanisms of acupuncture therapy for insulin resistance. *Zhen Ci Yan Jiu* **2019**, *44*, 231–234. [PubMed]

24. Fan, X.L.; Yu, M.L.; Fu, S.P.; Zhuang, Y.; Lu, S.F. Effectiveness of Acupuncture in Treatment of Simple Obesity in Animal Models: A Systematic Review and Meta-Analysis. *Evid. Based Complement. Altern. Med.* **2019**, *2019*, 5459326. [CrossRef] [PubMed]

25. Wang, L.H.; Huang, W.; Wei, D.; Ding, D.G.; Liu, Y.R.; Wang, J.J.; Zhou, Z.Y. Mechanisms of Acupuncture Therapy for Simple Obesity: An Evidence-Based Review of Clinical and Animal Studies on Simple Obesity. *Evid. Based Complement. Altern. Med.* **2019**, *2019*, 5796381. [CrossRef] [PubMed]

26. Machado, M.V.; Cortez-Pinto, H. Non-alcoholic fatty liver disease: What the clinician needs to know. *World J. Gastroenterol.* **2014**, *20*, 12956–12980. [CrossRef] [PubMed]

27. Kubes, P.; Mehal, W.Z. Sterile inflammation in the liver. *Gastroenterology* **2012**, *143*, 1158–1172. [CrossRef]

28. Zhang, J.; Huang, K.; Zhong, G.; Huang, Y.; Li, S.; Qu, S.; Zhang, J. Acupuncture Decreases NF-kappaB p65, miR-155, and miR-21 and Increases miR-146a Expression in Chronic Atrophic Gastritis Rats. *Evid. Based Complement. Altern. Med.* **2016**, *2016*, 9404629. [CrossRef]

29. Kim, S.Y.; Jin, C.Y.; Kim, C.H.; Yoo, Y.H.; Choi, S.H.; Kim, G.Y.; Yoon, H.M.; Park, H.T.; Choi, Y.H. Isorhamnetin alleviates lipopolysaccharide-induced inflammatory responses in BV2 microglia by inactivating NF-kappaB, blocking the TLR4 pathway and reducing ROS generation. *Int. J. Mol. Med.* **2019**, *43*, 682–692.

30. Anderson, N.; Borlak, J. Molecular mechanisms and therapeutic targets in steatosis and steatohepatitis. *Pharmacol. Rev.* **2008**, *60*, 311–357. [CrossRef]

31. Park, J.W.; Jeong, G.; Kim, S.J.; Kim, M.K.; Park, S.M. Predictors reflecting the pathological severity of non-alcoholic fatty liver disease: comprehensive study of clinical and immunohistochemical findings in younger Asian patients. *J. Gastroenterol. Hepatol.* **2007**, *22*, 491–497. [CrossRef] [PubMed]

32. Da Silva, M.D.; Bobinski, F.; Sato, K.L.; Kolker, S.J.; Sluka, K.A.; Santos, A.R. IL-10 cytokine released from M2 macrophages is crucial for analgesic and anti-inflammatory effects of acupuncture in a model of inflammatory muscle pain. *Mol. Neurobiol.* **2015**, *51*, 19–31. [CrossRef] [PubMed]

33. Lee, F.Y.; Huo, Z.J.; Zhang, L.; Guo, J.; Chen, H.; Liu, T.; Peng, B.; Hong, P.X.; Peng, Y.Y.; Fan, Y.F.; et al. The Effects of Needling Fenglong (ST40) and Neiguan (PC6) on IL-17 of ApoE-Gene-Knockout Mice's Liver. *Evid. Based Complement. Altern. Med.* **2014**, *2014*, 691863. [CrossRef] [PubMed]

34. Browning, J.D.; Horton, J.D. Molecular mediators of hepatic steatosis and liver injury. *J. Clin. Investig.* **2004**, *114*, 147–152. [CrossRef] [PubMed]

35. Koo, S.H. Nonalcoholic fatty liver disease: Molecular mechanisms for the hepatic steatosis. *Clin. Mol. Hepatol.* **2013**, *19*, 210–215. [CrossRef]

36. Yamaguchi, K.; Yang, L.; McCall, S.; Huang, J.; Yu, X.X.; Pandey, S.K.; Bhanot, S.; Monia, B.P.; Li, Y.X.; Diehl, A.M. Inhibiting triglyceride synthesis improves hepatic steatosis but exacerbates liver damage and fibrosis in obese mice with nonalcoholic steatohepatitis. *Hepatology* **2007**, *45*, 1366–1374. [CrossRef]

37. Caballero, F.; Fernandez, A.; De Lacy, A.M.; Fernandez-Checa, J.C.; Caballeria, J.; Garcia-Ruiz, C. Enhanced free cholesterol, SREBP-2 and StAR expression in human NASH. *J. Hepatol.* **2009**, *50*, 789–796. [CrossRef]

38. Donnelly, K.L.; Smith, C.I.; Schwarzenberg, S.J.; Jessurun, J.; Boldt, M.D.; Parks, E.J. Sources of fatty acids stored in liver and secreted via lipoproteins in patients with nonalcoholic fatty liver disease. *J. Clin. Investig.* **2005**, *115*, 1343–1351. [CrossRef]

39. Bell, M.; Wang, H.; Chen, H.; McLenithan, J.C.; Gong, D.W.; Yang, R.Z.; Yu, D.; Fried, S.K.; Quon, M.J.; Londos, C.; et al. Consequences of lipid droplet coat protein downregulation in liver cells: Abnormal lipid droplet metabolism and induction of insulin resistance. *Diabetes* **2008**, *57*, 2037–2045. [CrossRef]

40. Basaranoglu, M.; Kayacetin, S.; Yilmaz, N.; Kayacetin, E.; Tarcin, O.; Sonsuz, A. Understanding mechanisms of the pathogenesis of nonalcoholic fatty liver disease. *World J. Gastroenterol.* **2010**, *16*, 2223–2226. [CrossRef]

41. Tessari, P.; Coracina, A.; Cosma, A.; Tiengo, A. Hepatic lipid metabolism and non-alcoholic fatty liver disease. *Nutr. Metab. Cardiovasc. Dis.* **2009**, *19*, 291–302. [CrossRef] [PubMed]

42. Tan, R.; He, Y.; Zhang, S.; Pu, D.; Wu, J. Effect of transcutaneous electrical acupoint stimulation on protecting against radiotherapy- induced ovarian damage in mice. *J. Ovarian Res.* **2019**, *12*, 65. [CrossRef] [PubMed]

43. Li, T.; Xu, X.; Chen, B.; Rong, J.; Jiang, H. Photoacoustic imaging of acupuncture effect in small animals. *Biomed. Opt. Express* **2015**, *6*, 433–442. [CrossRef] [PubMed]

44. Zhang, J.; Guo, X.; Hamada, T.; Yokoyama, S.; Nakamura, Y.; Zheng, J.; Kurose, N.; Ishigaki, Y.A.-O.; Uramoto, H.; Tanimoto, A.; et al. Protective Effects of Peroxiredoxin 4 (PRDX4) on Cholestatic Liver Injury. *Int. J. Mol. Sci.* **2018**, *19*, 2509. [CrossRef] [PubMed]

45. Nabeshima, A.; Yamada, S.; Guo, X.; Tanimoto, A.; Wang, K.Y.; Shimajiri, S.; Kimura, S.; Tasaki, T.; Noguchi, H.; Kitada, S.; et al. Peroxiredoxin 4 protects against nonalcoholic steatohepatitis and type 2 diabetes in a nongenetic mouse model. *Antioxid Redox Signal* **2013**, *19*, 1983–1998. [CrossRef] [PubMed]

46. Guo, X.; Noguchi, H.; Ishii, N.; Homma, T.; Hamada, T.; Hiraki, T.; Zhang, J.; Matsuo, K.; Yokoyama, S.; Ishibashi, H.; et al. The Association of Peroxiredoxin 4 with the Initiation and Progression of Hepatocellular Carcinoma. *Antioxid. Redox Signal.* **2019**, *30*, 1271–1284. [CrossRef]

11

Proton NMR Enables the Absolute Quantification of Aqueous Metabolites and Lipid Classes in Unique Mouse Liver Samples

Aurélien Amiel [1,2], Marie Tremblay-Franco [1,2], Roselyne Gautier [1,2], Simon Ducheix [1], Alexandra Montagner [1], Arnaud Polizzi [1], Laurent Debrauwer [1,2], Hervé Guillou [1], Justine Bertrand-Michel [3] and Cécile Canlet [1,2,*]

[1] Toxalim-Research Centre in Food Toxicology, Toulouse University, INRAE UMR 1331, ENVT, INP-Purpan, Paul Sabatier University, F-31027 Toulouse, France; aurelien.amiel@yahoo.fr (A.A.); marie.tremblay-franco@inra.fr (M.T.-F.); roselyne.gautier@inra.fr (R.G.); simon.ducheix@univ-nantes.fr (S.D.); alexandra.montagner@inserm.fr (A.M.); arnaud.polizzi@inra.fr (A.P.); laurent.debrauwer@inra.fr (L.D.); herve.guillou@inra.fr (H.G.)

[2] Metatoul-AXIOM platform, National Infrastructure for Metabolomics and Fluxomics, MetaboHUB, Toxalim, INRAE UMR 1331, F-31027 Toulouse, France

[3] Metatoul-Lipidomic Core Facility, MetaboHUB, I2MC U1048, INSERM, F-31432 Toulouse, France; justine.bertrand-michel@inserm.fr

* Correspondence: cecile.canlet@inra.fr

Abstract: Hepatic metabolites provide valuable information on the physiological state of an organism, and thus, they are monitored in many clinical situations. Typically, monitoring requires several analyses for each class of targeted metabolite, which is time consuming. The present study aimed to evaluate a proton nuclear magnetic resonance (^{1}H-NMR) method for obtaining quantitative measurements of aqueous and lipidic metabolites. We optimized the extraction protocol, the standard samples, and the organic solvents for the absolute quantification of lipid species. To validate the method, we analyzed metabolic profiles in livers of mice fed three different diets. We compared our results with values obtained with conventional methods and found strong correlations. The ^{1}H-NMR protocol enabled the absolute quantification of 29 aqueous metabolites and eight lipid classes. Results showed that mice fed a diet enriched in saturated fatty acids had higher levels of triglycerides, cholesterol ester, monounsaturated fatty acids, lactate, 3-hydroxy-butyrate, and alanine and lower levels of glucose, compared to mice fed a control diet. In conclusion, proton NMR provided a rapid overview of the main lipid classes (triglycerides, cholesterol, phospholipids, fatty acids) and the most abundant aqueous metabolites in liver.

Keywords: metabolomics quantitative profiling; lipidomics; ^{1}H-NMR spectroscopy; liver; steatosis

1. Introduction

The liver is among the most metabolically diverse organs of the body, and it is involved in many metabolic processes. The liver plays a central physiological role in lipid metabolism; e.g., it hosts cholesterol synthesis, cholesterol degradation to bile acids, triglyceride production, and lipoprotein synthesis. The liver may be affected by many pathological aggressions. Associated with the obesity epidemic, Non Alcoholic Fatty Liver Diseases (NAFLD) is currently a major public health concern [1]. NAFLD ranges from benign fat accumulation to inflammatory steatohepatitis that may promote irreversible damage [1]. The current methods of diagnostic mostly rely on liver biopsies [2]. However, metabolomic approaches are extensively used for biomarker identification as well as for identification of metabolic pathways involved in the progression of lipid accumulation [3,4]. Therefore, there is a lot of interest in methods allowing the integration of both soluble metabolites and lipids from a single sample.

Metabolomics is currently established as a powerful investigation tool that provides rich information on metabolic disturbances in human disease. Mass spectrometry (MS) and nuclear magnetic resonance (NMR) are the two most widely used techniques in metabolomics. NMR spectroscopy has several advantages over MS, including high reproducibility, non-destructive analysis, a simple quantification approach, and minimal sample preparation [5]. ^{1}H-NMR-based metabolomics is currently widely used to gain insights into liver disease mechanisms [6,7] or to evaluate drug hepatotoxicity [8,9] and environmental contaminants [10]. In most studies that used proton NMR-based metabolomics for liver samples, analyses have been performed on either aqueous extracts or lipidic extracts. Those analyses employed spectral binning, followed by multivariate statistical analyses to highlight changes in metabolite composition due to disease [11–14], alcohol consumption [15–17], or contaminant exposure [18].

Lipids are a diverse, ubiquitous group of compounds, which have many key biological functions. Many diseases alter lipid metabolism; thus, a better understanding of these pathologies can be gained by analyzing lipid composition. Due to the structural diversity among lipid molecules, lipidomic profiling is complex. For the least abundant lipids (i.e., free fatty acids, cholesterol, oxylipids), we typically choose powerful, targeted, but time-consuming approaches, like liquid chromatography (LC) or gas chromatography (GC) coupled to mass spectrometry (MS) techniques (i.e., LC-MS or GC-MS), which can provide absolute quantitative results, under certain conditions [19]. However, to evaluate the most abundant lipids (i.e., phospholipids, sphingolipids, and triacylglycerides), we typically use LC-MS approaches that are not targeted, even though they do not provide quantitative results [20]. NMR is an alternative method that provides rapid, and in particular, quantitative analyses of hepatic lipids. Some studies have analyzed intact liver samples (biopsies) with high-resolution magic angle spinning (HR-MAS) NMR spectroscopy to study metabolic disruptions in human chronic hepatitis and cirrhosis [21] or to study non-alcoholic fatty liver disease (NAFLD) in murine models [22]. Those studies were carried out directly in the solid tissues, without any extraction. With HR-MAS, both lipid and aqueous metabolites can be simultaneous observed in the same spectrum, but the resolution is low, and absolute quantification is complex, due to overlapping signals. Other studies have performed metabolic analyses on tissue extracts to study human hepatocellular carcinoma (HCC) associated with NAFLD or cirrhosis [23] or to study the progression from hepatic steatosis to nonalcoholic steatohepatitis (NASH) in mouse models [24]. NMR analyses of tissue extracts require sample processing and separate analyses for lipidic and aqueous extracts. However, liquid state NMR provides spectra with a better resolution than those recorded with the HRMAS technique, and absolute quantification can be performed when a standard is used at a known concentration. Only a few studies have reported the absolute quantification of lipidic metabolites in liver samples, based on ^{1}H-NMR spectroscopy [24]. Indeed, lipid species contain many long-chain fatty acids, and therefore, many overlapping proton signals (e.g., $(CH_2)_n$ in fatty acids), which makes a detailed characterization of lipid species unfeasible. However, with ^{1}H NMR spectroscopy, it is possible to identify and quantify different classes of lipids, such as cholesterol, triglycerides, phospholipids, mono-unsaturated fatty acids (MUFAs), and poly-unsaturated fatty acids (PUFAs).

The present study aimed to evaluate ^{1}H-NMR spectroscopy for the identification and absolute quantification of polar and non-polar metabolites in the same liver sample. First, we compared two extraction methods to optimize aqueous and lipidic metabolite extractions. Then, we optimized the absolute quantification of lipid species on mixtures of lipid standards, by comparing internal vs. external standards and various organic solvents. Finally, the optimized method was applied to investigate the effects of a diet deficient in essential fatty acids on liver mouse metabolism. Hepatic lipids were quantified with both ^{1}H-NMR spectroscopy and conventional methods to compare the results and validate the methodology.

2. Results

2.1. Comparison of Extraction Methods

Sample preparation represents a crucial step in metabolomic studies. In this study, we aimed to obtain the best preparation for both polar and lipid molecules. Several classical solvent systems have been developed for liver extractions [25]. Among the various possibilities, we chose Bligh and Dyer [26] and Folch [27] extractions, because these two methods resulted in a biphasic solvent system. Moreover, these were the main extraction methods used in our lab for targeted lipidomics, performed with conventional methods, and for NMR-based metabolomics [28]. With these extraction methods, the upper phase contained the polar (aqueous) fraction, and the bottom phase contained the lipids. When we tested the Bligh and Dyer extraction method with 50 mg of liver, we noticed the presence of an emulsion, which made it difficult to separate the aqueous and organic phases. With the Folch extraction method, the organic phase was washed with a saturated NaCl solution, and the phases were well separated.

A visual assessment of the ^{1}H-NMR spectra revealed that the two extraction procedures produced similar peak coverages and intensities for the extracted lipids (Figure 1). For the aqueous extracts, the intensities were higher in the aromatic region (δ 9.0–6.0 ppm) with the Folch extraction method than with the Bligh and Dyer method (Figure 2).

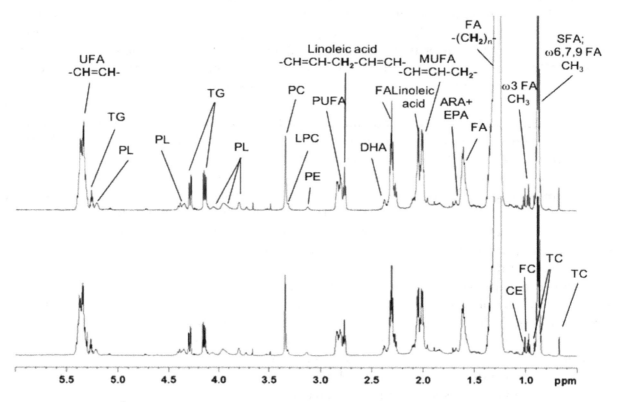

Figure 1. 600 MHz ^{1}H-NMR spectra of lipophilic extracts from mouse liver samples. The Folch extraction method (top) and the Bligh and Dyer extraction method (bottom) show the same peaks. The peaks are labeled in only one panel for clarity, as follows: FC, free cholesterol; CE, cholesterol ester; TC, total cholesterol; FA, fatty acids; SFA, saturated fatty acids; ARA, arachidonic acid; EPA, eicosapentaenoic acid; MUFA, monounsaturated fatty acids; DHA, docosahexaenoic acid; PUFA, polyunsaturated fatty acid; PE, phosphatidylethanolamine; LPC, lysophosphatidylcholine; PC, phosphatidylcholine; PL, phospholipids; TG, triglycerides; UFA, unsaturated fatty acids.

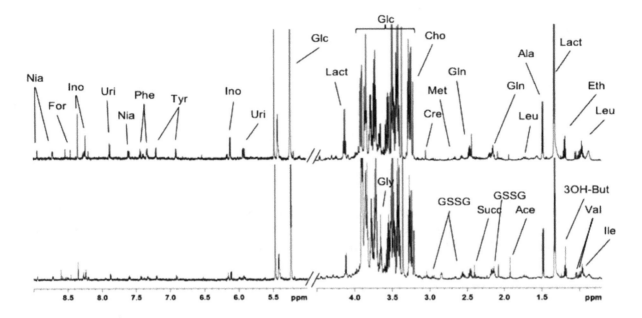

Figure 2. 600 MHz ^{1}H-NMR spectra of aqueous extracts from mouse liver samples. The Folch extraction method (top) revealed more peaks than the Bligh and Dyer extraction method (bottom). The peaks are labeled in only one panel for clarity, as follows: Ile, isoleucine; Val, valine; 3OH-But, 3-hydroxybutyrate; Ace, acetate; GSSG, glutathione oxidized; Succ, succinate; Gly, glycine; Leu, leucine; Eth, ethanol; Lact, lactate; Ala, alanine; Gln, glutamine; Met, methionine; Cre, creatine; Cho, choline; Glc, glucose; Uri, uridine; Ino, inosine; Tyr, tyrosine; Phe, phenylalanine; Nia, niacinamide; For, formate.

For each method, the buckets representing metabolites with signal-to-noise ratios above 10 (SNR > 10) were annotated by comparing the chemical shifts in the 1D ^{1}H-NMR spectra with those of reference spectra recorded under the same conditions and reference spectra deposited in the Biological Magnetic Resonance Databank [29] and the Human Metabolome Database [30]. We could identify 29 metabolites present in the polar fraction and eight lipid classes present in the non-polar fraction. ^{1}H-NMR resonance assignments of aqueous and lipidic metabolites are shown in Tables S1 and S2, respectively, with the chemical shifts, multiplicity, and coupling constants of the signals elucidated in the ^{1}H-NMR spectra for both the water- and lipid-soluble extracts from mouse liver. For the lipidic extracts, among the selected 52 buckets, 50 were detected with an SNR > 10 with both extraction methods, which suggested that there was no significant difference between the two extraction methods, based on this criterion. For the aqueous extracts, among the selected 80 buckets, 40 and 58 were detected with an SNR > 10 with the Bligh and Dyer and the Folch extraction methods, respectively. This finding confirmed that the Folch method provided better extraction of the aqueous metabolites.

We performed a multivariate analysis combined with a principal component analysis (PCA) of the NMR buckets that described components of the extracts from both methods. We found that, for lipidic extracts, the two extraction methods were separated along the second principal component, which explained 11% of the variability. For aqueous extracts, the samples were separated along the first principal component, which explained 72.1% of the variability. These results suggested that the aqueous metabolites extracted were significantly different between these two extraction methods (Figure 3). The loading plot for aqueous liver extracts showed signals that contributed to the separation between extraction methods (Figure 4). Taurine, lactate, glucose, choline, alanine, glutathione and others amino acids are elevated in Folch extraction, and glycogen and adenosinemonophosphate (AMP) are elevated in Blye and Dyer extraction.

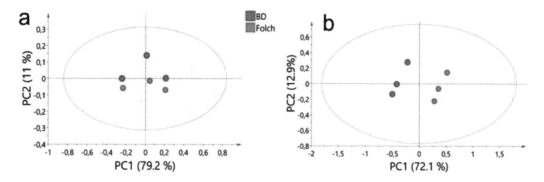

Figure 3. Principal component analysis score plot of the two extraction methods. (**a**) Liver lipidic extracts (*n* = 3); (**b**) liver aqueous extracts (*n* = 3). BD = Bligh and Dyer extraction method (red); Folch = Folch extraction method (green). Ellipses indicate the 95% confidence region.

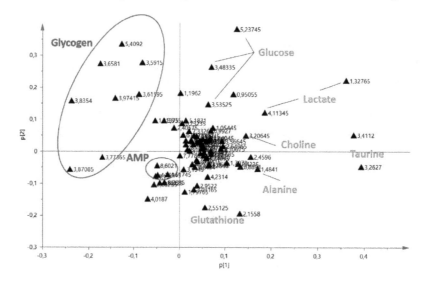

Figure 4. Principal component analysis loading plot of the two extraction methods for aqueous liver extracts. NMR buckets with the highest absolute loadings contributed the most to the separation between the two extraction methods and were annotated. Metabolites in red were elevated in Blye and Dyer extraction and metabolites in green were elevated in Folch extraction.

Generally, when the two classical Bligh and Dyer and Folch lipid extraction methods were used, most studies focused either on the analysis of lipid extracts using MS techniques [31] or on the analysis of aqueous extracts by NMR spectroscopy [32,33], but few studied reported the analysis of both extracts. Our results showed that, in this case, the Folch extraction method was more efficient in extracting aqueous metabolites than the Bligh and Dyer method, but the two extraction methods showed no differences in extracting lipidic metabolites. The variability was similar with both extraction methods. Therefore, we selected the Folch extraction method for all subsequent analyses in this study.

2.2. Absolute Quantification of Lipidic and Aqueous Metabolites

In NMR, absolute quantification requires the use of an internal or external standard at a known concentration. A number of reference compounds are available for quantitative NMR analysis. The most widely used reference compounds for chemical shift referencing and quantitative analysis are tetramethylsilane (TMS, organic solubility), 3-(trimethylsilyl)-1-propane sulfonic acid sodium salt (DSS, aqueous solubility), and 3-(trimethylsilyl)propionic acid sodium salt (TSP, aqueous solubility) [34]. In this study, for aqueous extracts, we used TSP as an internal standard, TSP was directly dissolved in the sample. Signals used for absolute quantification of aqueous metabolites were indicated in bold in Table S1. For lipid quantifications, TMS was directly dissolved in the sample as an internal standard; as an external standard, TSP was dissolved in deuterated water (D_2O) in a coaxial capillary tube for mixtures of lipid standards. The final solvent in an NMR experiment is another key point: in the literature, deuterated chloroform ($CDCl_3$) and a mixture of $CDCl_3$ and deuterated methanol (CD_3OD) are mostly used for lipidomic analyses. In the present study, we tested both pure deuterated chloroform ($CDCl_3$) and a 4:1 (*v/v*) mixture of $CDCl_3$ and CD_3OD for the final solvent. The lipid extracts and standards were dissolved in these solvents.

The metabolites were quantified according to the following expression:

$$Cx = \frac{\frac{Ix \times Cs}{Nx}}{\frac{Is}{Ns}} \times \frac{V}{M} \tag{1}$$

where Cx is the metabolite concentration, Ix is the integral of the metabolite proton peak, Nx is the number of protons in the metabolite proton peak, Cs is the standard concentration, Is is the integral of the standard proton peak, Ns is the number of protons in the standard proton peak, V is the volume of the analyzed extract, and M is the weight of liver tissue analyzed.

The quantification of lipid species was simple for isolated peaks without any signal overlapping, such as the total cholesterol (TC, singlet, 3H, 0.68 ppm), ω-3 fatty acids (ω-3 FAs, triplet, 3H, 0.97 ppm), arachidonic and eicosapentaenoic acids (ARA+EPA, multiplet, 2H, 1.68 ppm), MUFAs (multiplet, 4H, 2.01 ppm), docosahexaenoic acid (DHA, multiplet, 4H, 2.38 ppm), linoleic acid (triplet, 2H, 2.27 ppm), phosphatidylethanolamine (PE, multiplet, 2H, 3.12 ppm), phosphatidylcholine and lysophosphatidylcholine (PC+LPC, singlet, 9H, 3.20 ppm), triglycerides (doublet of doublets, 2H, 4.29 ppm), and sphingomyelin (SM, multiplet, 1H, 5.70 ppm). Free cholesterol (FC) and cholesterol ester (CE) could be quantified based on the signals at 1.01 and 1.02 ppm, respectively, with the deconvolution algorithm available in Topspin software (Bruker, Rheinstetten, Germany). PUFAs could not be quantified directly, because the number of protons that corresponded to the signals at 2.82 ppm could not be determined precisely. As previously mentioned by Vidal et al. [35], it was possible to determine the molar percentage of unsaturated fatty acids (UFA) with the following equation:

$$UFA\ (\%) = \frac{100 \times ((2 \times A7) + A9))}{((2 \times A9) + (4 \times A8))} \tag{2}$$

where $A7$ is the signal integration between 1.92 and 2.15 ppm corresponding to the functional group $-CH_2-CH=CH-$ acyl group except for $-CH_2-$ of DHA acyl group; $A8$ is the signal integration between 2.25 and 2.36 ppm corresponding to the functional group $-OCO-CH_2-$ acyl group except for DHA; and $A9$ is the signal integration between 2.36 and 2.42 ppm corresponding to the functional group $-OCO-CH_2-CH_2-$ of DHA acyl group.

The total fatty acid concentration could be determined as the sum of the signals at 0.97 ppm (ω-3 FAs) and 0.88 ppm. From this value, we could calculate the concentrations of UFAs, saturated fatty acids (SFAs), and PUFAs.

To validate our quantification method, we analyzed five mixtures of five lipid standards (triglycerides C17:0; FC; oleate cholesterol; DHA; and linoleic acid) and five mixtures of three phospholipid standards (PC, PE, and SM) at different concentrations (Table S3). These 10 mixtures represented most of the common signals in ^1H NMR spectra of lipophilic extracts from liver samples. Annotated NMR spectra of mixture of lipid standards (mix3) and mixture of phospholipid standards (mix6) are presented in Figures S1 and S2 respectively. The concentrations of lipid species were determined by calibrating to the internal and external standards in the two organic solvents. Tables 1 and 2 list the correlations between the concentrations obtained with NMR signal integration and their respective real concentrations, obtained by internal or external standard calibrations. The corresponding scatter plots and linear regressions are available in Figures S3 and S4 (TSP and $CDCl_3$), Figures S5 and S6 (TMS and $CDCl_3$), Figures S7 and S8 (TSP and $CDCl_3$-CD_3OD mixture), and

Figures S9 and S10 (TMS and CDCl$_3$-CD$_3$OD mixture). All hypotheses underlying the linear regression (linearity, independence, homogeneity) were validated by the residue analysis. The results showed that the external standard and the solvent mixture CDCl$_3$/CD$_3$OD (4:1) provided the best correlations (r > 0.9) and linearity in the regression analyses (i.e., slopes that approximated 1).

Table 1. Pearson's r correlations and regression slopes indicate the similarity between NMR quantifications and real lipid concentrations for lipid mixtures dissolved in the solvent, CDCl$_3$.

Lipid Species	External Standard (TSP)			Internal Standard (TMS)		
	Pearson's r	p-value [a]	Slope	Pearson's r	p-value [a]	Slope
Total FA	0.98	0.002	1.3	0.82	0.089	0.8
Saturated FA	0.98	0.002	1.2	0.97	0.006	1.0
ω-3 FA	0.98	0.002	1.0	0.94	0.019	1.8
MUFA	0.98	0.001	1.2	0.93	0.019	2.0
PUFA	0.92	0.03	0.8	0.95	0.015	1.7
UFA	0.94	0.017	0.8	0.95	0.014	1.7
DHA	0.99	0.0001	1.1	0.93	0.024	1.9
Linoleic acid	0.98	0.002	0.9	0.93	0.025	1.7
TC	0.99	0.0003	1.2	0.89	0.04	2.5
FC	0.95	0.011	1.0	0.89	0.04	1.7
CE	0.99	0.00007	0.8	0.98	0.004	1.4
Triglycerides	0.99	0.001	1.2	0.98	0.004	1.0
PC	0.95	0.012	1.2	0.96	0.009	1.2
PE	0.55	0.33	0.1	0.99	0.0001	0.2
SM	0.94	0.018	0.8	0.98	0.002	0.9
Total PL	0.91	0.03	0.9	0.95	0.015	1.0

[a] p value of the Pearson test (H0: $r = 0$); Abbreviations: TSP, 3-(trimethylsilyl)propionic acid sodium salt; TMS, tetramethylsilane; FA, fatty acids; MUFA, monounsaturated fatty acids; PUFA, monounsaturated fatty acids; UFA, unsaturated fatty acids; DHA, docosahexaenoic acid; TC, total cholesterol; FC, free cholesterol; CE, cholesterol ester; PC, phosphatidylcholine; PE, phosphatidylethanolamine; SM, sphingomyelin; PL, phospholipids.

Table 2. Pearson's r correlations and regression slopes indicate the similarity between NMR quantifications and real lipid concentrations for lipid mixtures dissolved in the mixture of solvents, CDCl$_3$/CD$_3$OD (4:1).

Lipid Species	External Standard (TSP)			Internal Standard (TMS)		
	Pearson's r	p-value [a]	Slope	Pearson's r	p-value [a]	Slope
Total FA	0.99	5×10^{-5}	1.0	0.98	2×10^{-3}	1.2
Saturated FA	0.99	2×10^{-5}	1.0	0.98	2×10^{-3}	1.2
ω-3 FA	0.99	5×10^{-5}	1.0	0.98	2×10^{-3}	1.0
MUFA	0.99	3×10^{-5}	1.1	0.99	4×10^{-4}	1.0
PUFA	0.99	5×10^{-4}	1.0	0.97	6×10^{-3}	1.5
UFA	0.99	3×10^{-4}	1.0	0.97	5×10^{-3}	1.4
DHA	0.99	1×10^{-5}	1.1	0.99	4×10^{-5}	0.7
Linoleic acid	0.99	8×10^{-6}	0.9	0.99	2×10^{-4}	1.0
TC	0.98	2×10^{-3}	1.1	0.96	9×10^{-3}	1.6
FC	0.99	6×10^{-4}	1.0	0.93	2×10^{-2}	1.5
CE	0.99	8×10^{-4}	0.9	0.98	2×10^{-3}	0.9
Triglycerides	0.99	3×10^{-6}	1.0	0.99	7×10^{-4}	1.0
PC	0.99	5×10^{-5}	1.2	0.99	2×10^{-4}	1.1
PE	0.98	3×10^{-3}	0.6	0.91	3×10^{-2}	0.5
SM	0.99	8×10^{-4}	0.9	0.96	8×10^{-3}	0.8
Total PL	0.99	3×10^{-5}	1.0	0.99	2×10^{-5}	1.2

[a] pvalue of the Pearson test (H0: $r = 0$); Abbreviations: TSP, 3-(trimethylsilyl)propionic acid sodium salt; TMS, tetramethylsilane; FA, fatty acids; MUFA, monounsaturated fatty acids; PUFA, monounsaturated fatty acids; UFA, unsaturated fatty acids; DHA, docosahexaenoic acid; TC, total cholesterol; FC, free cholesterol; CE, cholesterol ester; PC, phosphatidylcholine; PE, phosphatidylethanolamine; SM, sphingomyelin; PL, phospholipids.

These results also suggested that TMS was unsuitable for quantitative analyses and that the nature of the solvent was important. Phospholipids contain polar headgroups and nonpolar fatty acyl residues, which lead to line broadening in ^{1}H-NMR spectroscopy; thus, the quantification was not accurate. Accordingly, we used an external standard and the solvent mixture, $CDCl_3/CD_3OD$ (4:1 v/v), for the biological study.

2.3. Analytical Validation with Liver Samples in a Dietary Intervention Study

We evaluated the use of ^{1}H-NMR spectroscopy for quantifying aqueous and lipidic metabolites in liver samples from mice fed the following diets: COCO (deficient in essential fatty acids, with 5% saturated FA-rich oil), REF (balanced diet with 5% REF oil), and FISH (n-3 PUFA-enriched diet, with 5% PUFA-rich oil). Lipids were quantified with ^{1}H-NMR spectroscopy and an external standard dissolved in the mixture of solvents, $CDCl_3/CD_3OD$ (4:1 *v/v*).

2.3.1. Comparison with GC-FID Data

We compared ^{1}H-NMR spectroscopy results to those obtained with GC with a flame ionization detector (GC-FID). We took the GC-FID data as the reference method for quantifying fatty acids and neutral lipids. Table 3 shows the correlation between NMR quantifications (expressed in nmol/mg of liver) and GC-FID quantifications. The correlations were good for all tested lipids ($r > 0.8$, $p < 0.01$), except for ARA+EPA.

Table 3. Pearson's r correlations indicate the similarity between NMR and GC-FID quantifications of lipid concentrations in livers of mice in the dietary study.

Lipid Species	Pearson's r	*p*-value [a]
Total FA	0.93	8.8×10^{-8}
Saturated FA	0.85	1.43×10^{-5}
ω-3 FA	0.80	1.1×10^{-4}
MUFA	0.96	4.5×10^{-10}
PUFA	0.80	9.6×10^{-5}
ARA+EPA	0.69	2×10^{-3}
DHA	0.95	3.4×10^{-9}
Linoleic acid	0.96	6.7×10^{-10}
MUFA/PUFA	0.89	1.3×10^{-6}
Total cholesterol	0.99	1.2×10^{-14}
Free cholesterol	0.91	1.3×10^{-6}
Cholesterol ester	0.98	6.6×10^{-12}
Triglycerides	0.98	7.7×10^{-12}

[a] p value of the Pearson test (H0: $r = 0$); Abbreviations: FA, fatty acids; MUFA, monounsaturated fatty acids; PUFA, polyunsaturated fatty acids; DHA, docosahexaenoic acid.

2.3.2. Comparison with LC-MS Data

The quantification of phospholipids with LC-MS provided relative values, due to the unavailability of standards for calibrating LC-MS quantifications. Thus, for phospholipids, we could only compare relative differences between diets. Table 4 shows the ratios of phospholipid concentrations between the test and reference diets. These ratios were calculated with results from the ^{1}H-NMR and LC-MS analyses to compare the two methods. The relative error between LC-MS and NMR values were smaller than 6% for PE, PC+LPC and total PC except for SM (10%). We can assume that the quantification ratios provided by the ^{1}H-NMR analyses were similar to the quantification ratios provided by the LC-MS analyses. For SM ratio, the relative error was larger because the NMR signal was weak.

Table 4. Comparison between ^{1}H-NMR and LC-MS methods for determining ratios of phospholipid concentrations in livers from mice fed different diets in the dietary study.

Concentration Ratio	PE		PC + LPC		SM		Total PL, Except LPC	
	LC-MS	NMR	LC-MS	NMR	LC-MS	NMR	LC-MS	NMR
COCO/REF	0.94	0.95	1.07	1.01	0.90	0.81	1.05	1.03
FISH/REF	1.24	1.17	1.13	1.06	1.00	1.10	1.12	1.08

Abbreviations: COCO, a diet with 5% saturated FA-rich oil; REF: a diet with 5% reference oil (control); FISH: a diet with 5% n-3 long-chain PUFA-rich oil; PE, phosphatidylethanolamine; PC, phosphatidylcholine; LPC, lysophosphatidylcholine; PL, phospholipids;.

2.3.3. Comparison with LipSpin Results

LipSpin is a bioinformatic tool for the automatic quantification of lipid species, which uses ^{1}H-NMR spectra of biological matrices [36]. Lipid quantifications rely on line-shape fitting analyses of spectral regions, from which individual signal areas are obtained. The user can select a signal pattern optimized for blood serum, which is provided by the algorithm; however, we designed our own signal pattern and imported our standard spectra, because our experimental conditions were different (i.e., solvents and acquisition parameters). This tool is user-friendly, fast, and requires only the import of NMR spectra. LipSpin provided the integration values for SFA, ω-3 FA, MUFA, ARA+EPA, linoleic acid, FC, EC, triglyceride, PL, PE, SM, PC, and LPC signals. The concentration was calculated for each lipid species based on the total cholesterol concentration determined with GC-FID. Table 5 shows the correlations between LipSpin quantifications (expressed in nmol/mg liver) and our NMR quantifications. We found good correlations for ω-3 FA, MUFA, linoleic acid, EC, and triglycerides ($r > 0.8$, $p < 0.01$), but low correlation values were obtained for other lipid species.

Table 5. Pearson's r correlations between LipSpin and NMR quantifications of lipid concentrations in livers from mice fed different diets in the dietary study.

Lipid Species	Pearson's r	p-value [a]
Saturated FA	0.66	5.7×10^{-3}
ω-3 FA	0.98	7.4×10^{-12}
MUFA	0.97	3.0×10^{-10}
ARA+EPA	0.001	0.99
DHA	0.31	0.24
Linoleic acid	0.95	2.8×10^{-8}
Free cholesterol	0.54	0.031
Esterified cholesterol	0.80	1.8×10^{-4}
Triglycerides	0.97	9.2×10^{-10}
Total phospholipids	0.27	0.32
PE	0.58	0.017
SM	0.14	0.59
PC+LPC	0.37	0.15

[a] p value of the Pearson test (H0: $r = 0$); Abbreviations: FA, fatty acids; MUFA, monounsaturated fatty acids; ARA, arachidonic acid; EPA, eicosapentaenoic acid; DHA, docosahexaenoic acid; PE, phosphatidylethanolamine; SM, sphingomyelin; PC, phosphatidylcholine; LPC, lysophosphatidylcholine.

2.3.4. Biological Results

Figure 5 shows the mean concentrations of lipid species in the livers of mice fed each diet obtained from ^{1}H-NMR spectra. Lipid modifications were in good agreement with the results previously obtained with the standard GC-FID method [37]. The ^{1}H-NMR and GC-FID methods also showed comparable significant increases in triglycerides and CE in mice fed the COCO diet compared to mice fed the REF diet. In addition, the ^{1}H-NMR method highlighted significant increases in fatty acids, MUFAs, and SFAs, and significant decreases in PUFAs (DHA, EPA, linoleic acid, and ω-3 FA) in mice fed the COCO diet compared to mice fed the REF diet. Moreover, we observed significant increases in DHA and ω-3 FAs in mice fed the FISH diet compared to mice fed the REF diet. Although we did not compare the results on aqueous metabolites with results obtained with other methods, we found no significant changes in aqueous metabolites among the three diets, based on absolute concentrations.

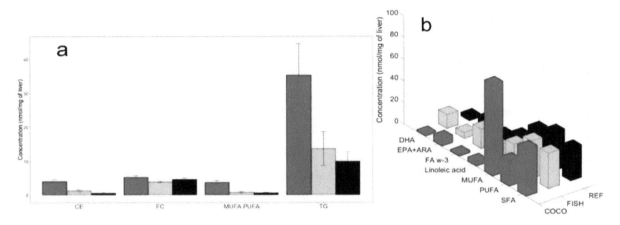

Figure 5. The quality of dietary fatty acids (FAs) affected hepatic lipid composition. Mouse liver lipid compositions were measured after 12-week diets of COCO (red) or FISH (green), compared to a reference (black) diet as revealed by ^{1}H-NMR spectra. (**a**) Liver cholesterol (CE and FC) contents, triglyceride (TG) contents, and MUFA/PUFA ratios. (**b**) Liver fatty acid contents. Abbreviations: COCO, a diet with 5% saturated FA-rich oil; REF, a diet with 5% reference oil; FISH, a diet with 5% n-3 long-chain PUFA-rich oil; CE, cholesterol ester; FC, free cholesterol; MUFA, monounsaturated FAs; PUFA, polyunsaturated FAs; TG, triglycerides; DHA, docosahexaenoic acid; EPA, eicosapentaenoic acid; ARA, arachidonic acid; FA w-3, omega-3 FAs; SFA, saturated FAs.

Absolute quantification of metabolites (i.e., both aqueous and lipidic metabolites) requires knowing the number of protons under each signal, which is given after all NMR signals are identified. Thus, it is important to work with well-resolved signals with no overlap to ensure the integration of pure signals. Because it was difficult to identify all the signals in a NMR spectrum of a biological sample, due to numerous potential line overlaps, we applied the binning method to NMR data, so as to use the entire spectrum to compare metabolic profiles between the three groups of animals.

To compare the metabolic profiles of livers from mice fed different diets, we performed a partial least squares-discriminant analysis (PLS-DA), based on the ^{1}H-NMR spectra. Mice were fed COCO, REF, and FISH diets. For the lipidic extracts, mice fed the COCO diet were well separated on the first component from mice fed the REF and FISH diets (Figure 6a). This component could explain 47.7% of the variability. In addition, mice fed the FISH diet were separated from mice fed the REF diet on the second component, which explained 38.9% of the variability. For aqueous extracts, prior to PLS-DA modeling, we applied an orthogonal signal correction to the data to filter out variations that were unrelated to the diet. Figure 6b shows that mice fed the COCO or FISH diets were clearly separated from mice fed the REF diet on the first component, which explained 42.1% of the variability. We found eight lipid species and fifteen aqueous metabolites that were responsible for the separation between diets (Table 6). From binning data, we observed significant increases in triglyceride, and MUFA levels in mice fed the COCO diet compared to mice fed the REF diet. We also observed changes in aqueous metabolites between the COCO and REF diets. Compared to the REF diet, the COCO diet caused significant increases in 3-hydroxybutyrate, alanine, glycerophosphocholine, inosine, lactate, leucine, phenylalanine, succinate, threonine, tyrosine, and valine and a significant decrease in glucose (Table 6).

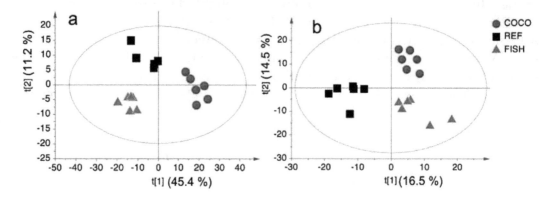

Figure 6. Partial Least Squares-Discriminant Analysis score plot for ^{1}H-NMR data. (**a**) Liver lipidic extracts (R^2 = 98.5%; Q^2 = 0.884); (**b**) liver aqueous extracts (orthogonal signal correction filtration, 53.4% of the remaining variability, R^2 = 98.7%; Q^2 = 0.883). Ellipses indicate the 95% confidence regions. Abbreviations: COCO, a diet with 5% saturated FA-rich oil; REF, a diet with 5% reference oil; FISH, a diet with 5% n-3 long-chain PUFA-rich oil.

Table 6. Fold-change of discriminants metabolites from binning data in mouse liver extracts induced by the COCO and FISH diets compared to the REF diet.

Metabolites [a]	FC [b] COCO	FC [b] FISH
FA $(CH_2)_n$	0.71 *	0.82
EPA+ARA	0.67 *	0.80
FA CH3	0.73 *	0.80
Linoleic acid	0.28 *	0,92
MUFA	1.99 *	0.84
PC+LPC+SM	0.61 *	0.94
PL (Except LPC)	0.65 *	1.15
TG	1.63 *	0.98
3-Hydroxybutyrate	1.21 *	1.10
Alanine	1.30 *	0.97
Choline	1.02	1.68 *
Glucose	0.88 *	0.88 *
Glutamine	1	1.18 *
Glutathione	1.07	1.30 *
GPC	1.39 *	1.61 *
Inosine	1.24 *	1
Lactate	1.27 *	1.14 *
Leucine	1.23 *	1.11 *
Phenylalanine	1.32 *	1.15
Succinate	1.50 *	1.38 *
Threonine	1.28 *	1.03
Tyrosine	1.47 *	1.28 *
Valine	↑1.21 *	1.07

[a] Metabolites that were significantly different between groups; relative integrations of buckets were compared between groups with the Kruskal-Wallis test and a multiple test correction ($p < 0.05$). [b]FC, Fold Change = test diet/control diet. * indicates a significative difference between diets. Abbreviations: COCO, a diet with 5% saturated FA-rich oil; REF, a diet with 5% reference oil; FISH, a diet with 5% n-3 long-chain PUFA-rich oil; FA, fatty acids; EPA, eicosapentaenoic acid; ARA, arachidonic acid; MUFA, monounsaturated FAs; PC, phosphatidylcholine; LPC, lysophosphatidylcholine; SM, sphingomyelin; PL, phospholipids; TG, triglycerides; GPC, glycerophosphocholine.

3. Discussion

3.1. Lipid Quantification: Comparison to Other Methods

In this study, we evaluated the usefulness of an NMR method for quantifying lipid species, based on peak integration and a linear combination of integrals with a standard. We started by optimizing the standard (either internal or external), the organic solvent in which the lipid species would be dissolved, and a mixture of standard lipids. We found that an external standard, TSP, dissolved in D_2O in a coaxial tube provided better results than the internal standard, which was TMS dissolved in the sample. Because TMS is a volatile compound, it was difficult to determine its exact concentration after completing the sample preparation process. With an external standard, quantification was more accurate, because there was no interaction between the standard solution in the coaxial tube and the molecules in the sample. In previous studies, several organic solvents were used to analyze lipidic extracts with NMR, including $CDCl_3$ alone [38] or mixtures of solvents, such as $CDCl_3/CD_3OD$ [17] or $CDCl_3/CD_3OD/D_2O$-EDTA [39]. Because phospholipids contain polar headgroups and nonpolar fatty acyl residues, they form bilayers in an aqueous environment and 'inverse' micelles in an organic solvent, which are characterized by line broadening in ^{1}H-NMR spectroscopy. When a solvent mixture contains both nonpolar and polar solvents, stable micelles are formed, which results in well resolved NMR signals and more accurate quantification [39].

The NMR method developed here for lipid quantification provided good correlations with the quantifications of different lipid classes determined with GC-FID and LC-MS. Both GC-FID and LC-MS are time-consuming, because they require an extraction and analysis method per class of lipids, as well as calibration curves for absolute quantification. In ^{1}H-NMR spectroscopy, deconvolution or line fitting is useful for overlapping signals. We compared our ^{1}H-NMR spectroscopy method with the LipSpin method for the quantification of lipid species [36]. The LipSpin tool is user-friendly, fast, requires only the import of NMR spectra, and it automatically provides the integration value for each lipid species. We obtained good correlations between our method and the LipSpin method for ω-3 FA, MUFA, linoleic acid, EC, and triglycerides. For the other lipid species, the correlations between quantification values obtained with the two methods were not very good, likely due to the lower resolution of our spectra; indeed, some peaks, like PC, LPC, and SM, were not well resolved. In addition, we had not optimized all the parameters available in the LipSpin tool.

3.2. Metabolic Differences between Livers of Mice Fed an Essential Fatty Acid-Deficient Diet or a Control Diet

In this study, we investigated the metabolic disturbances that occurred during the development of steatosis induced by an essential PUFA deficiency. Deficiencies in essential fatty acids are well-known to promote de novo lipogenesis through transcriptional processes [40] involving the transcription factors, SREBP1c [41], ChREBP [42], and LXR [37]. These processes increase the expression and activity of hepatic enzymes involved in de novo lipogenesis (ACC, FAS), elongation (ELOVL6), and desaturation (SCD1). In turn, the elevated activities of these enzymes cause an increase in triglycerides enriched in MUFAs, such as oleic acid (C18:1n-9). Our metabolomics approach revealed that, with the COCO diet, liver triglycerides and MUFAs were up-regulated, as expected, but we also observed up-regulated levels of liver CEs, 3-hydroxybutyrate, alanine, glycerophosphocholine, inosine, lactate, leucine, phenylalanine, succinate, threonine, tyrosine, and valine, compared to mice fed the REF diet. In addition, we observed down-regulated levels of phospholipids and glucose in livers of mice fed the COCO diet compared to mice fed the REF diet. A similar increase in CE was previously reported in lipidic extracts of livers from mice with NASH [43]. That study also highlighted a reduced PUFA to MUFA ratio in NASH, but they observed no difference in triglyceride levels, compared to healthy mice. A reduced PUFA/MUFA ratio is considered a marker of lipid peroxidation in association with oxidative stress. In cancer tissues, such as HCC, a glycolytic shift was observed, with high levels of lactate and low levels of glucose [23,44]. Liver mitochondria produce 3-hydroxybutyrate during fatty acid oxidation. High levels of 3-hydroxybutyrate were also found in human HCC tissues. The aromatic amino acids, phenylalanine and tyrosine, are oxidized in the TCA cycle, after conversion into fumarate. Therefore, accumulations of aromatic amino acids and 3-hydroxybutyrate suggested that mitochondrial function and inflammatory status were impaired in the livers of mice fed the COCO diet.

The present study also revealed changes in amino acid metabolism associated with the COCO diet. Previous studies have shown that changes in branched chain amino acid levels in human liver occurred in hepatic pathologies, such as NASH or alcohol-related liver damage [45]. We observed elevated hepatic concentrations of leucine, and valine, consistent with previous reports that hepatic amino acid metabolism was abnormally regulated, and branched chain amino acid oxidation was reduced in these pathologies. Elevations in alanine were also described in hepatic pathologies [6].

3.3. Advantages and Limitations of ^{1}H-NMR Spectroscopy for Metabolic Profiling in Liver

We evaluated a simple protocol for the simultaneous characterization of lipidic and aqueous metabolic profiles in mouse liver tissues. We used NMR spectroscopy to identify and quantify both polar and non-polar metabolites. ^{1}H-NMR spectroscopy is often used to quantify aqueous metabolites in metabolomic studies, but it has rarely been used for quantifying lipid species. Currently, there is much interest in using this technique for obtaining absolute quantifications of complex lipids, such as phospholipids or sphingolipids, which cannot be obtained with MS. Furthermore, NMR is a non-destructive technique; therefore, the analyzed sample can subsequently be used in MS analyses, which can provide a molecular species characterization for each family. ^{1}H NMR has some drawbacks, such as low sensitivity, signal overlapping, and low resonance discrimination. Nevertheless, this technique can provide a rapid quantitative overview of the major lipid classes (fatty acids, triglycerides, phospholipids, and cholesterol) with a simple, single extraction, without extensive sample preparation, and due to its spectral linearity, without the need of multiple internal standards for quantitative estimations.

4. Materials and Methods

4.1. Animals

In vivo studies were conducted under E.U. guidelines for the use and care of laboratory animals, and they were approved by an independent Ethics Committee (TOXCOM/0043/NL AP). To address the relative contribution of the quantity and quality of dietary FAs to triglyceride accumulation, we fed 6-week old male C57BL6 mice (Charles River, Les Oncins, France) different diets for 12 weeks ($n = 6$ in each group). The diets were as follows: one contained 5% saturated FA-rich oil (COCO), a second contained 5% reference oil (REF), and a third contained 5% n-3 long-chain PUFA-rich oil (FISH) [37]. At sacrifice, the liver was collected and immediately cut into samples that were snap-frozen in liquid nitrogen and stored at −80 °C until use for NMR and GC analysis.

4.2. Extraction Procedure

Liver samples (100–120 mg) were homogenized in 1.2 mL methanol in the Fastprep-24 homogenizer (MP Biomedicals, Irvine, CA, USA). For the comparison of extraction methods, a homogenate that corresponded to 50 mg of tissue was extracted, with modifications, according to the method described by Bligh and Dyer [26], in dichloromethane/methanol/water (2.5:2.5:2.1, v/v/v), and a second homogenate from the same sample that corresponded to 50 mg of tissue was extracted according to the method described by Folch [27] in dichloromethane/ methanol/NaCl 0.9% in water (2:1:0.2, v/v/v). After centrifugation (1000× g, 15 min, 4 °C), the solutions separated into an upper methanol/water phase (with polar metabolites) and a lower dichloromethane phase (with lipophilic compounds), with an intermediate phase of protein and cellular debris. The aqueous and organic phases were collected and evaporated to dryness. Chloroform was replaced by dichloromethane for security reason [46]. For the dietary intervention study, liver samples (100–120 mg) were homogenized in 1.2 mL methanol in a Fastprep-24 homogenizer (MP Biomedicals, Irvine, CA, USA). A homogenate that corresponded to

50 mg of tissue was extracted as described above for NMR analysis, and two homogenates from the same sample that corresponded to 1 mg of tissue were extracted for GC and LC-MS analyses.

4.3. GC Analysis of Neutral Lipids and Fatty Acids

To analyze neutral lipids, we introduced three internal standards (3 μg of stigmasterol, 3 μg of cholesteryl heptadecanoate, and 15 μg of glyceryl trinonadecanoate) before extracting lipids from the homogenates. The dichloromethane phases were evaporated to dryness and dissolved in 20 μL ethyl acetate. Then, 1 μL of the lipid extract was analyzed with GC on a FOCUS-FID system (Thermo Electron, Waltham, MA, USA) equipped with a Zebron-1 fused silica capillary column (Phenomenex, Torrance, CA, USA; 5 m × 0.32 mm i.d., 0.50 μm film thickness) [47]. The oven temperature was programmed to increase from 200 °C to 350 °C at a rate of 5 °C per min, and the carrier gas was hydrogen (0.5 bar). The injector and detector were maintained at 315 °C and 345 °C, respectively.

To analyze fatty acid methyl ester (FAME), we introduced the internal standard, glyceryl tri heptadecanoate (2 μg), before extracting lipids from the homogenates. The lipid extracts were hydrolyzed in KOH (0.5 M in methanol) at 50 °C for 30 min, and transmethylated in a 10% boron trifluoride methanol solution (1 mL, Sigma-Aldrich, St. Louis, MO, USA) and hexane (1 mL) at 80 °C for one hour. After adding water (1 mL) to the crude solution, FAMEs were extracted with hexane (3 mL), evaporated to dryness, and dissolved in ethyl acetate (20 μL). FAMEs (1 μL) were analyzed with gas-liquid chromatography [48] on a Clarus 600-FID system (Perkin Elmer, Waltham, MA, USA) equipped with a Famewax fused silica capillary column (RESTEK, Lisses, France; 30 m × 0.32 mm i.d. 0.25 μm film thickness). The oven temperature was programmed to increase from 130 °C to 220 °C at a rate of 2 °C per min, and the carrier gas was hydrogen (0.5 bar). The injector and the detector were maintained at 225 °C and 245 °C, respectively.

4.4. HPLC-MS Analysis of Phospholipids

Lipids were extracted from 1 mg of liver with a method adapted from that described by Bligh and Dyer [26]. Extractions were performed in dichloromethane/methanol (2% acetic acid)/water (2.5:2.5:2 v/v/v), in the presence of six internal standards, including ceramides (Cer, d18:1/15:0, 16 ng); phosphatidylethanolamine (PE 12:0/12:0, 180 ng); phosphatidylcholine (PC, 13:0/13:0, 16 ng); SM (d18:1/12:0, 16 ng); phosphatidylinositol (PI, 16:0/17:0, 30 ng); and phosphatidylserine (PS, 12:0/12:0, 156.25 ng). The solution was centrifuged at 1500 rpm for 3 min. The organic phase was collected and dried under nitrogen, then dissolved in 50 μl methanol. The extract (5 μL) was analyzed with an Agilent 1290 UPLC system coupled to a G6460 triple quadrupole spectrometer (Agilent Technologies, Santa Clara, CA, USA) and equipped with MassHunter software, for data acquisition and analysis. A Kinetex HILIC column (Phenomenex, 50 × 4.6 mm, 2.6 μm) was used for LC separations. The column temperature was controlled at 40 °C. The flow rate of the mobile phase was 0.3 mL/min. The mobile phase contained two parts: A was acetonitrile; and B was 10 mM ammonium formate in water, pH 3.2. The gradient was prepared with the following specifications: from 10% to 30% B in 10 min; 10–12 min in 100% B; and then, at 13 min, back to 10% B for 1-min re-equilibrium, prior to the next injection. An electrospray source was employed in positive ion mode for Cer, PE, PC, and SM analyses and in negative ion mode for PI and PS analyses. The collision gas was nitrogen. The needle voltage was set at +4000 V. Several scan modes were used. First, to obtain the natural masses of different species, we analyzed cellular lipid extracts with precursor ion scans of 184 m/z, 241 m/z, and 264 m/z for PC/SM, PI, and Cer, respectively; and neutral loss scans of 141 and 87 for PE and PS, respectively. The collision energy optimums for Cer, PE, PC, SM, PI, and PS were 25 eV, 20 eV, 30 eV, 25 eV, 45 eV, and 22 eV, respectively. Then, the corresponding SRM transitions were used to quantify different phospholipid species in each class. Two MRM acquisitions were necessary, due to important differences between phospholipid classes. Data were analyzed with QqQ Quantitative (vB.05.00) and Qualitative analysis software (vB.04.00).

4.5. ^{1}H-NMR Measurements

All NMR experiments were performed on a Bruker Avance spectrometer (Bruker Biospin, Rheinstetten, Germany), operating at a proton frequency of 600.13 MHz, with an inverse detection 5-mm ^{1}H-^{13}C-^{15}N cryoprobe attached to a Cryoplatform (the preamplifier unit).

Dry lipid extracts were reconstituted in 500 µl CDCl$_3$/CD$_3$OD (4:1, *v/v*) and transferred into 5-mm NMR tubes. ^{1}H-NMR spectra were recorded in the presence of a reusable coaxial capillary tube that contained 120 µl TSP (1.17 mM) in D$_2$O, which also served as an internal standard for quantitative estimations. Dry aqueous extracts were reconstituted in 600 µl D$_2$O containing TSP (0.70 mM) and transferred into 5-mm NMR tubes.

A T1 (spin-lattice relaxation) measurement experiment was performed on the entire liver lipid extract (with TSP solution in the coaxial capillary as reference) in a sealed tube using an inversion-recovery sequence. The T1 values for TC (0.68 ppm), FC (1.01 ppm), CE (1.02 ppm), TG (5.27 ppm), TG (4.16 and 4.32 ppm), PL (5.23 ppm), UFA (5.35 ppm), linoleic acid (2.76 ppm), PUFA (2.82 ppm), FA (0.88 ppm), w3 UFA (0.98 ppm), MUFA (2.02 ppm), ARA+EPA (2.10 ppm), DHA (2.38 ppm) and TSP were 0.792, 0.792, 0.792, 1.44, 0.576, 1.44, 2.88, 1.58, 1.73, 3.17, 3.17, 1.44, 1.44, 1.15 and 3.45 s, respectively.

^{1}H-NMR spectra of liver lipid extracts were obtained with a one-pulse sequence, with a spectral width of 10 ppm, and the time domain data had 32,000 data points. The flip angle of the radio-frequency pulse was 30°, and the total relaxation delay was 15 s to ensure complete recovery of the magnetization between scans of the lipid components and for the external reference TSP. For each sample, 256 scans were accumulated, and data were Fourier-transformed, after multiplying by an exponential window function with a line-broadening function of 0.3 Hz to the free induction decays (FIDs).

^{1}H-NMR spectra of aqueous liver extracts were acquired at 300 K with a conventional presaturation pulse sequence for water suppression, based on the first increment of the nuclear Overhauser effect spectroscopy (NOESY) pulse sequence. Solvent presaturation was applied during a recycling delay and mixing time (100 ms) to suppress residual water. A total of 256 transients were collected into 32,000 data points with a spectral width of 12 ppm and a relaxation delay of 15 s. Prior to the Fourier transform procedure, we applied an exponential line-broadening of 0.3 Hz to the FIDs.

4.6. Data Processing and Multivariate Analysis

NMR spectra were phase- and baseline-corrected, then calibrated (TSP, 0.0 ppm for aqueous extracts and TC, 0.68 ppm for lipidic extracts) with Topspin software (version 2.1, Bruker). Next, NMR data were reduced with AMIX software (version 3.9, Bruker) to integrate 0.01 ppm-wide regions that corresponded to the δ 10.0–0.5 ppm and the δ 6.4–0.6 ppm regions for aqueous and lipidic extracts, respectively. The 5.1–4.5 ppm region, which included water resonance, was excluded in the NMR spectra of aqueous extracts. We included 757 and 552 NMR buckets in the data matrices for aqueous and lipidic extracts, respectively. To account for differences in sample volumes, each integration region was normalized to the total spectral area.

Multivariate pattern-recognition techniques were applied to study the effects of diet on the metabolome. First, we performed a PCA to reveal intrinsic clusters and detect eventual outliers. We then performed a PLS-DA to model the relationship between diet and NMR data. For aqueous extracts, prior to PLS-DA modeling, we applied orthogonal signal correction [49] to remove confounding variability; i.e., variability that was not linked to the diet (e.g., physiological, experimental, or instrumental variability). Data were Pareto-scaled (the square root of the standard deviation is used as the scaling factor). For all plots of scores, we performed Hotelling's T2 statistics to construct 95% confidence ellipses. The R^2Y parameter represented the explained variance. Seven-fold cross validation was used to determine the number of latent variables that should be included in the PLS-DA model and to estimate the predictive ability (or predicted variance, Q^2 parameter) of the fitted model. PLS-DA models with Q^2 values higher than 0.4 were considered valid [50]. In addition, the robustness of PLS-DA models was assessed with a permutation test (number of permutations = 200). In the permutation plot, a Q^2 intercept < 0.05 indicated a robust model [51]. Discriminant variables were determined with the Variable Importance in the Projection (VIP) value, a global measure of the influence of each variable in the PLS components. Variables with VIPs > 1 were considered discriminants. Finally, we tested the significance of relative integration differences between groups, based on the non-parametric Kruskal-Wallis test. The false discovery rate (FDR) was applied to account for multiple testing. NMR variables that showed FDR-adjusted p-values < 0.05 were considered significantly different. We used SIMCA-P software (V13, Umetrics, Umea, Sweden) to perform the multivariate analyses, and we used R (https://www.r-project.org/) for univariate testing.

4.7. Statistical Analysis

We performed analytical validations of ^{1}H-NMR lipid quantifications by comparing the results with analogous measurements obtained with other methods. Comparisons were performed with linear regression and Pearson's (r) correlation.

Linear regression analyses were used to compare known concentrations of lipidic species and signal integrations obtained with ^{1}H-NMR. A known concentration was used as the independent variable, and the NMR-predicted concentration was used as the response variable. Hypotheses of linear regression were assessed based on the residuals: the Durbin-Watson, Shapiro-Wilks, and Breush-Pagan tests were applied, respectively, to test for the independence, normality, and homogeneity of residuals.

Pearson's correlation was used to compare LipSpin-computed and NMR-computed quantifications of lipids and to compare GC-FID-computed and NMR-computed quantifications. We set 0.05 as the threshold for significance. Univariate analyses were performed with R software (https://www.r-project.org/).

5. Conclusions

The current study showed the potential and limitations of ^{1}H-NMR spectroscopy for quantifying aqueous, and specially, lipid metabolites in the liver. We demonstrated that ^{1}H-NMR spectra could provide a rapid overview of the major lipid classes and the most abundant aqueous metabolites. To achieve better extractions of aqueous and lipid metabolites and more accurate quantifications, we recommend the Folch extraction method, an external standard, and the CDCl$_3$/CD$_3$OD mixture of solvents. We found that LipSpin was a good alternative for lipid quantification, but the parameters must be optimized. Our metabolomics analysis allowed us to discriminate between livers of mice fed a diet deficient in essential fatty acids from livers of mice fed a balanced diet. The COCO dietary challenge was mainly associated with disturbances in lipid and energy metabolism, accompanied by altered amino acid metabolism.

Supplementary Materials: Table S1: Compounds identified in the polar extract of mouse liver tissue from NMR data: assigned chemical shifts and multiplicities, Table S2: Compounds identified in the non-polar extract of mouse liver tissue from NMR data: assigned chemical shifts and multiplicities, Table S3: Composition of lipid mixtures, Table S4: real lipid concentrations and concentrations computed from NMR data for lipid mixtures of Table S3, Table S5: lipid concentrations computed from GC and NMR data in mice livers, Table S6: NMR bucketing table for aqueous liver samples, Table S7: NMR bucketing table for lipidic liver samples, Figure S1: 600 MHz ^{1}H-NMR spectrum of a mixture of five lipid standards (TG C17:0; FC; oleate cholesterol; DHA; linoleic acid), Figure S2: 600 MHz ^{1}H-NMR spectrum of a mixture of three lipid standards (PC, PE, SM), Figure S3: Scatter plot and linear regressions of NMR quantifications and lipid concentrations in lipid mixtures of Table S3 dissolved in CDCl$_3$ and using an external standard (TSP) for neutral lipids and phospholipids, Figure S4: Scatter plot and linear regressions of NMR quantifications and lipid concentrations in lipid mixtures of Table S3 dissolved in CDCl3 and using an external standard (TSP) for fatty acids, Figure S5: Scatter plot and linear regressions of NMR quantifications and lipid concentrations in lipid mixtures of Table S3 dissolved in CDCl$_3$ and using an internal standard (TMS) for neutral lipids and phospholipids, Figure S6: Scatter plot and linear regressions of NMR quantifications and lipidconcentrations in lipid mixtures of Table S3 dissolved in CDCl $_3$ and using an internal standard (TMS) for fatty acids, Figure S7: Scatter plot and linear regressions of NMR quantifications and lipid concentrations in lipidmixtures of Table S3 dissolved in CDCl $_3$-CD$_3$OD mixture and using an external standard (TSP) for neutral lipids and phospholipids, Figure S8: Scatter plot and linear regressions of NMR quantifications and lipid concentrations lipid mixtures of Table S3 dissolved in CDCl^3-CD^{3}OD mixture and using an external standard (TSP) for fattyacids, Figure S9: Scatter plot and linear regressions of NMR quantifications and lipid concentrations in lipid mixtures of Table S1 dissolved in CDCl₃-CD₃OD mixture and using an internal standard (TMS) for neutral lipids and phospholipids, Figure S10: Scatter plot and linear regressions of NMR quantifications and lipid concentrations in lipid mixtures of Table S1 dissolved in CDCl₃-CD₃OD mixture and using an internal standard (TMS) for neutral lipids and phospholipids.

Author Contributions: Conceptualization, L.D., J.B.-M., and H.G.; methodology, C.C.; validation, C.C.; formal analysis, A.A. and M.T.-F.; investigation, A.A., R.G., and C.C.; resources, S.D., A.M., A.P., and H.G.; data curation, A.A. and C.C.; writing—original draft preparation, C.C.; writing—review and editing, H.G., J.B.-M., L.D., M.T.-F., A.M; supervision, L.D.; project administration, L.D. All authors have read and agreed to the published version of the manuscript. All authors have read and agreed to the published version of the manuscript.

References

1. Friedman, S.L.; Neuschwander-Tetri, B.A.; Rinella, M.; Sanyal, A.J. Mechanisms of NAFLD development and therapeutic strategies. *Nat. Med.* **2018**, *24*, 908–922. [CrossRef] [PubMed]
2. Younossi, Z.; Tacke, F.; Arrese, M.; Chander Sharma, B.; Mostafa, I.; Bugianesi, E.; Wai-Sun Wong, V.; Yilmaz, Y.; George, J.; Fan, J.; et al. Global Perspectives on Nonalcoholic Fatty Liver Disease and Nonalcoholic Steatohepatitis. *Hepatology* **2019**, *69*, 2672–2682. [CrossRef] [PubMed]
3. Dumas, M.-E.; Kinross, J.; Nicholson, J.K. Metabolic phenotyping and systems biology approaches to understanding metabolic syndrome and fatty liver disease. *Gastroenterology* **2014**, *146*, 46–62. [CrossRef] [PubMed]
4. Mardinoglu, A.; Bjornson, E.; Zhang, C.; Klevstig, M.; Söderlund, S.; Ståhlman, M.; Adiels, M.; Hakkarainen, A.; Lundbom, N.; Kilicarslan, M.; et al. Personal model-assisted identification of NAD+ and glutathione metabolism as intervention target in NAFLD. *Mol. Syst. Biol.* **2017**, *13*, 916. [CrossRef] [PubMed]
5. Emwas, A.-H.; Roy, R.; McKay, R.T.; Tenori, L.; Saccenti, E.; Gowda, G.A.N.; Raftery, D.; Alahmari, F.; Jaremko, L.; Jaremko, M.; et al. NMR Spectroscopy for Metabolomics Research. *Metabolites* **2019**, *9*, 123. [CrossRef] [PubMed]
6. Le Moyec, L.; Triba, M.N.; Nahon, P.; Bouchemal, N.; Hantz, E.; Goossens, C.; Amathieu, R.; Savarin, P. Nuclear magnetic resonance metabolomics and human liver diseases: The principles and evidence associated with protein and carbohydrate metabolism. *Biomed. Rep.* **2017**, *6*, 387–395. [CrossRef] [PubMed]
7. Amathieu, R.; Triba, M.N.; Goossens, C.; Bouchemal, N.; Nahon, P.; Savarin, P.; Le Moyec, L. Nuclear magnetic resonance based metabolomics and liver diseases: Recent advances and future clinical applications. *World J. Gastroenterol.* **2016**, *22*, 417–426. [CrossRef]
8. Jiang, L.; Si, Z.H.; Li, M.H.; Zhao, H.; Fu, Y.H.; Xing, Y.X.; Hong, W.; Ruan, L.Y.; Li, P.M.; Wang, J.S. 1H NMR-based metabolomics study of liver damage induced by ginkgolic acid (15:1) in mice. *J. Pharm. Biomed. Anal.* **2017**, *136*, 44–54. [CrossRef]
9. Dagla, I.; Benaki, D.; Baira, E.; Lemonakis, N.; Poudyal, H.; Brown, L.; Tsarbopoulos, A.; Skaltsounis, A.L.; Mikros, E.; Gikas, E. Alteration in the liver metabolome of rats with metabolic syndrome after treatment with Hydroxytyrosol. A Mass Spectrometry and Nuclear Magnetic Resonance-based metabolomics study. *Talanta* **2018**, *178*, 246–257. [CrossRef]
10. Bonvallot, N.; Canlet, C.; Blas-Y-Estrada, F.; Gautier, R.; Tremblay-Franco, M.; Chevolleau, S.; Cordier, S.; Cravedi, J.P. Metabolome disruption of pregnant rats and their offspring resulting from repeated exposure to a pesticide mixture representative of environmental contamination in Brittany. *PLoS ONE* **2018**, *13*, e0198448. [CrossRef]
11. Chen, M.; Zheng, H.; Xu, M.; Zhao, L.; Zhang, Q.; Song, J.; Zhao, Z.; Lu, S.; Weng, Q.; Wu, X.; et al. Changes in hepatic metabolic profile during the evolution of STZ-induced diabetic rats via an 1H NMR-based metabonomic investigation. *Biosci. Rep.* **2019**, *39*. [CrossRef] [PubMed]
12. Ghosh, S.; Sengupta, A.; Sharma, S.; Sonawat, H.M. Metabolic fingerprints of serum, brain, and liver are distinct for mice with cerebral and noncerebral malaria: A ¹H NMR spectroscopy-based metabonomic study. *J. Proteome Res.* **2012**, *11*, 4992–5004. [CrossRef] [PubMed]
13. Ruiz-Rodado, V.; Nicoli, E.R.; Probert, F.; Smith, D.A.; Morris, L.; Wassif, C.A.; Platt, F.M.; Grootveld, M. 1H NMR-Linked Metabolomics Analysis of Liver from a Mouse Model of NP-C1 Disease. *J. Proteome Res.* **2016**, *15*, 3511–3527. [CrossRef] [PubMed]

14. Zheng, H.; Cai, A.; Shu, Q.; Niu, Y.; Xu, P.; Li, C.; Lin, L.; Gao, H. Tissue-Specific Metabolomics Analysis Identifies the Liver as a Major Organ of Metabolic Disorders in Amyloid Precursor Protein/Presenilin 1 Mice of Alzheimer's Disease. *J. Proteome Res.* **2019**, *18*, 1218–1227. [CrossRef] [PubMed]

15. Fernando, H.; Bhopale, K.K.; Kondraganti, S.; Kaphalia, B.S.; Ansari, G.A.S. Lipidomic Changes in Rat Liver after Long-Term Exposure to Ethanol. *Toxicol. Appl. Pharmacol.* **2011**, *255*, 127–137. [CrossRef]

16. Fernando, H.; Bhopale, K.K.; Kondraganti, S.S.; Kaphalia, B.S.; Ansari, G.A.S. Alcohol-Induced Hepatic Steatosis: A Comparative Study to Identify Possible Indicator(s) of Alcoholic Fatty Liver Disease. *J. Drug Alcohol Res.* **2018**, *7*. [CrossRef]

17. Fernando, H.; Kondraganti, S.; Bhopale, K.K.; Volk, D.E.; Neerathilingam, M.; Kaphalia, B.S.; Luxon, B.A.; Boor, P.J.; Ansari, G.A.S. 1H and 31P NMR Lipidome of Ethanol-Induced Fatty Liver. *Alcohol. Clin. Exp. Res.* **2010**, *34*, 1937–1947. [CrossRef]

18. Cabaton, N.J.; Poupin, N.; Canlet, C.; Tremblay-Franco, M.; Audebert, M.; Cravedi, J.P.; Riu, A.; Jourdan, F.; Zalko, D. An Untargeted Metabolomics Approach to Investigate the Metabolic Modulations of HepG2 Cells Exposed to Low Doses of Bisphenol A and 17β-Estradiol. *Front. Endocrinol.* **2018**, *9*, 571. [CrossRef]

19. Wei, F.; Lamichhane, S.; Orešič, M.; Hyötyläinen, T. Lipidomes in health and disease: Analytical strategies and considerations. *TrAC Trends Anal. Chem.* **2019**, *120*, 115664. [CrossRef]

20. Khoury, S.; Canlet, C.; Lacroix, M.Z.; Berdeaux, O.; Jouhet, J.; Bertrand-Michel, J. Quantification of Lipids: Model, Reality, and Compromise. *Biomolecules* **2018**, *8*, 174. [CrossRef]

21. Martínez-Granados, B.; Morales, J.M.; Rodrigo, J.M.; Del Olmo, J.; Serra, M.A.; Ferrández, A.; Celda, B.; Monleón, D. Metabolic profile of chronic liver disease by NMR spectroscopy of human biopsies. *Int. J. Mol. Med.* **2011**, *27*, 111–117. [CrossRef] [PubMed]

22. Cobbold, J.F.L.; Anstee, Q.M.; Goldin, R.D.; Williams, H.R.T.; Matthews, H.C.; North, B.V.; Absalom, N.; Thomas, H.C.; Thursz, M.R.; Cox, R.D.; et al. Phenotyping murine models of non-alcoholic fatty liver disease through metabolic profiling of intact liver tissue. *Clin. Sci. Lond. Engl.* **2009**, *116*, 403–413. [CrossRef] [PubMed]

23. Teilhet, C.; Morvan, D.; Joubert-Zakeyh, J.; Biesse, A.S.; Pereira, B.; Massoulier, S.; Dechelotte, P.; Pezet, D.; Buc, E.; Lamblin, G.; et al. Specificities of Human Hepatocellular Carcinoma Developed on Non-Alcoholic Fatty Liver Disease in Absence of Cirrhosis Revealed by Tissue Extracts 1H-NMR Spectroscopy. *Metabolites* **2017**, *7*, 49. [CrossRef] [PubMed]

24. Vinaixa, M.; Rodríguez, M.A.; Rull, A.; Beltrán, R.; Bladé, C.; Brezmes, J.; Cañellas, N.; Joven, J.; Correig, X. Metabolomic assessment of the effect of dietary cholesterol in the progressive development of fatty liver disease. *J. Proteome Res.* **2010**, *9*, 2527–2538. [CrossRef] [PubMed]

25. Lin, C.Y.; Wu, H.; Tjeerdema, R.S.; Viant, M.R. Evaluation of metabolite extraction strategies from tissue samples using NMR metabolomics. *Metabolomics* **2007**, *3*, 55–67. [CrossRef]

26. Bligh, E.G.; Dyer, W.J. A rapid method of total lipid extraction and purification. *Can. J. Biochem. Physiol.* **1959**, *37*, 911–917. [CrossRef]

27. Folch, J.; Lees, M.; Sloane Stanley, G.H. A simple method for the isolation and purification of total lipides from animal tissues. *J. Biol. Chem.* **1957**, *226*, 497–509.

28. Beckonert, O.; Keun, H.C.; Ebbels, T.M.D.; Bundy, J.; Holmes, E.; Lindon, J.C.; Nicholson, J.K. Metabolic profiling, metabolomic and metabonomic procedures for NMR spectroscopy of urine, plasma, serum and tissue extracts. *Nat. Protoc.* **2007**, *2*, 2692–2703. [CrossRef]

29. Ulrich, E.L.; Akutsu, H.; Doreleijers, J.F.; Harano, Y.; Ioannidis, Y.E.; Lin, J.; Livny, M.; Mading, S.; Maziuk, D.; Miller, Z.; et al. BioMagResBank. *Nucleic Acids Res.* **2008**, *36*, D402–D408. [CrossRef]

30. Wishart, D.S.; Tzur, D.; Knox, C.; Eisner, R.; Guo, A.C.; Young, N.; Cheng, D.; Jewell, K.; Arndt, D.; Sawhney, S.; et al. HMDB: The Human Metabolome Database. *Nucleic Acids Res.* **2007**, *35*, D521–D526. [CrossRef]

31. Reis, A.; Rudnitskaya, A.; Blackburn, G.J.; Mohd Fauzi, N.; Pitt, A.R.; Spickett, C.M. A comparison of five lipid extraction solvent systems for lipidomic studies of human LDL. *J. Lipid Res.* **2013**, *54*, 1812–1824. [CrossRef] [PubMed]

32. Wu, H.; Southam, A.D.; Hines, A.; Viant, M.R. High-throughput tissue extraction protocol for NMR-and MS-based metabolomics. *Anal. Biochem.* **2008**, *372*, 204–212. [CrossRef] [PubMed]

33. Viant, M.R.; Ebbels, T.M.D.; Beger, R.D.; Ekman, D.R.; Epps, D.J.T.; Kamp, H.; Leonards, P.E.G.; Loizou, G.D.;

MacRae, J.I.; van Ravenzwaay, B.; et al. Use cases, best practice and reporting standards for metabolomics in regulatory toxicology. *Nat. Commun.* **2019**, *10*, 1–10. [CrossRef] [PubMed]

34. Bharti, S.K.; Roy, R. Quantitative 1H NMR spectroscopy. *TrAC Trends Anal. Chem.* **2012**, *35*, 5–26. [CrossRef]

35. Vidal, N.P.; Manzanos, M.J.; Goicoechea, E.; Guillén, M.D. Quality of farmed and wild sea bass lipids studied by (1) H NMR: Usefulness of this technique for differentiation on a qualitative and a quantitative basis. *Food Chem.* **2012**, *135*, 1583–1591. [CrossRef] [PubMed]

36. Barrilero, R.; Gil, M.; Amigó, N.; Dias, C.B.; Wood, L.G.; Garg, M.L.; Ribalta, J.; Heras, M.; Vinaixa, M.; Correig, X. LipSpin: A New Bioinformatics Tool for Quantitative 1H NMR Lipid Profiling. *Anal. Chem.* **2018**, *90*, 2031–2040. [CrossRef]

37. Ducheix, S.; Montagner, A.; Polizzi, A.; Lasserre, F.; Marmugi, A.; Bertrand-Michel, J.; Podechard, N.; Al Saati, T.; Chétiveaux, M.; Baron, S.; et al. Essential fatty acids deficiency promotes lipogenic gene expression and hepatic steatosis through the liver X receptor. *J. Hepatol.* **2013**, *58*, 984–992. [CrossRef]

38. Jiang, C.; Yang, K.; Yang, L.; Miao, Z.; Wang, Y.; Zhu, H. A 1H NMR-Based Metabonomic Investigation of Time-Related Metabolic Trajectories of the Plasma, Urine and Liver Extracts of Hyperlipidemic Hamsters. *PLoS ONE* **2013**, *8*, e66786. [CrossRef]

39. Li, J.; Vosegaard, T.; Guo, Z. Applications of nuclear magnetic resonance in lipid analyses: An emerging powerful tool for lipidomics studies. *Prog. Lipid Res.* **2017**, *68*, 37–56. [CrossRef]

40. Botolin, D.; Wang, Y.; Christian, B.; Jump, D.B. Docosahexaneoic acid (22:6, n-3) regulates rat hepatocyte SREBP-1 nuclear abundance by Erk-and 26S proteasome-dependent pathways. *J. Lipid Res.* **2006**, *47*, 181–192. [CrossRef]

41. Jump, D.B. Fatty acid regulation of hepatic lipid metabolism. *Curr. Opin. Clin. Nutr. Metab. Care* **2011**, *14*, 115–120. [CrossRef] [PubMed]

42. Dentin, R.; Benhamed, F.; Pégorier, J.P.; Foufelle, F.; Viollet, B.; Vaulont, S.; Girard, J.; Postic, C. Polyunsaturated fatty acids suppress glycolytic and lipogenic genes through the inhibition of ChREBP nuclear protein translocation. *J. Clin. Investig.* **2005**, *115*, 2843–2854. [CrossRef] [PubMed]

43. Klein, M.S.; Dorn, C.; Saugspier, M.; Hellerbrand, C.; Oefner, P.J.; Gronwald, W. Discrimination of steatosis and NASH in mice using nuclear magnetic resonance spectroscopy. *Metabolomics* **2011**, *7*, 237–246. [CrossRef]

44. Yang, Y.; Li, C.; Nie, X.; Feng, X.; Chen, W.; Yue, Y.; Tang, H.; Deng, F. Metabonomic studies of human hepatocellular carcinoma using high-resolution magic-angle spinning 1H NMR spectroscopy in conjunction with multivariate data analysis. *J. Proteome Res.* **2007**, *6*, 2605–2614. [CrossRef]

45. Schofield, Z.; Reed, M.A.; Newsome, P.N.; Adams, D.H.; Günther, U.L.; Lalor, P.F. Changes in human hepatic metabolism in steatosis and cirrhosis. *World J. Gastroenterol.* **2017**, *23*, 2685–2695. [CrossRef]

46. Chen, I.S.; Shen, C.S.J.; Sheppard, A.J. Comparison of methylene chloride and chloroform for the extraction of fats from food products. *J. Am. Oil Chem. Soc.* **1981**, *58*, 599–601. [CrossRef]

47. Barrans, A.; Collet, X.; Barbaras, R.; Jaspard, B.; Manent, J.; Vieu, C.; Chap, H.; Perret, B. Hepatic lipase induces the formation of pre-beta 1 high density lipoprotein (HDL) from triacylglycerol-rich HDL2. A study comparing liver perfusion to in vitro incubation with lipases. *J. Biol. Chem.* **1994**, *269*, 11572–11577.

48. Lillington, J.M.; Trafford, D.J.; Makin, H.L. A rapid and simple method for the esterification of fatty acids and steroid carboxylic acids prior to gas-liquid chromatography. *Clin. Chim. Acta Int. J. Clin. Chem.* **1981**, *111*, 91–98. [CrossRef]

49. Wold, S.; Antti, H.; Lindgren, F.; Öhman, J. Orthogonal signal correction of near-infrared spectra. *Chemom. Intell. Lab. Syst.* **1998**, *44*, 175–185. [CrossRef]

50. McCombie, G.; Browning, L.M.; Titman, C.M.; Song, M.; Shockcor, J.; Jebb, S.A.; Griffin, J.L. omega-3 oil intake during weight loss in obese women results in remodelling of plasma triglyceride and fatty acids. *Metab. Off. J. Metab. Soc.* **2009**, *5*, 363–374. [CrossRef]

51. Lapins, M.; Eklund, M.; Spjuth, O.; Prusis, P.; Wikberg, J.E. Proteochemometric modeling of HIV protease susceptibility. *BMC Bioinform.* **2008**, *9*, 181. [CrossRef] [PubMed]

Permissions

The contributors of this book come from diverse backgrounds, making this book a truly international effort. This book will bring forth new frontiers with its revolutionizing research information and detailed analysis of the nascent developments around the world.

We would like to thank all the contributing authors for lending their expertise to make the book truly unique. They have played a crucial role in the development of this book. Without their invaluable contributions this book wouldn't have been possible. They have made vital efforts to compile up to date information on the varied aspects of this subject to make this book a valuable addition to the collection of many professionals and students.

This book was conceptualized with the vision of imparting up-to-date information and advanced data in this field. To ensure the same, a matchless editorial board was set up. Every individual on the board went through rigorous rounds of assessment to prove their worth. After which they invested a large part of their time researching and compiling the most relevant data for our readers.

The editorial board has been involved in producing this book since its inception. They have spent rigorous hours researching and exploring the diverse topics which have resulted in the successful publishing of this book. They have passed on their knowledge of decades through this book. To expedite this challenging task, the publisher supported the team at every step. A small team of assistant editors was also appointed to further simplify the editing procedure and attain best results for the readers.

Apart from the editorial board, the designing team has also invested a significant amount of their time in understanding the subject and creating the most relevant covers. They scrutinized every image to scout for the most suitable representation of the subject and create an appropriate cover for the book.

The publishing team has been an ardent support to the editorial, designing and production team. Their endless efforts to recruit the best for this project, has resulted in the accomplishment of this book. They are a veteran in the field of academics and their pool of knowledge is as vast as their experience in printing. Their expertise and guidance has proved useful at every step. Their uncompromising quality standards have made this book an exceptional effort. Their encouragement from time to time has been an inspiration for everyone.

The publisher and the editorial board hope that this book will prove to be a valuable piece of knowledge for researchers, students, practitioners and scholars across the globe.

List of Contributors

Federica Belmonte, Antonella Bisogno, Luca Pierri, Antonella Di Nuzzi, Laura Di Michele, Anna Pia Delli Bovi and Salvatore Guercio Nuzio
Department of Medicine and Surgery and Dentistry, "Scuola Medica Salernitana", Pediatrics Section University of Salerno, 84081 Baronissi (Salerno), Italy

Angelo Colucci
Department of Medicine and Surgery and Dentistry, "Scuola Medica Salernitana", Pediatrics Section University of Salerno, 84081 Baronissi (Salerno), Italy
Theoreo srl, Via degli Ulivi 3, 84090 Montecorvino Pugliano (SA), Italy

Jacopo Troisi
Department of Medicine and Surgery and Dentistry, "Scuola Medica Salernitana", Pediatrics Section University of Salerno, 84081 Baronissi (Salerno), Italy
Theoreo srl, Via degli Ulivi 3, 84090 Montecorvino Pugliano (SA), Italy
European Biomedical Research Institute of Salerno (EBRIS), Via S. de Renzi, 3, 84125 Salerno, Italy
Hosmotic srl, Via R. Bosco 178, 80069 Vico Equense (NA), Italy

Giovanni Scala
Hosmotic srl, Via R. Bosco 178, 80069 Vico Equense (NA), Italy

Pierpaolo Cavallo
Department of Physics, University of Salerno, 84084 Fisciano (Salerno), Italy

Claudia Mandato
Department of Pediatrics, Children's Hospital Santobono-Pausilipon, 80129 Naples, Italy

Pietro Vajro
Department of Medicine and Surgery and Dentistry, "Scuola Medica Salernitana", Pediatrics Section University of Salerno, 84081 Baronissi (Salerno), Italy
European Laboratory of Food Induced Intestinal Disease (ELFID), University of Naples Federico II, 80100 Naples, Italy

Futaba Shoji, Midori Maruyama and Kumi Suzuki
Institute for Advanced Biosciences, Keio University, Tsuruoka, Yamagata 997-0052, Japan

Hitoshi Ozawa, Akiyoshi Hirayama, Tomoyoshi Soga and Masaru Tomita
Institute for Advanced Biosciences, Keio University, Tsuruoka, Yamagata 997-0052, Japan

Systems Biology Program, Graduate School of Media and Governance, Keio University, Fujisawa, Kanagawa 252-0882, Japan

Hisami Yamanaka-Okumura
Department of Clinical Nutrition and Food Management, Graduate School of Biomedical Sciences, Tokushima University Graduate School, Tokushima 770-8503, Japan

Hiroshi Tatano
Department of Clinical Nutrition and Food Management, Graduate School of Biomedical Sciences, Tokushima University Graduate School, Tokushima 770-8503, Japan
Department of Health and Nutrition, Faculty of Nursing and Nutrition, The University of Shimane, Izumo, Shimane 693 -8550, Japan

Yuji Morine and Mitsuo Shimada
Department of Digestive and Pediatric Surgery, Graduate School of Medical Sciences, Tokushima University, Tokushima 770-8503, Japan

Sandra Steensels, Jixuan Qiao and Baran A. Ersoy
Joan & Sanford I. Weill Department of Medicine, Weill Cornell Medical College, New York, NY 10021, USA

Diren Beyoğlu and Jeffrey R. Idle
Arthur G. Zupko's Division of Systems Pharmacology and Pharmacogenomics, Arnold & Marie Schwartz College of Pharmacy and Health Sciences, Long Island University, 75 Dekalb Avenue, Brooklyn, NY 11201, USA

Vivaldy Prinville, Leanne Ohlund and Lekha Sleno
Department of Chemistry, Université du Québec à Montréal (UQAM), Montreal, QC H3C 3P8, Canada

Lorraine Smith, Joran Villaret-Cazadamont, Cécile Canlet, Hervé Guillou, Nicolas J. Cabaton and Sandrine Ellero-Simatos
Toxalim (Research Center in Food Toxicology), Université de Toulouse, INRAE, ENVT, INP-Purpan, UPS, 31300 Toulouse, France

Sandrine P. Claus
LNC Therapeutics, 17 place de la Bourse, 33076 Bordeaux, France

Manuel García-Jaramillo
Nutrition Program, School of Biological and Population Health Sciences, Oregon State University, Corvallis, OR 97331, USA
Department of Chemistry, Oregon State University, Corvallis, OR 97331, USA
The Linus Pauling Institute, Oregon State University, Corvallis, OR 97331, USA

Kelli A. Lytle, Melinda H. Spooner and Donald B. Jump
Nutrition Program, School of Biological and Population Health Sciences, Oregon State University, Corvallis, OR 97331, USA
The Linus Pauling Institute, Oregon State University, Corvallis, OR 97331, USA

Adrian Covaci
Toxicological Centre, University of Antwerp, Universiteitsplein 1, 2610 Wilrijk, Belgium

Robim Marcelino Rodrigues and Tamara Vanhaecke
Research Group In Vitro Toxicology and Dermato-Cosmetology (IVTD), Vrije Universiteit Brussel, Laarbeeklaan 103, 1090 Jette, Belgium

Matthias Cuykx
Toxicological Centre, University of Antwerp, Universiteitsplein 1, 2610 Wilrijk, Belgium
Research Group In Vitro Toxicology and Dermato-Cosmetology (IVTD), Vrije Universiteit Brussel, Laarbeeklaan 103, 1090 Jette, Belgium

Charlie Beirnaert and Kris Laukens
Department of Mathematics & Computer Science, University of Antwerp, Middelheimlaan 1, 2020 Antwerp, Belgium
Biomedical Informatics Network Antwerpen (Biomina), University of Antwerp, Middelheimlaan 1, 2020 Antwerp, Belgium

Maria Guarino
Hepatology, Department for BioMedical Research, University of Bern, 3008 Bern, Switzerland
Gastroenterology, Department of Clinical Medicine and Surgery, University of Naples Federico II, 80131 Naples, Italy

Jean-François Dufour
Hepatology, Department for BioMedical Research, University of Bern, 3008 Bern, Switzerland
University Clinic of Visceral Surgery and Medicine, Inselspital Bern, 3008 Bern, Switzerland

Jing Zhang
Department of Pathology and Laboratory Medicine, Kanazawa Medical University, 1-1 Daigaku, Uchinada, Kahoku, Ishikawa 920-0293, Japan

Junji Moriya and Junji Kobayashi
Department of General Internal Medicine, Kanazawa Medical University, Ishikawa 920-0293, Japan

Xiangjin Meng
Department of Pathology and Laboratory Medicine, Kanazawa Medical University, 1-1 Daigaku, Uchinada, Kahoku, Ishikawa 920-0293, Japan
Department of General Internal Medicine, Kanazawa Medical University, Ishikawa 920-0293, Japan

Xin Guo and Sohsuke Yamada
Department of Pathology and Laboratory Medicine, Kanazawa Medical University, 1-1 Daigaku, Uchinada, Kahoku, Ishikawa 920-0293, Japan
Department of Pathology, Kanazawa Medical University Hospital, Ishikawa 920-0293, Japan

Reimon Yamaguchi
Department of Dermatology, Kanazawa Medical University, Ishikawa 920-0293, Japan

Simon Ducheix, Alexandra Montagner, Arnaud Polizzi and Hervé Guillou
Toxalim-Research Centre in Food Toxicology, Toulouse University, INRAE UMR 1331, ENVT, INP-Purpan, Paul Sabatier University, F-31027 Toulouse, France

Aurélien Amiel, Marie Tremblay-Franco, Roselyne Gautier, Laurent Debrauwer and Cécile Canlet
Toxalim-Research Centre in Food Toxicology, Toulouse University, INRAE UMR 1331, ENVT, INP-Purpan, Paul Sabatier University, F-31027 Toulouse, France
Metatoul-AXIOM platform, National Infrastructure for Metabolomics and Fluxomics, MetaboHUB, Toxalim, INRAE UMR 1331, F-31027 Toulouse, France

Justine Bertrand-Michel
Metatoul-Lipidomic Core Facility, MetaboHUB, I2MC U1048, INSERM, F-31432 Toulouse, France

Index